CONTRAST ECHOCARDIOGRAPHY

DEVELOPMENTS IN CARDIOVASCULAR MEDICINE

VOLUME 15

Other volumes in this series:

1. Lancée CT, ed: Echocardiology. 1979. ISBN 90-247-2209-8.
2. Baan J, Arntzenius AC, Yellin EL, eds: Cardiac dynamics. 1980. ISBN 90-247-2212-8.
3. Thalen HJT, Meere CC, eds: Fundamentals of cardiac pacing. 1979. ISBN 90-247-2245-4.
4. Kulbertus HE, Wellens HJJ, eds: Sudden death. 1980. ISBN 90-247-2290-X.
5. Dreifus LS, Brest AN, eds: Clinical applications of cardiovascular drugs. 1980. ISBN 90-247-2295-0.
6. Spencer MP, Reid JM, eds: Cerebrovascular evaluation with Doppler ultrasound. 1981. ISBN 90-247-2384-1.
7. Zipes DP, Bailey JC, Elharrar V, eds: The slow inward current and cardiac arrhythmias. 1980. ISBN 90-247-2380-9.
8. Kesteloot H, Joossens JV, eds: Epidemiology of arterial blood pressure. 1980. ISBN 90-247-2386-8.
9. Wackers FJT, ed: Thallium-201 and technetium-99m-pyrophosphate myocardial imaging in the coronary care unit. 1980. ISBN 90-247-2396-5.
10. Maseri A, Marchesi C, Chierchia S, Trivella MG, eds: Coronary care units. 1981. ISBN 90-247-2456-2.
11. Morganroth J, Moore EN, Dreifus LS, Michelson EL, eds: The evaluation of new antiarrhythmic drugs. 1981. ISBN 90-247-2474-0.
12. Alboni P: Intraventricular conduction disturbances. 1981. ISBN 90-247-2483-X.
13. Rijsterborgh H, ed: Echocardiology. 1981. ISBN 90-247-2491-0.
14. Wagner GS, ed: Myocardial infarction measurement and intervention. 1982. ISBN 90-247-2513-5.

series ISBN 90-247-2336-1

CONTRAST ECHOCARDIOGRAPHY

edited by

RICHARD S. MELTZER

THORAXCENTER, ERASMUS UNIVERSITY, ROTTERDAM

Present address: Mt. Sinai Medical Center, New York

and

JOS ROELANDT

THORAXCENTER, ERASMUS UNIVERSITY, ROTTERDAM

1982

MARTINUS NIJHOFF PUBLISHERS

THE HAGUE / BOSTON / LONDON

Distributors:

for the United States and Canada

Kluwer Boston, Inc.
190 Old Derby Street
Hingham, MA 02043
USA

for all other countries

Kluwer Academic Publishers Group
Distribution Center
P.O. Box 322
3300 AH Dordrecht
The Netherlands

Library of Congress Cataloging in Publication Data   CIP
Main entry under title:

Contrast echocardiography.

  (Developments in cardiovascular medicine;
v. 15)
  Includes index.
  1. Ultrasonic cardiography.   I. Meltzer,
Richard S.   II. Roelandt, Jos.   III. Series.
[DNLM: 1. Echocardiography.   W1 DE99 7VME v. 15 / WG
141.5.E2 C759]
RC683.5.U5C66   616.1′207543   81-18949
                               AACR2

ISBN 90-247-2531-3 (this volume)
ISBN 90-247-2336-1 (series)

PRINTED IN THE NETHERLANDS

To our parents

To Collette, Eva, Martine,
    Michelle, Piet, Raf and Sara

CONTENTS

C. Future prospects

FOREWORD

Why a book on contrast echocardiography? Over the past dozen years enough experience has accumulated to warrant a more extensive treatment of this method. Furthermore, there are new developments that suggest increased clinical utility for contrast echocardiography in the future. This book aims to summarize the "state of the art" for those interested in echocardiography – presumably mainly cardiologists, but here and there those of a more technical bent will find useful information as well. We feel that a more basic understanding of microbubble dynamics is necessary to advance research for such applications as transmission through the lungs, videodensitometric quantitation of cardiac output, intracardiac shunts, etc. All of these topics are extensively dealt with.

The reader will note that many of the clinical chapters are written by pediatric cardiologists. This is only natural, since shunt detection and analysis of flow relationships are relatively more important in congenital heart diseases, and currently represent the most important uses for contrast echocardiography in day-to-day practice.

We would like to point out that the information content of contrast echocardiograms is frequently much greater than appreciated. The only information that many echocardiographers currently obtain from contrast studies is limited to a "yes–no" answer as to the presence or absence of a shunt or the proper identification of a structure. Systematic analysis of contrast echocardiograms reveals much more, however. For example, the slope of an individual trajectory on M-mode contrast echocardiography can yield similar information to that obtained by Doppler echocardiography: both yield the component of blood flow velocity towards or away from the ultrasonic transducer. A multigate Doppler system has even been developed at the University of Washington in Seattle that is capable of color-coding the Doppler signal and inserting it as a sort of contrast into an M-mode tracing. Thus, contrast can give "Doppler information" (velocity) and Doppler can be used to insert "contrast-like information" into an echocardiographic tracing! Contrast and Doppler echocardiography are likely to interact in a more direct manner as well: microbubbles are very strong contrast agents for Doppler ultrasound and may improve its signal-to-noise ratio. Contrast studies using microbubbles have just begun in Doppler echocardiography.

The past development of echocardiography has concentrated first of all on anatomy and only later on physiology as deduced from motion of the anatomic structures. Ultrasonic cardiac diagnosis has been limited to cardiac imaging. Cardiologists would like to have further levels of information potentially available when investigating the cardiovascular system. Flows and pressures are the traditional variables considered, since they have been available for measurement over the past decades. In the future ultrasonic diagnosis will be increasingly able to address the many levels of information needs of the practicing cardiologist. In addition to anatomic information, physiologic information on flows and velocities is now available. It is even possible that pressure measurements may be attainable in the future. Perhaps some of this physiologic information will be somewhat difficult to relate directly to former modes of thinking for a cardiologist, since a parameter such as flow velocity has not been intensively investigated and is not integrated into the classical decision-making process. It is therefore too early to know whether this parameter will be very helpful clinically. Other ways of looking at tissue perfusion and even tissue characterization are being investigated. Whether these will reach any clinical utility is difficult to assess. We can envisage a multipurpose instrument that not only images cardiac anatomy with the high time resolution necessary for cardiac motion studies, but that can also be used to interrogate specific parts of the heart with respect to flow, pressure, tissue characteristics (ischemia, scar, etc.). It is our belief that contrast studies will have an increasingly important part in the more physiologically oriented aspects of echocardiography in the 1980s and 1990s.

Occasionally contradictions between different chapters may be noticed. We have not tried to remove these, since each chapter is written by an authority, and the contradictions reflect current areas of dispute or uncertainty in this developing field.

Of the many individuals who have helped and encouraged us in our studies on contrast echocardiography, we would first of all like to thank Prof. Paul G. Hugenholtz, the director of the Thoraxcenter. We also wish to thank all the people in the animal and echo departments of the Thoraxcenter and at the Delft Engineering School who have directly or indirectly helped us. We appreciate the stimulating interest in our endeavors of Dr. Richard Popp. Finally, Dr. Meltzer wishes to acknowledge support for research in the field of contrast echocardiography from the American Heart Association, in the form of a Clinician-Scientist Award.

Richard S. Meltzer and Jos Roelandt

CONTRIBUTORS

Allen, H.D., Department of Pediatrics, University of Arizona, Health Sciences Center, Tucson, AZ 85724, USA

Armstrong, B.E., Division of Pediatric Cardiology, Department of Pediatrics, Box 3090, Duke University Medical Center, Durham, NC 27710, USA

Bommer, W., Section of Cardiovascular Medicine, School of Medicine TB172, University of California, Davis, CA 95616, USA

DeMaria, A.N., Department of Medicine, University of Kentucky, College of Medicine, Lexington, KY 40506, USA

Feigenbaum, H., Krannert Institute of Cardiology, Department of Medicine, Indiana University School of Medicine and the Veterans Administration Medical Center, 1100 West Michigan Street, Indianapolis, IN 46223, USA

Fox, W.W., Division of Neonatology, Children's Hospital of Philadelphia, School of Medicine, Philadelphia, PA, USA

Gewitz, M.H., Division of Cardiology, Children's Hospital of Philadelphia, School of Medicine, Philadelphia, PA, USA

Goldberg, J., Department of Pediatrics, University of Arizona, Health Sciences Center, Tucson, AZ 85724, USA

Goldstein, J.A., University of California Hospital, San Francisco, CA 94143, USA

Gramiak, R., Department of Radiology, Strong Memorial Hospital, University of Rochester, School of Medicine and Dentistry, Rochester, NY 14642, USA

Hagler, D.J., Mayo Medical School, Division of Pediatric Cardiology, Mayo Clinic, Rochester, MN 55901, USA

Harinck E., Department of Paediatric Cardiology, Wilhelmina Children's Hospital, University of Utrecht, Nieuwe Gracht 137, 3512 LK Utrecht, The Netherlands

Hunter, S., Regional Cardiothoracic Center, Freeman Hospital, Newcastle upon Tyne, UK

Jones, M., National Institutes of Health, Building 10, Room 6N252, Bethesda, MD 20205, USA

Kisslo, J., Duke University Medical Center, P.O. Box 3818, Durham, NC 27710, USA

Kronik, G., First Department of Internal Medicine, Cardiology Division, University of Vienna, Lazarettgasse 9, A 1090 Vienna, Austria

Lancée, T., Thoraxcenter, Erasmus University, P.O. Box 1738, 3000 DR Rotterdam, The Netherlands

Mackay,R.S., Department of Biology, Boston University, Boston, MA 02215, USA

Martin, R.P., Division of Cardiology, Medical Center, Box 468, University of Virginia, Charlottesville, VA 22908, USA

Mason, D.T., Section of Cardiovascular Medicine, School of Medicine TB172, University of California, Davis, CA 95616, USA

McGhie, J., Thoraxcenter, Erasmus University, P.O. Box 1738, 3000 DR Rotterdam, The Netherlands

Meltzer, R.S., Thoraxcenter, Erasmus University, P.O. Box 1738, 3000 DR Rotterdam, The Netherlands

Meijboom, E.J., Division of Pediatric Cardiology, University of Groningen Hospital, Groningen, The Netherlands

Mill, G.J., van, Department of Paediatric Cardiology, Wilhelmina Children's Hospital, University of Utrecht, Nieuwe Gracht 137, 3512 LK Utrecht, The Netherlands

Moulaert, A.J., Department of Paediatric Cardiology, Wilhelmina Children's Hospital, Nieuwe Gracht 137, 3512 LK Utrecht, The Netherlands

Pieroni, D.R., Children's Hospital of Buffalo, Department of Cardiology, 219 Bryant Street, Buffalo, NY 14222, USA

Pizzuto, F., Malattie dell' Apparato Cardiovascolare, Cattedra II, Università di Roma, Policlinico Umberto I, 00161 Rome, Italy

Popp, R.L., Stanford University Medical School, Stanford, CA 94305, USA

Preis, L.K., JR., East Jefferson Hospital, Cardiology Consultants of Louisiana, 4200 Houma Boulevard, Metaire, LA 70011, USA

Reale, A., Malattie dell' Apparato Cardiovascolare, Cattedra II, Università di Roma, Policlinico Umberto I, 00616 Rome, Italy

Rasor, J., Ultra Med, Inc., 253 Humboldt Ct., Sunnyvale, CA 94086, USA

Ritman, E.L., Mayo Medical School, Department of Physiology and Biophysics, Mayo Clinic, Rochester, MN 55901, USA

Roelandt, J., Thoraxcenter, Erasmus University, P.O. Box 1738, 3000 DR Rotterdam, The Netherlands

Roland, J.-M.A., Children's Hospital of Buffalo, Department of Cardiology, 219 Bryant Street, Buffalo, NY 14222, USA

Rubissow, G.J., 47 Rue Boileau, 75016 Paris, France *and* 66 Ivy Drive, Ross, CA 94957, USA

Sahn,D.J., Department of Pediatrics, University of Arizona, Health Sciences Center, Tucson, AZ 85724, USA

Schiller, N.B., Cardiology Division, University of California Hospital, San Francisco, CA 94143, USA

Serruys,P.W., Thoraxcenter, Erasmus University, P.O. Box 1738, 3000 DR Rotterdam, The Netherlands

Serwer, G.A., Division of Pediatric Cardiology, Department of Pediatrics, Box 3090, Duke University Medical Center, Durham, NC 27710, USA

Seward, J.B., Mayo Medical School, Division of Cardiovascular Diseases and Internal Medicine, *and of* Pediatric Cardiology, Mayo Clinic, Rochester, MN 55901, USA

Shematek, J.P., Clinic of Surgery, National Heart, Lung and Blood Institute, Bethesda, MD 20205, USA

Sutherland, G.R., Regional Cardiothoracic Center, Freeman Hospital, Newcastle upon Tyne, UK

Tajik, A.J., Mayo Medical School, Division of Cardiovascular Diseases and Internal Medicine, *and of* Pediatric Cardiology, Mayo Clinic, Rochester, MN 55901, USA

Tickner, E.G., Ultra Med, Inc., 253 Humboldt Court, Sunnyvale, CA 94086, USA

Tucker, C.R., Stanford University, Stanford, CA 95305, USA

Valdes-Cruz, L.M., Department of Pediatrics, University of Arizona, Health Sciences Center, Tucson, AZ 85724, USA

Weyman, A.E., Cardiac Ultrasound Laboratory, Massachusetts General Hospital, Harvard Medical School, Boston, MA 02114, USA

Wood, D.C., Division of Cardiology, Children's Hospital of Philadelphia, School of Medicine, Philadelphia, PA, USA

1. AN INTRODUCTION TO CONTRAST ECHOCARDIOGRAPHY

HARVEY FEIGENBAUM

Contrast echocardiography started when Dr. Gramiak and his colleagues at the University of Rochester noted that the intracardiac injection of indocyanine green dye produced a cloud of echoes on the M-mode echocardiogram [1]. Subsequently, it was noted that the injection of almost any liquid through a small bore needle or catheter would produce this contrast effect. One possibility was that the echo-producing microbubbles were forming at the tip of the needle or catheter by cavitation. It was also suspected that many of the microbubbles were suspended in the liquid prior to the injection [1,2]. Indocyanine green dye appeared to give the best contrast effect principally because of its surface tension permitting the development of very small microbubbles which would stay in suspension for longer periods of time [2]. Thus, indocyanine green dye has been the standard contrast agent, although many echocardiographers have used saline, 5% water, and even the patient's blood.

From an historical point of view, the original use for contrast echocardiography was the identification of structures within the heart [1, 3]. This technique proved to be vital in the early days of echocardiography when we attempted to prove the identity of certain echoes on the echocardiogram. Gramiak and his coworkers identified many cardiac structures using this technique [1] and we at Indiana used this approach principally to identify the various echoes originating from the left ventricle [3]. Virtually every part of the echocardiogram has been identified with the use of contrast echocardiography. We have even used this technique to verify the identity of the left main coronary artery [4].

The next clinical use for contrast echocardiography was in the detection of right-to-left shunts [5–7]. It became apparent that the contrast producing microbubbles were too large to traverse the capillaries. As a result, an injection of contrast on the right side of the heart would remain on the right side unless there was a right-to-left shunt which bypassed the pulmonary capillaries. The abnormal flow need not only be at the intracardiac level. The technique could demonstrate right-to-left shunting through a pulmonary arteriovenous shunt [8, 9]. Patients with predominant left-to-right shunts through an atrial septal defect frequently have a small right-to-left shunt [10,11]. Thus, in many patients with an atrial septal defect and a left-to-right shunt one could see some microbubbles traverse the septum from the right atrium to the left atrium.

The other contrast technique used for the detection of left-to-right shunts was the concept of negative contrast echocardiography [12]. With a left-to-right shunt there was a jet of non-contrast containing blood which would produce an echo-free area within the chamber filled with contrast. This negative contrast effect was first reported in patients with atrial septal defects [12]. However, this same phenomenon has been noted with left-to-right shunts at the ventricular level [13].

Although most echocardiographers limit the contrast injections to peripheral venous or right sided injections, several investigators have utilized contrast echocardiography at the time of cardiac catheterization [5, 14]. The advantages of the contrast echocardiography in this setting is the elimination of cineangiography. A situation whereby selective contrast echocardiography may be useful is in infants with a patent ductus arteriosus who already have an arterial catheter in place. A contrast injection directly into the aorta via the catheter provides a very sensitive means of detecting a left-to-right shunt through a patent ductus arteriosus [15].

Another clinical application for contrast echocardiography has been the detection of tricuspid regurgitation [16]. This technique is based upon the fact that with tricuspid regurgitation contrast will be seen in the inferior vena cava and hepatic veins with ventricular systole as regurgitant blood passes from the right ventricle into the right atrium. Thus, the clinical uses of contrast echocardiography at the present time are limited primarily to the detection of tricuspid regurgitation, right-to-left shunts and, to a lesser extent, left-to-right shunts. Some echocardiographers use contrast echocardiography in an invasive manner and the technique is still being used to help identify cardiac structures as we continue to explore new areas of the heart with echocardiography.

The future of contrast echocardiography is almost unlimited. As this book indicates, there is a vast amount of interest and research currently being done with regard to contrast echocardiography. Probably the most exciting aspect of this research is the development of new contrast producing agents [17–21]. The use of indocyanine green dye or saline is certainly useful and relatively benign for the patient; however, the contrast effect is not uniform and one cannot quantitate such injections. A whole host of new contrast producing agents are being studied. These include the injection of carbon dioxide gas, Ringer's lactate, hydrogen peroxide, gelatin encapsulated microbubbles, and sugar encapsulated microbubbles. All of these agents have significant advantages over the current contrast techniques. It is going to be exciting to see how these various agents develop. Hopefully, one or more of these new agents will be able to traverse the capillaries so that one can visualize the left side of the heart with a peripheral venous injection.

These new contrast agents open new possibilities for the technique of contrast echocardiography. One now has the theoretical possibility of measuring hemodynamics, especially on the right side of the heart. Cardiac output, and hopefully even intracardiac pressure, can be measured using these new contrast agents. Another potential application is that of myocardial perfusion. Such an application might require an injection in the root of the aorta, which is not exactly noninvasive, but is not much more invasive than an arterial line which is routinely done in almost all intensive care units.

The future of echocardiography is extremely exciting. One important aspect of this future is the development of contrast echocardiography. If and when the new contrast agents become clinically useful, they will undoubtedly have a big impact on the practice of echocardiography.

REFERENCES

1. Gramiak R, PM Shah, DH Kramer: Ultrasound cardiography: contrast studies in anatomy and function. Radiology 92:929, 1969.
2. Meltzer R, G. Tickner, T Sahines, RL Popp: The source of ultrasonic contrast effect. J Clin Ultrasound 8:121, 1980.
3. Feigenbaum H, JM Stone, DA Lee, WK Nasser, S Chang: Identification of ultrasound echoes from the left ventricle using intracardiac injections of indocyanine green. Circulation 41:615, 1970.
4. Weyman AE, H Feigenbaum, JC Dillon, KW Johnston, RC Eggleton: Noninvasive visualization of the left main coronary artery by cross-sectional echocardiography. Circulation 54:169, 1976.
5. Seward JB, AJ Tajik, JG Spangler, DG Ritter: Echocardiographic contrast studies: initial experience. Mayo Clin Proc 50:163, 1975.
6. Valdes-Cruz LM, DR Pieroni, J-MA Roland, PJ Varghese: Echocardiographic detection of intracardiac right-to-left shunts following peripheral vein injections. Circulation 54:558, 1976.
7. Serruys PW, M VanDenBrand, PG Hugenholtz, J Roelandt: Intracardiac right-to-left shunts demonstrated by two-dimensional echocardiography after peripheral vein injection. Br Heart J 42:429, 1979.
8. Seward JB, AJ Tajik, DJ Hagler, DG Ritter: Peripheral venous contrast echocardiography. Am J Cardiol 39:202, 1977.
9. Hernandez A, AW Strauss, R McKnight, AF Hartman Jr: Diagnosis of pulmonary arteriovenous fistula by contrast echocardiography. J Pediatr 93:258, 1978.
10. Fraker TD, PJ Harris, VS Behar, JA Kisslo: Detection and exclusion of interatrial shunts by two-dimensional echocardiography and peripheral venous injection. Circulation 59:379, 1979.
11. Kronik G, J Slany, H Moesslacher: Contrast M-mode echocardiography in diagnosis of atrial septal defect in acyanotic patients. Circulation 59:372, 1979.
12. Weyman AE, LS Wann, RL Caldwell, RA Hurwitz, JC Dillon, H Feigenbaum: Negative contrast echocardiography: a new method for detecting left-to-right shunts. Circulation 59:498, 1979.
13. Feigenbaum H: Echocardiography, 3rd edn, p 362. Lea & Febiger, Philadelphia, 1981.
14. Paquet M, H Gutgesell: Echocardiographic features of total anomalous pulmonary venous connection. Circulation 51:599, 1975.
15. Allen HD, DJ Sahn, SJ Goldberg: New serial contrast technique for assessment of left-to-right shunting patent ductus arteriosus in the neonate. Am J Cardiol 41:288, 1978.
16. Lieppe W, VS Behar, R Scallion, JA Kisslo: Detection of tricuspid regurgitation with two-dimensional echocardiography and peripheral vein injections. Circulation 57:128, 1978.
17. Bommer WJ, DT Mason, AN DeMaria: Studies in contrast echocardiography: development of new agents with superior reproducibility and transmission through lungs. Circulation (Suppl II) 60:17, 1979 (Abstract).

4

18. Bommer WJ, et al: Development of a new echocardiographic contrast agent capable of pulmonary transmission and left heart opacification following peripheral venous injection. Circulation (Suppl II) 62:17, 1979.
19. Imai Y, et al: A study of the contrast echoes: in regard to the method with a solution containing carbon dioxide microbubbles. Jpn J Med Ultrason 6:179, 1979.
20. Meltzer RS, EG Tickner, RL Popp: Clinical note. Why do the lungs clear ultrasonic contrast? Ultrasound Med Biol 6:263, 1980.
21. Meltzer RS et al: Intravenous carbon dioxide as an echocardiographic contrast agent. J Clin Ultrasound 9:127, 1981.

A. PHYSICAL PROPERTIES AND THEORETIC CONSIDERATIONS

2. THE SOURCE OF ECHOCARDIOGRAPHIC CONTRAST

RICHARD S. MELTZER, E. GLENN TICKNER, RICHARD L. POPP, and JOS ROELANDT

INTRODUCTION

In the mid-1960s Joyner first noted ultrasonic contrast effect and he was acknowledged in the first publication on this subject by Gramiak et al. in 1968 [1]. Within a short time a similar contrast effect was noted using several different unrelated biologically compatible solutions, and it was suggested that the source of the contrast effect was microbubbles of air caused by cavitation at the catheter tip during injection [2–4]. Catheter tip cavitation had just been described in the radiologic literature [5]. The most important argument in favor of the microbubble origin of ultrasonic contrast was that its intensity decreased in water tank experiments when increased pressure was placed on the fluid. Such behavior would be expected of a bubble of air, but not of a solid or liquid ultrasonic reflector. However, this in vitro observation by no means proved that the contrast seen in vivo necessarily is made of microbubbles of gas – only that the microbubbles are one possible source. For example it has been suggested that the spontaneous contrast occasionally observed in patients with mitral prosthetic valves might be due to particulate matter such as platelets or fibrin or fine pieces of the cloth sewing ring of the prostheses [6]. We thus decided to study the source of ultrasonic contrast effect directly and performed the following studies [7, 8].

METHODS

Visual and microscopic inspection

The following different test ultrasonic contrast agents were examined:
a. Tap water allowed to stand overnight
b. Warm tap water recently agitated in a syringe
c. Indocyanine green dye solution (1.25 mg/ml) allowed to stand overnight
d. Indocyanine green solution (1.25 mg/ml) freshly prepared and agitated
e. Carbonated water
f. Precision sized microbubbles suspended in a gelatin matrix (Rasor Associates, Sunnyvale, Calif.).

Each solution was examined visually in a syringe, with particular attention to the gross air content and microbubble content in the form of foam. A few drops were

8

then placed on a glass slide and examined microscopically. Surface tension studies were performed on the indocyanine green dye solution and gelatin using the standard platinum wire ring technique [9].

Ultrasonic tests

To test whether microbubbles could be ultrasonically imaged using commercially available echocardiographic equipment, a suspension of very small microbubbles (range of diameters from 2 to 20 μm) in gelatin was placed at the bottom of a beaker filled with water degassed by prolonged boiling. These were imaged using a Smith Kline Ekoline 20A echocardiograph with a focused 2.25 MHz transducer. The experimental set up is illustrated in Figure 1. The rates of rise of the microbubbles were calculated by measuring their slopes as recorded on hardcopy at a speed of 50 mm/s.

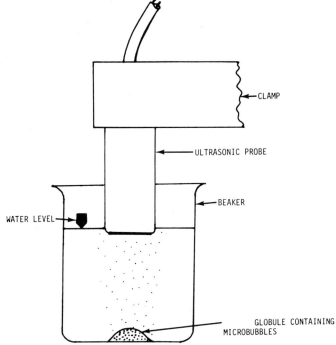

Figure 1. Setup for bubble rise experiments. A globule containing the precision microbubbles to be studied is placed at the bottom of a beaker filled with water that has been degassed by boiling. The ultrasonic transducer is fixed just below the water level by a clamp. Reproduced by permission of Ultrasound in Medicine and Biology.

Using the same echocardiographic instrument, we examined the six test fluids listed above for their ultrasonic contrast properties. Each fluid was injected into a tube inside a silastic chamber submerged in a tank of degassed water. Contrast intensity was judged not only by the density of the printout from the intraluminal echoes so created, but also by the amount of decrease of the posterior wall echoes as

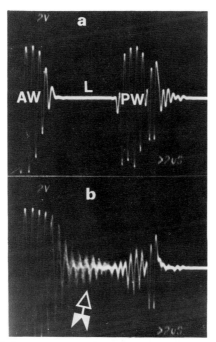

Figure 2. Preprocessed radiofrequency signal of silastic chamber in water tank. a) Signal with only degassed water in chamber lumen (L). AW: anterior wall, PW: posterior wall. b) A few seconds later, after injection of microbubbles into chamber lumen. Note appearance of echoes in the previously echo-free lumen (arrow), and decrease in amplitude of the posterior wall echo. Reproduced by permission of J Clin Ultrasound.

a result of absorption and scattering. This decrease is due to ultrasonic reflection and scattering from the intraluminal contrast, so that insufficient acoustic energy remains in the beam to reflect from the posterior wall, repass the intraluminal microbubbles, and reach the transducer. Further, this effect was quantitatively studied by obtaining the preprocessed radiofrequency signal of the posterior wall echo (Figure 2) and by determining how it varied over a wide range of intraluminal concentrations of a suspension of precision microbubbles. In theory, reflective characteristics of such a suspension are determined by the individual microbubble properties (type of gas, diameter) as well as their concentration and geometric distribution. In this experiment we held the type of microbubble constant and varied only their intraluminal concentration. With the test apparatus and machine settings unchanged, the posterior wall echo amplitude resulting from each different concentration of precision microbubbles was measured.

Cavitation was tested in a large tank of degassed water by visual observation using a bright sidelight and by ultrasound. The same commercially available echocardiographic instrument was used, and the transducer was fixed just under the surface of the water. It was aimed at an area containing the jet resulting from forceful injections 3–10 cm distal to the needle or catheter. Forceful hand injections were repeatedly made by each of two observers through 19-gauge, 7/8 in. long and

23-gauge, 3/4 in. long needles. Mechanical injections were performed using a power injector employed for angiography in the catheterization laboratory.

To test the hypothesis that injections below the cavitation threshold can cause echocardiographic contrast in vitro, we used a Krautkramer-Branson 3.5 MHz transducer sutured directly to the left ventricular epicardium in open-chested anesthetized pigs. Injections of physiologic saline were made through a catheter directly into the left ventricle in 20 pigs, using the same injection technique as that used clinically to obtain echo contrast in our noninvasive laboratory, with one important difference in technique: the hand injections were performed very slowly, at rates less than $0.3 \, cm^3/s$, which were well below the threshold for cavitation of the system. Results were monitored using an Organon Teknika Echocardiovisor SE M-mode instrument.

RESULTS

Visual and microscopic observations

The following fluids had visually evident bubbles of air or foam: agitated tap water, freshly prepared and agitated indocyanine green dye solution, carbonated water, and the precision microbubbles in gelatin. The tap water and indocyanine green solution which had remained in open beakers overnight had no visually apparent bubbles of air or foam.

The freshly prepared indocyanine green solution, recently agitated tap water, and carbonated water all had rapidly changing amounts and sizes of gas bubbles, both in the syringe and under the microscope. Bubbles in the tap water rapidly coalesced and rose to the upper surface of the syringe, until there was only a single large gas bubble or a small number of large bubbles, with few or no small bubbles at the upper surface and with no bubbles apparent in the fluid phase below. Carbonated water showed the continual creation of small bubbles which grew and rose to the surface when large enough – a phenomenon familiar to anyone who has observed carbonated beverages in glass bottles after opening. As with the bubbles in tap water, these bubbles coalesced when reaching the gas–liquid interface in the syringe, leaving few small bubbles and no foam. The indocyanine green solution was qualitatively different, since the bubbles were smaller, rose more slowly, remained predominantly in a foam, and only partly coalesced into large bubbles. Serial photographs of syringe contents are really necessary to convey this dynamic bubble behavior, but an idea of the difference between different fluids can be obtained by examining Figure 3, which shows syringes with the four test fluids containing microbubbles several seconds after agitation, placed horizontally for photography.

This dynamic behavior of microbubbles was also observed under the microscope and recorded on videotape. The tap water solution contained no microscopically apparent bubbles, since these all rose to the surface between the time the syringe was agitated and the microscope could be focused on the drop of water on the glass slide.

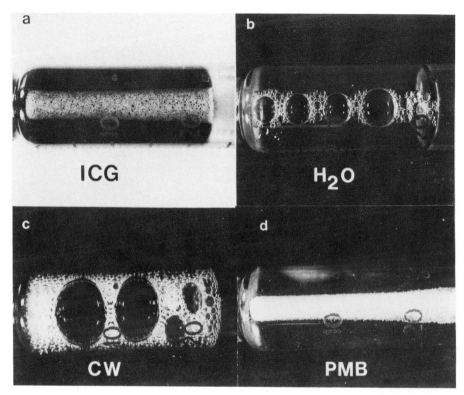

Figure 3. Photographs of syringes with different test solutions several seconds after agitation, placed horizontally. a) Indocyanine green solution, b) tap water, c) carbonated water, d) precision microbubbles in gelatin. Reproduced by permission of J Clin Ultrasound.

Bubbles from the indocyanine green solution (Figure 4, upper panel) and from the carbonated water were quite apparent microscopically, and continued to move and coalesce. The precision microbubbles in gelatin were the most stable microscopically, and also the most uniform (Figure, lower panel). They did not change size or coalesce during the five minutes microscopic observation period. As predicted previously [8], microbubbles in indocyanine green solutions dissolved and thus shrank slowly, seeming to accelerate as their diameter fell below 20 μm with total dissolution occurring in under 2 s from the time a diameter of 20 μm had been reached. Bubbles larger than 60–80 μm in diameter changed little for the several minute observation period.

Surface-tension measurements on indocyanine green and on gelatin solutions showed that both had low surface-tension properties (43 dynes/cm^2, or 0.6 relative to water).

Ultrasonic tests

Precision microbubbles in gelatin ranging from 2 to 20 μm in diameter were placed

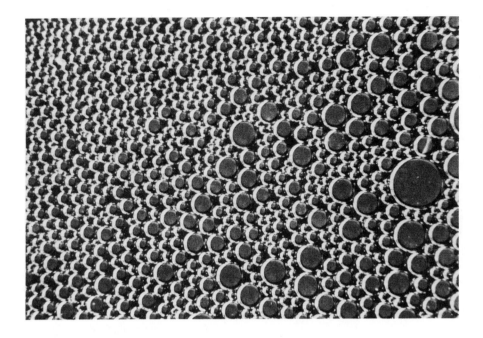

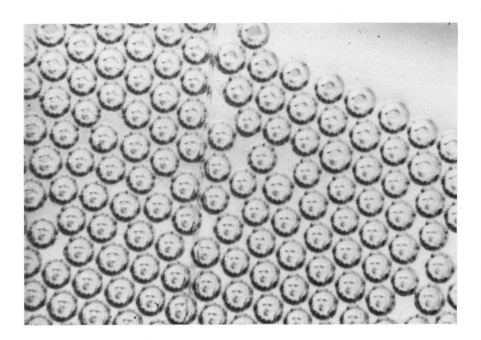

Figure 4. Upper panel: microscopic view of indocyanine green foam under cover slip. There is a considerable variability in bubble size. Lower panel: precision microbubbles in gelatin. Note uniformity of size.

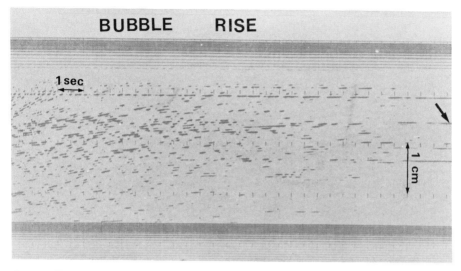

Figure 5. Tracing resulting from experimental setup illustrated in Figure 1. A smaller bubble rises more slowly and yields a flatter trajectory (arrow at right of tracing). Reproduced by permission of Ultrasound in Medicine and Biology.

at the bottom of a beaker as illustrated in Figure 1, and a resulting M-mode tracing is shown in Figure 5. This experiment allowed definite identification of microbubbles as the source of the observed contrast, for their rate of rise as calculated from the slope of the trajectories from M-mode tracings corresponded to the calculated rate of rise of microbubbles based on Stokes's law for frictional resistance [10]. No particulate matter was seen microscopically in the gelatin-microbubble preparation. In addition, this would not be expected to rise spontaneously in a beaker of water. Using the silastic chamber inside a water tank, the test fluids were rated as follows with respect to intensity of ultrasonic contrast effect:

a. No contrast effect: water and indocyanine green solution that had been in open beakers overnight

b. Moderate contrast effect (intraluminal contrast without abolishing posterior wall echo): freshly agitated saline and the fluid phase of freshly agitated indocyanine green solution

c. Strong contrast effect (intraluminal contrast and complete abolishment of posterior wall echo due to "overload" effect): foam from freshly agitated indocyanine green solution, carbonated water, precision microbubble infusion.

Since it is at present impossible to quantify the number and size of microbubbles in a given volume of fluid being sampled ultrasonically, we cannot further compare the ultrasonic signal for different contrast agents resulting from the same concentration of microbubbles, or the same total volume of gas, etc. Using infusions at varying rates of a known concentration of precision microbubbles, we were able to observe a progressive decrease in the amplitude of the preprocessed radio frequency echo from the silastic tube posterior wall with increasing intraluminal bubble concentration (Figure 6).

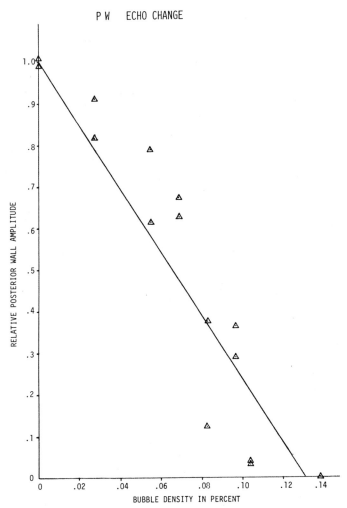

Figure 6. Decrease in posterior wall echo amplitude as seen in Figure 2 (mean of largest three peak-to-peak cycles) with varying intraluminal concentrations of precision microbubbles. Reproduced by permission of the Journal of Clinical Ultrasound.

Cavitation occurred both ultrasonically and visually in a water tank when injections through a 19-gauge, 7/8 in. long needle exceeded flow rates of 10 cm³/s, both by hand and by using a mechanical injector. Through a 23-gauge, 3/4 in. long needle cavitation occurred above flow rates of 3 cm³/s. For these flow rates and tube sizes a cavitation number of 0.16 and 0.27 Thoma units can be calculated, and since these are below the critical number of 0.35, cavitation would be expected [4, 5, 7]. Cavitation was always seen at higher flow rates and never at flow rates below these threshold values. These flow rates were at the upper limit of maximal hand injection through the respective needles, and were higher than that used during our clinical contrast echocardiographic studies. On the basis of our experience we judged that such force would be likely to cause peripheral vein rupture or intravenous infiltration. We therefore felt that the cavitation effect that could be observed in water tanks probably was not the cause of the ultrasonic contrast observed in our patients.

Further testing of the importance of cavitation was carried out in 20 anesthetized pigs with open thorax and with epicardial echo transducers using direct left ventricular catheter injections. Physiologic saline was drawn up in a $10 cm^3$ syringe, agitated, and gross air excluded, as is our practice in clinical contrast echocardiographic injections. This was then slowly infused at a rate far below the cavitation threshold (less than $0.3 cm^3/s$). All 20 pigs had excellent left ventricular opacification by contrast.

DISCUSSION

These studies establish that microbubbles are a source of ultrasonic contrast effect, but do not exclude the possibility that other sources may occasionally yield echocardiographic contrast. Especially intriguing in this respect is the rare observation of "spontaneous" contrast – in the lack of vessel invasion, decompression, infection, obstetric accidents, etc. – both on the left side of the heart [6, 11, 12] and right side of the heart [13, 14]. Particulate matter, absorption of gas from the gut in the portal system, liberation of oxygen due to hemolysis, and spontaneous cavitation caused by the low local pressures in a regurgitant jet of blood due to the Bernoulli principle, have all been suggested as possible mechanisms.

Our finding that clinical ultrasonic contrast is likely due to microbubbles of air already present in the injectate rather than needle tip cavitation has clinical implications regarding the method used to attain ultrasonic contrast. It suggests that more attention should be focused on the contrast agent and its preparation and gas content, and less on the geometric form of the injection apparatus: stopcocks, right-angle connections, orifice size, etc. If a standardized and reproducible contrast injection is to be attained in the future, it will thus have to have a standard microbubble content rather than a standard injection pressure or flow rate. High flows are probably important to flush a bolus of contrast along a vein into the central circulation without "margination", but seem unnecessary in central catheter injections.

An implication of microbubbles as the source of ultrasonic contrast is that the physical properties of microbubbles and their dynamic behavior in the circulation must be studied in order to explain the behavior of the contrast effect observed clinically. We believe this sort of knowledge has helped to explain why the lungs remove ultrasound contrast normally (Chapter 4), has suggested methods of causing transmission of echocardiographic contrast through the lungs (Chapters 10, 11 and 25), and may help to elucidate the mechanisms of spontaneous echocardiographic contrast [6, 12, 14] and decompression sickness (Chapter 5) [8, 15].

REFERENCES

1. Gramiak R, PM Shah: Echocardiography of the aortic root. Invest Radiol 3:356–366, 1968.
2. Gramiak R, PM Shah, DH Kramer: Ultrasound cardiography: contrast studies in anatomy and function. Radiology 92:939–948, 1969.
3. Kremkau FW, R Gramiak, EL Carstensen, PM Shah, DH Kramer: Ultrasonic detection of cavitation at catheter tips. Am J Roentgenol 3:159, 1968.
4. Ziskin MC, A Bonakdarpour, DP Weinstein, et al: Contrast agents for diagnostic ultrasound. Invest Radiol 7:500–505, 1972.
5. Bove AA, DF Adams, AE Hugh, PR Lynch: Cavitation at catheter tips. A possible cause of air embolus. Invest Radiol 3:159–164, 1968.
6. Schuchman H, H. Feigenbaum, JE Dillon, et al: Intracavitary echoes in patients with mitral prosthetic valves. J Clin Ultrasound 3:107–110, 1975.
7. Meltzer RS, EG Tickner, TP Sahines, RL Popp: The source of ultrasound contrast effect. J Clin Ultrasound 8:121–127, 1980.
8. Meltzer RS, EG Tickner, RL Popp: Why do the lungs clear ultrasonic contrast? Ultrasound Med Biol 6:263–269, 1980.
9. Adam NK: The Physics and Chemistry of Surfaces. Dover, NY 1968.
10. Happle J, H Brenner: Low Reynolds Number Hydrodynamics. Prentice-Hall, Englewood Cliffs, NJ, 1965.
11. Gramiak R, NC Nanda: Structure identification in echocardiography. In: Gramiak R, RC Waag (eds) Cardiac Ultrasound, pp 29–46. CV Mosby, St. Louis, 1975.
12. Preis LK, JP Hess, JL Austin, GB Craddock, LB McGuire, RP Martin: Left ventricular microcavitations in patients with Beall valves. Am J Cardiol 45: 402, 1980 (abstract).
13. Finberg HJ: Ultrasonic visualization of in vivo flow phenomena without injected contrast material. In: Proc 25th Meeting Am Inst Ultrasound Med, p 17. New Orleans, 1980.
14. Meltzer RS, CT Lancée, GR Swart, J Roelandt: "Spontaneous" echo contrast on the right side of the heart. J Clin Ultrasound (in press).
15. Meltzer RS, OEH Sartorius, CT Lancée, PW Serruys, PD Verdouw, C Essed, J Roelandt: Transmission of echocardiographic contrast through the lungs. Ultrasound Med Biol 7: 377–384, 1981.

3. CONTRAST AGENTS FOR DIAGNOSTIC ULTRASOUND

RAYMOND GRAMIAK

A recognized advantage of ultrasound over radiologic techniques is its inherent natural contrast which differentiates solid structures of the heart from blood-filled cavities and from great vessels without an exogenous contrast material. However, the need for such a contrast material became apparent early in our experience, since the M-mode display, in itself, did not provide recognizable or familiar anatomic images from which structure identity could be deduced. As a result, our initial publication [1] dealt with contrast injections as markers for cavity or valve identification; and to a lesser extent for the description of normal intracardiac flow patterns, for the recognition of aortic regurgitation, and for the validation of systolic anterior motion of the mitral valve as well as mid-systolic preclosure of the aortic valve in IHSS. Demonstration of intracardiac shunts was also included, and it was observed that the contrast effect was not recirculated and was probably filtered by the pulmonary and systemic capillary beds.

Our initial contrast successes were with indocyanine green, but it soon became apparent that a similar contrast effect was also obtained from saline, 5% dextrose in water, or even the patient's own blood, which suggested that indocyanine green was not vital to the contrast effect. The likelihood that microbubbles represented the echo sources was first suggested when small amounts of foam were noted in syringes of indocyanine green which had been allowed to stand prior to use. We were almost certain of the bubble hypothesis when hand injections of tap water into tap water produced an ultrasonic contrast effect that was associated with a hazy, light-scattering flow stream emanating from the syringe.

Professor Edwin Carstensen and his graduate student, Fred Kremkau [2], conceived an experimental system, which featured a fluid-filled transparent chamber with an inflow catheter tip connected to a mechanical injector and an outflow portion leading to a reservoir, through which the ambient pressure within the chamber could be raised. Provision was made for an ultrasound transducer on the end of the chamber facing the flow from the catheter tip. M-mode studies of the ultrasonic signals were recorded on 35 mm film, along with a marker for the precise moment of injection, and a display of any audible sounds produced within the chamber. Various fluids were injected at different velocities and under different conditions of pressurization. These investigations revealed that injections of water, sucrose, or saline solution into water at atmospheric pressure produced echoes only when the injection velocity exceeded the threshold for transient cavitation. During

these injections, an intense light-scattering jet was observed in the chamber at the catheter tip and there was a distal diffusion of a less intense cloudlike swirl of light-scattering particles. On the M-mode recordings, the injections were seen as a contrast stream moving toward the probe followed by filling of the entire chamber with echo sources. The presence of cavitation was documented by a strong cavitation hiss during the injections. When the injections were repeated at cavitation velocities with superimposed pressures of 20–25 lbs/square inch; no echoes, visible light-scattering, or cavitation hiss could be detected. It appeared to be an inescapable conclusion that the pressure-sensitive, light-scattering particles present only during conditions of transient cavitation could only be microbubbles and that these represented the source of contrast echoes.

Injections of blood into blood were also investigated in our laboratory using the pressurized chamber. It was possible to produce echoes in the chamber at velocities which were much lower than those required to cavitate water. The echo sources persisted for a much longer time in blood and could be observed floating upward in the chamber. Calculations based on their rate of rise indicated the presence of bubbles with a diameter of about 400 μm [3]. The mechanism for the production of bubbles during injection probably differs when clear, especially degassed, fluids are used as compared to injections involving blood. With degassed, clear liquids higher jet velocities are required to create regions of low pressure of such a magnitude that the fluid is probably vaporized. Once the injection stops or the velocity drops below the cavitation threshold, the bubble formation ceases; hence the name transient cavitation. During the phase of active injection, bubbles which move out of low pressure regions collapse rapidly producing shock waves, giving rise to the hiss of transient cavitation.

In gas-rich media, such as blood, cavitation occurs at much lower flow rates. The bubbles that are produced persist considerably longer than those produced with transient cavitation; hence the name stable cavitation. They also do not collapse suddenly, so a cavitation hiss is not produced.

Others have also become interested in the source of the contrast effect. Most recently, Meltzer et al. [4] injected degassed water into degassed water using syringes and needles commonly employed clinically. They were able to observe cavitation by seeing light-scattering at a flow rate of 10 cm^3/s through a 19-gauge, 2.2 cm long needle and at 3 cm^3/s through a 23-gauge, 1.9 cm long needle, rates which were at the upper limit of maximum hand injection using 10 cm^3 and 20 cm^3 plastic syringes. The force required to produce cavitation was judged to be greater than that used clinically through butterfly needles. Cavitation in blood was not studied.

Investigations to date have shown that the source of contrast effect has been the microbubble and that these bubbles could be injected directly, or produced by transient or stable cavitation. Whether one mechanism or another predominates in patient examinations is probably of little significance when one examines the shortcomings of the method. Injections into peripheral veins produce a varied contrast response ranging from nonvisualization of the injection to good filling of right heart

cavities. Variability in the injection rate, number and volume of bubbles, and transit time through the venous system, all will influence the intensity of the contrast effect. Gravitational trapping of bubbles in the major veins of the arm, shoulder, or neck is very difficult to control and could conceivably delay microbubbles long enough for the bubbles to collapse completely by diffusion. Control of the variables in contrast injection should provide consistent patterns of chamber filling and emptying with a constant intensity, which can be quantitated for the development of indicator dilution techniques or for the calculation of the volume of a shunt. It is probably important to note that quantitation of contrast intensity would not only require a standard amount of the agent, but would probably also depend heavily on the range of scatterer sizes, since large scatterers reflect more of the ultrasonic energy and would also interfere with those more deeply placed, because of acoustic attenuation.

Some improvement in achieving a standardized "dose" of ultrasonic contrast has recently been achieved by the use of medically pure carbon dioxide [5] in volumes of $1-3 \, cm^3$ agitated with $5-8 \, cm^3$ of 5% dextrose in water. When the echocardiographic recordings made with CO_2 were compared to those obtained with 5% dextrose in water alone; it was clearly shown that a more reproducible contrast effect was obtained with intravenous CO_2-enriched injection than was possible with the unenriched medium.

Ziskin [6] compared the effectiveness of carbon dioxide to other agents by injecting them intra-arterially in dogs and measuring the amplitude of a Doppler-shifted audio signal. Both carbonated water and direct injection of carbon dioxide were among the most effective agents surpassed only by ether, which boils at body temperature. Both ether and carbon dioxide are attractive, since their gas content or gas-producing ability can be readily allocated at the time of injection. However, it may be quite difficult to control bubble size, since carbon dioxide solutions have been shown to be relatively unstable with rapidly changing bubble size and eventual coalesence into macrobubbles [4]. Similarly, bubble size control may be extremely difficult with an agent such as ether.

Hydrogen peroxide has enjoyed a period of intravascular use as an adjunctive source of oxygen for the anoxic or ischemic heart [7], in the treatment of the atherosclerotic process [8], and the potentiation of the effects of radiation on malignant tumors [9]. Hydrogen peroxide reacts with peroxidase and catalase enzyme systems in the blood producing oxygen and water. Arterial infusion of a 0.5% or less solution appears to be safe. In one series, $250 \, cm^3$ of 0.24 or 0.48% hydrogen peroxide was injected intra-arterially over 30 or 40 minutes in 37 patients with no apparent adverse effect [10].

In 1970, Dr. Robert Merin, Dr. Andrew Neal (then a medical student) and the present author used a 0.3% solution of hydrogen peroxide in saline in animal experiments with mongrel dogs. When $5 \, cm^3$ of the diluted solution was injected into a peripheral vein, an excellent contrast effect filled the right atrium and ventricle completely. A catheter injection of $5 \, cm^3$ of a 0.3% solution into the left atrium or left ventricle produced contrast filling that was judged to be too intense.

During these injections, the ECG and pressures in the right and left ventricle as well as in the left atrium were monitored and no change was evident. We did not extend these studies to humans, since we were unable to obtain an FDA approved source of injectable hydrogen peroxide.

Dr. Wang Xinfang and colleagues at Wuhan Medical College in Wuhan, China reported on the use of hydrogen peroxide as a contrast agent in humans [11]. In 100 patients, there were 420 injections with doses ranging from 0.5 to 1.0 ml of a 2–3% solution, which was injected in 1–2 s, preceded and followed by a saline flush. The echocardiographic studies indicated good results in 94% of the patient studies. Failures were attributed to insufficient peroxide concentration. Side effects related to the injection were noted in 11% and consisted of minor complaints of cough, abdominal pain, hemoptysis (on the day following the study in a patient with rheumatic heart disease), transient chest oppression and dizziness. No major problems were encountered. An interval of 5 min between injections with a maximum of 5 per study was recommended. The authors comment that hydrogen peroxide contrast echocardiography produced the best and most constant contrast effects with stronger and more persistent echoes. In fact, bubbles were still detectable in the heart on an average of 77.4 s in normals and 198 s in individuals with heart failure.

The observation of spontaneous, or in situ contrast in the heart or major blood vessels may offer a clue to other potential mechanisms for the generation of intracardiac contrast.

We became interested in direct imaging of intracardiac blood flow patterns when we noted that M-mode echocardiograms contained signals within heart cavities that were cardiac cycle related and changed with the phase of respiration as well as with altered cardiac function in disease states [12]. It seemed that only microbubbles could be generated and absorbed so rapidly and also be influenced by ambient pressure changes related to respirations. In addition, we encountered a patient with mitral prolapse who filled his left ventricular outflow tract with dense, transient contrast effect during the performance of a vigorous Valsalva maneuver. We postulated that severe turbulence developed during the Valsalva and that microbubbles were generated as the result of stable cavitation.

There can be little doubt that circulating blood has intrinsic echogenic properties, regardless of their origin, that could eventually provide a basis for real-time imaging of flow patterns. It is relatively common to see small bright particles in the inferior vena cava or in the portal system during routine abdominal real-time-B-scanning [13]. These punctate echoes appear to flow with the blood stream and are accelerated or decelerated by respirations. Those moving within the inferior vena cava also display a pattern of motion which appears to correspond to the hemodynamics of the right atrium.

Blood echoes are seen most readily in young, asthenic individuals and do not appear related to the time of day or to the state of digestive activity. Though the mechanism of the contrast effect has not been elucidated, it would appear that instruments with greater sensitivity and a higher signal-to-noise ratio could improve

the direct demonstration of blood flow in major vessels and probably in the heart as well.

Other observations of spontaneous intracardiac contrast serve to direct attention toward the development of other approaches which will require further investigation to establish their potential utility. The Indianapolis group [14] observed small, bright, particulate echo sources originating from a prosthetic mitral valve. Their clinical investigations led to the conclusion that the particles originated in fibrin deposits on the cage of the prosthesis. In an unrelated study, Ophir [15] and associates demonstrated that collagen (a strong reflector of ultrasound) in the form of 2 μm microspheres produced a tissue-staining effect and enhanced the ultrasonic reflection from liver. They also noted that in vitro comparison of the collagen particles to blood produced a strong contrast effect.

Fatty particles probably are not suitable for blood flow imaging with current instrumentation despite the fact that the characteristic impedance of fat differs more from that of blood than any other soft tissue. Ziskin's early work included intra-arterial infusion of milk at 2 ml/s with no significant enhancement of ultrasonic reflectivity [6]. We tried the intravenous injection of 15 cm^3 boluses of a 10% fat emulsion composed of 0.5 μm fatty particles (Intralipid 10%) in dogs. Real-time observation of right and left heart cavities did not reveal a recognizable change in the reflectivity of the blood stream.

Though it is clear that cavitation associated with high flow velocities can release gas from the circulating blood, another possible mechanism for this same effect has come to our attention. A patient with a malfunctioning mitral prosthesis and with clinical evidence of hemolysis demonstrated discrete echo sources which originated in the prosthesis and floated upward in the left ventricular outflow tract much like microbubbles. We filled our acoustically-monitored experimental chamber with blood and injected small amounts of Zaponin, which is a potent hemolytic agent. Echo sources could be observed floating upward in the chamber, but these could not be duplicated with subsequent injections of Zaponin in the presence of a chamber pressure of 20 lbs/square inch. It appears therefore that hemolysis is associated with the release of blood gas in a molecular form.

Hemolysis can also be produced by ultrasonic energy. Wong and Watmaugh [16] exposed blood samples to 750 kHz ultrasound at intensities ranging from 0.25 to 3.0 W/cm^2. Hemolysis could be detected in the blood samples and was related to cavitation induced by the ultrasonic energy. When the hearts of rats were exposed for 5 min to the same range of intensities, hemolysis was observed. The authors mention that acoustically-induced gas bubbles were probably present and played a role in this process. Certainly, the use of acoustic energy to cavitate the blood in either atrial cavity could provide a useful clinical tool if the energy could be delivered in a very short burst, so highly focused that tissues in the path receive no damage, and controlled with real-time observation to insure accurate confinement of the cavitating energy.

Recently, the group at Davis, California headed by DeMaria and working in conjunction with Rasor Associates of Sunnyvale, California has reported a contrast technique which represents a substantial breakthrough in the recognized problems of contrast echocardiography. These investigators have reported the use of $2-10\ \mu m$ gas-containing microballoons in a liquid suspension for the production of left heart contrast [17]. Intravenous injections in animals resulted in left heart opacification and left atrial injection filled right heart cavities indicating passage through both the pulmonary and systemic capillary beds. Preliminary work on myocardial staining [18] and on determination of cardiac output by indicator dilution techniques [19] has also been reported. The key to human applications would appear to lie in the stability of the microballoons, and the acceptability of the encapsulating material and its suspending liquid for intravascular use.

The future course of development of ultrasonic contrast agents will depend heavily on their ability to obtain the important clinical data which appears to be feasible with our present perception of contrast techniques. It will also be influenced by the emergence of direct imaging of blood flow patterns, further extension of Doppler technology, and the refinement of processing methods from which more information about the physical status of tissue can be derived – the so-called tissue signatures.

On the surface, the need for structure validation does not appear great except for the instances when bizarre anomalies are present. In these cases, a flow marker which allows recognition of right and left heart chamber filling sequences should be sufficient for anatomic validation. On the other hand, the endocardium of the left ventricular cavity is an excellent example of a weakly echoing source, which cannot be continuously imaged in all patients; thereby detracting from our ability to quantitate left ventricular cavity size. The small, omnidirectional scatterers, which constitute the currently successful contrast agents, should provide a marker for the endocardial limits in all patients and remove the element of ambiguity from left ventricular function studies. Furthermore, the reflections from the contrast material should be sufficiently unique in their shape, position, and reflectivity to make automated border finding algorithms relatively easy to implement from which global and segmental function could be automatically derived.

The anticipated tissue-staining qualities of ultrasonic contrast agents might be similarly applied to the evaluation of left ventricular function, but could also serve to identify perfusion deficits, infarcts, laminated clots, or intracardiac tumors in which neovascularity has developed.

Expectations are high that contrast agents with controlled particle size and volume will be highly useful in the development of indicator dilution studies for quantitation of valvular regurgitation, intracardiac shunts, and cardiac output.

How threatened is the whole concept of exogenous contrast echocardiography by the exciting possibilities of direct blood flow imaging or Doppler detection and characterization of flow parameters? The improvement in instrumentation which appears to be related to blood flow imaging will also be beneficial to the detection of contrast echoes. This could reduce the degree of impedance mismatch necessary for intracardiac contrast and allow the use of simpler or less expensive contrast media. Certainly, the imaging of a circulating bolus of contrast will have some practical advantages as compared to direct imaging, since the former will clearly indicate the sequence of chamber and great vessel filling where this may be more difficult to detect and decode when all flow signals have a common appearance and are not sequentially separated.

Doppler processing of echoes is still in its infancy and the potential of real-time, two-dimensional flow display has not been reached. Contrast agents could play an important role, since the contrast particles are much more reflective than red blood cells and offer the advantage of instrumentation operating at a much more advantageous signal-to-noise ratio. Combined imaging of soft tissue motion and blood circulation would be much more practical under these conditions.

The widespread efforts of investigators to provide a method for the analysis of tissue structure also represents a source of potential support for the extraction of data derived from contrast methods. Availability of highly detailed, time-varying changes in the distribution of intracardiac echo sources should provide a description of eddies and vortices from which a more quantitative characterization of turbulence can be derived. This should be useful in assessing the severity of hemodynamic abnormalities.

The initial benefit derived from ultrasonic contrast injections was the validation of structures which eliminated the uncertainty and provided a valuable stimulus to the attainment of clinical credibility for M-mode echocardiography in the early 1970s. Today's two-dimensional imaging systems provide relatively easy anatomic orientation and are poised on the brink of another sonic boom which, undoubtedly, will be based on functional data derived from blood flow imaging.

REFERENCES

1. Gramiak R, PM Shah, DH Kramer: Ultrasound cardiography: contrast studies in anatomy and function. Radiology 92:939–948, 1969.
2. Kremkau FW, R Gramiak, EL Carstensen, PM Shah, DH Kramer: Ultrasonic detection of cavitation at catheter tips. Am J Roentgenol 110:177–183, 1970.
3. Kremkau FW, EL Carstensen, R Gramiak: Ultrasonic detection of cavitation at catheter tips. Electrical Engineering Technical Report GM09933, University of Rochester, Department of Electrical Engeneering, Rochester, New York, March 1969.
4. Meltzer RS, EG Tickner, TP Sahines, RL Popp: The source of ultrasound contrast effect. J Clin Ultrasound 8:121–127, 1980.
5. Meltzer RS, PW Serruys, PG Hugenholtz, J Roelandt: Intravenous carbon dioxide as an echocardiographic contrast agent. J Clin Ultrasound 9:127–131, 1981.
6. Ziskin MC, A Bonakdarpour, DP Weinstein, PR Lynch: Contrast agents for diagnostic ultrasound. Invest Radiol 7:500–505, 1972.
7. Urschel HC, JW Finney, AR Morales, GA Balla, GJ Rage, JT Mallams: Cardiac resuscitation with hydrogen peroxide. Ann Thor Surg 2:665, 1966.
8. Finney JW, BE Jay, GJ Rage, HC Urschel, JT Mallams, GA Balla: Removal of choles-

24

terol and other lipids from experimental animal and human atheromatous arteries by dilute hydrogen peroxide. Angiol 17:223, 1966.

9. Mallams JT, GA Balla, JW Finney: Regional oxygenation and radiation. Current status. Am J Roentgenol Radium Ther Nucl Med 93:160, 1965.

10. Collier RE, GA Balla, JW Finney, AD D'Errico, JW Tomme, JE Miller, JT Mallams: Differential localization of isotopes in tumors through the use of intra-arterial hydrogen peroxide. Am J Roentgenol 94:789–797, 1965.

11. Xinfang W, W Jiaen, C Hanrong, L Chengfa: Contrast echocardiography with hydrogen peroxide. Chin Med J 92:693–702, 1979.

12. Gramiak R, PM Shah: Detection of intracardiac blood flow by pulsed echo-ranging ultrasound. Radiology 100:415–418, 1971.

13. Finberg HJ: Ultrasonic visualization of in vivo flow phenomena without introduced contrast material. Proc 25th Annu Convention Am Inst Ultrasound Med 17, 1980.

14. Schuchman H, H Feigenbaum, JC Dillon, S Chang: Intracavitary echoes in patients with mitral prosthetic valves. J Clin Ultrasound 3:107–110, 1975.

15. Ophir J, A Gobuty, RE McWhirt, NF Maklad: Ultrasonic backscatter from contrast producing collagen microspheres. Ultrasonic Imaging 2:67–77, 1980.

16. Wong YS, DJ Watmough: Haemolysis of red blood cells in vitro and in vivo caused by therapeutic ultrasound at 0.75 MHz. Proc Ultrasound Interaction Biol Med Int Symp, Castle Reinhardsbrunn, GDR, 10–14 November, 1980: C14.

17. Bommer WJ, EG Tickner, J Rasor, T Grehl, DT Mason, AN DeMaria: Development of a new echocardiographic contrast agent capable of pulmonary transmission and left heart opacification following peripheral venous injection. Circulation (Suppl III) 62: III-34, 1980.

18. DeMaria AN, WJ Bommer, K Riggs, A Dajee, M Keown, OL Kwan, DT Mason: Echocardiographic visualization of myocardial perfusion by left heart and intracoronary injections of echo contrast agents. Circulation (Suppl III) 62: III-143, 1980.

19. DeMaria AN, W Bommer, K Riggs, A Dajee, L Miller, DT Mason: In vivo correlation of cardiac output and densitometric dilution curves obtained by contrast two-dimensional echocardiography. Circulation (Suppl III) 62: III-101, 1980.

4. WHY CAPILLARY BEDS REMOVE ULTRASONIC CONTRAST

E. GLENN TICKNER and RICHARD S. MELTZER

INTRODUCTION

Ultrasonic contrast is an important part of ultrasonography because it improves identification of various interfaces. Complete definition without it is often difficult because only subtle dissimilarities in reflection characterictics exist. A good contrast agent has a vastly different acoustic impedance from the tissue with which it interfaces. Injectable contrast permits a clear partition between the contrast bearing fluid and its surroundings, and hence its diagnostic value. The acoustic impedance difference between injected ultrasonic contrast and surrounding tissue is due to microbubbles of gas [1–5]. Materials and substances other than bubbles have been studied [6, 7], but none have been found to be anywhere near as echogenic as microbubbles. This result may best be understood by inspecting the theoretical and experimental results of Lubbers and Van Den Berg [8] who examined the scattering from spheres for various excitation frequencies. For example, their results show that a 40 μm diameter microbubble excited by a 2 MHz frequency reflects 2×10^5 more signal than an equivalent size glass or steel sphere and nearly 4×10^5 times as much as an equivalent diameter red cell aggregate. This relative reflection ratio is even more pronounced for smaller bubbles. Microbubbles are thus superior ultrasonic contrast agents because they are superior reflectors: To say ultrasonic contrast is to say micobubbles. To ask the question, "Why do capillary beds remove ultrasonic contrast?" is really to ask the question, "Why do capillary beds remove microbubbles?" It is the latter question we wish to address in this chapter.

MICROBUBBLES

Meltzer et al. [5] showed that most commonly used contrast agents such as shaken saline, shaken indocyanine green, etc. have a spectrum of bubble sizes, and the great majority of these bubbles are larger than the pulmonary capillary diameter of about 8 μm [9]. If injected peripherally, these larger bubbles will be held up by the pulmonary vasculature, as if in a sieve. The smaller bubbles will pass through the lungs and shrink by dissolving along the way. The wedged bubbles probably stay at their blocking site until they dissolve sufficiently to pass to the next blockage point (bifurcation). Butler and Hills [10] slowly infused or bolus injected microbubbles

(14–189 μm) directly into the arterial and venous system and found in both cases that for normal systems the capillary beds removed all gas. They concluded that the lungs are superb filters for microbubbles.

Epstein and Plesset [11] examined low concentrations of gas bubbles dissolving in liquid solutions; their study found that bubbles will shrink and disappear by diffusion in both unsaturated and saturated solutions because of surface tension effects. Surface tension increases the pressure within a bubble above the local ambient pressure. This additional incremental internal pressure within a bubble p_i is given as

$$p_i = 4\,\sigma/d \tag{1}$$

where σ is the surface tension and d is the bubble diameter [12]. This greater pressure increases the gas concentration within the bubble and thus increases the diffusion rate. Gas loss causes a decreased bubble diameter and accelerates the dissolving

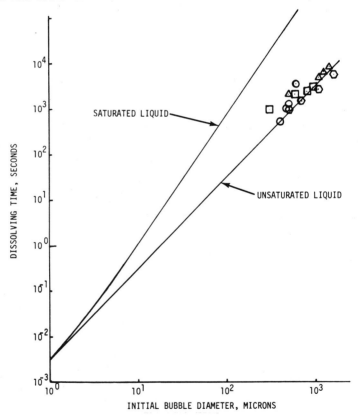

Figure 1. Log–log plot showing relationship between initial bubble diameter and time of total dissolution. Calculations based on theory presented by Epstein and Plesset [11], assuming nitrogen in degassed whole blood but not correction for flow effects. Data by Yang et al. [13] for unsaturated liquids given by the following symbols: ⊙, oxygen bubbles in human blood; ⊡, oxygen bubbles in canine blood; △, nitrogen bubbles in human plasma; and ⊙ oxygen bubbles in human plasma. Courtesy of Ultrasound in Medicine and Biology.

process until total dissolution occurs. The dissolving time for a single microbubble, taking into account the effects of surface tension, is presented in Figure 1 for both saturated and unsaturated solutions of infinite extent. Based on the results, an 8 μm nitrogen microbubble will completely dissolve between 190 and 550 ms depending upon the degree of saturation of the surrounding fluids. Carbon dioxide microbubbles, being more soluble in blood and body tissue, will dissolve even faster. Data from Yang et al. [13] also are presented in Figure 1 and indicate that nitrogen microbubbles in blood plasma dissolve as if in an unsaturated solution. Thus, the expected dissolving time will be close to 190 ms. All other effects, such as wiping away the diffusion boundary layer and using other gases, can decrease this time dramatically [14]. This figure should be considered conservative. Hamilton [15] gives a pulmonary capillary to left heart circulation time in humans of approximately two seconds or more. Hence, single 8 μm microbubbles dissolve completely in less than 190 ms and cannot appear in the left atrium.

Normally microbubbles are also not expected to survive the systemic capillarities. Hamilton [15] points out that normal systemic circulation times of more than 12 s are to be expected. Microbubbles injected into the arterial circulation cannot exist long enough to appear in the venous return flow. Systemic capillaries remove these bubbles as efficiently as pulmonary capillaries as verified by Butler and Hills.

Recent reports [16–19] have noted some obvious exceptions to the dissolving microbubble theory. Reale et al. [16] in Italy and Meltzer et al. [17] in the Netherlands reported left heart contrast following pulmonary wedge injections of carbon dioxide gas. Bommer et al. [18] observed left-sided contrast by peripherally injecting a saccharide microbubble dispersion.

It is not difficult to explain why pulmonary wedge injections yield left-sided contrast. Gas can be injected under pressure in large quantities at a rate greater than removal from the lungs. As a consequence, some of the gas is transported directly through the pulmonary circulation as a bolus to appear in the left heart. This procedure suffers from the necessity for wedge catheter placement, with all the associated risks and costs, and from the difficulty in standardizing the effect, that is in always obtaining the same contrast.

Bommer et al. reported left-heart contrast with peripherally injected contrast agents. This was done using a new, dense microbubble dispersion developed by Ultra Med, Inc. (formerly Rasor Associates) that was capable of passing through the entire pulmonary circulation. This material released over a million microbubbles whose mean diameter was 10 μm and size spectrum contained from 0.5 to 15 μm microbubbles. Some of these bubbles survived passage through the lungs. The question remains, "How can these microbubbles survive when others cannot?" The answers are quite complex and not completely understood at this time. One difference between the normally injected contrast, in which bubbles always dissolve, and this example wherein some survive, is bubble density.

If large concentration of noncoalescing microbubbles are brought together, dissolving may be reduced. The outermost bubbles tend to protect the inner ones because they are at the same gas concentration. Bubble dissolution is caused by a concentration gradient. If a gradient does not exist, dissolving does not occur. For the case of an assemblage of microbubbles, the outer bubbles eventually dissolve because they are only partially protected by the inner bubbles. The net result is that an assemblage of bubbles dissolves more slowly than individual bubbles.

If a train of packed microbubbles smaller than 8 μm enter a pulmonary capillary, a somewhat equivalent protective mechanism may exist. The bubbles still dissolve, but at reduced rates because the survivors within the train feed one another. The net effect is that some of the bubble train can emerge from the pulmonary circulation. It still must be shown if the process is quantifiable.

Preliminary calculations to verify these observations theoretically have shown that a bubble train model may allow a percentage of the bubbles within the train to pass through the pulmonary circulation as observed in reference [18]. A bubble train requires very special conditions, which normally are not met, to prevent complete dissolution. The first part of a train may increase the alveolar gas concentration to slow diffusion so that the remainder of the train can escape dissolution. Another important factor is that the saccharide coating protects the internal microbubble from normal fluid mechanical effects until it is partly dissolved.

SUMMARY

The microvasculature, both pulmonary and systemic, acts as a superb filter for microbubbles. Larger bubbles are held up at various bifurcations until they dissolve somewhat to pass downstream. Transit times across normal capillaries are long enough to allow bubbles of the size of these capillaries to dissolve completely before they can be detected at a downstream site. Consequently, they are eliminated from the circulation. In certain special circumstances, high concentrations of microbubbles have been observed to pass through the pulmonary circulation. It is suspected that the high density of bubbles provides limited self-protection to slow dissolution.

REFERENCES

1. Gramiak R, P Shah, D Kramer: Ultrasound cardiography: contrast studies in anatomy and function. radiology 92:939–948, 1969.
2. Kremkau FW, R Gramiak, E Carstensen, P Shah, H Kramer: Ultrasonic detection of cavitation at catheter tips. Am J Roentgenol 110:177–183, 1970.
3. Barrera J, P Fulkerson, SE Rittger, R Nerem: The nature of contrast echocardiographic "targets". Circulation (Suppl II) 58:II–233, 1978.
4. Seward JB, A Tajik, J Sprangler, D Ritter: Echographic contrast studies, initial experience. Mayo Clin Proc 50:163–192, 1975.
5. Meltzer R, EG Tickner, T Sahines, R Popp: The source of ultrasound contrast effect. J Clin Ultrasound 8:121–127, 1980.

6. Ophir J, R McWhirt, N Maklad: Aqueous solution as potential ultrasonic contrast agents. Ultrasonic Imaging 1:265–279, 1979.
7. Ophir J, A Gobuty, R McWhirt, N Maklad: Ultrasonic backscatter from contrast producing collagen microspheres. Ultrasonic Imaging 2:67–77, 1980.
8. Lubbers J, J Van den Berg: An ultrasonic detector for microgasemboli in a bloodflow line. Ultrasound Med Biol 2:301–310, 1976.
9. Weibel ER: Morphometry of the Human Lung, pp 78–82. Academic Press, N Y, 1975.
10. Butler B, B Hills: The lung as a filter for microbubbles. J Appl Physiol 47:537–543, 1979.
11. Epstein P, M Plesset: On the stability of gas bubbles in liquid-gas solutions. J Chem Phys 18:1505–1509,1950.
12. Vennard J, R Street: Elementary fluid mechanics, 5th Edn, p 25, John Wiley, 1975.
13. Yang W, R Echigo, D Molten, J Hwang: Experimental studies of the dissolution of gas bubbles in whole blood and plasma – I. Stationary bubbles. J Biomech 3:275–281, 1971.
14. Yang W, R Echigo, D Molten, J Hwang: Experimental studies of the dissolution of gas bubbles in whole blood and plasma – II. Moving bubbles. J Biomech 4:283–288, 1971.
15. Hamilton WF (ed): Handbook of Physiology, Vol 2, Sec 2 circ, p 1709. Am Physiol Soc, Washington, DC, 1963.
16. Reale A, F Pizzuto, P Gioffre, A Nigri, F Romeo, E Martuscelli, E Mangieri, G Scibilia: Contrast echocardiography:transmission of echos to the left heart across the pulmonary vascular bed. Eur Heart J 1:101–107, 1980.
17. Meltzer R, O Sartorius, C Lancée, P Serruys, P Verdouw, C Essed, J Roelandt: Transmission of ultrasonic contrast though the lungs. Ultrasound Med Biol 7: 377–384, 1981.
18. Bommer W, G Tickner, J Rasor, T Grehl, D Mason, A DeMaria: Development of a new echographic contrast agent capable of pulmonary transmission and left heart opacification following peripheral venous injection. Am J Cardiol, 1980 (abstract).

5. ULTRASONIC STUDIES DURING EXPERIMENTAL DECOMPRESSION

GEORGE J. RUBISSOW and R. STUART MACKAY

INTRODUCTION

Ultrasonic exploration is the method of choice in the study of tiny bubbles postulated to be the principle cause of decompression sickness (DS). These bubbles, which can occur when inert gas in blood and tissues exists in supersaturation during decompression following diving, are readily detected ultrasonically because small bubbles interact very strongly with sound waves. Over the last twenty years, a variety of ultrasonic techniques has been perfected and applied to DS studies [1, 2] as described briefly in this chapter.

These studies aimed at finding ways for the most rapid and safe decompression of divers, caisson workers, and others exposed to decompression. Since susceptibility to DS was found to vary considerably with divers, activity, and other factors, it was hoped that monitoring "silent bubbles", postulated to exist before clinical signs of DS appear, could be used to control the decompression profile to give an optimum safe ascent tailored to an individual, and to control treatment if symptoms developed. On a detailed level the central questions remained: where, when, and how do bubbles form, their size and physiological action, do they form in blood or in tissues and in which tissues, and how are gases exchanged between tissues and blood?

Nonpathological decompression is also a possible source of silent bubbles which could be used effectively as a contrast agent in ultrasonic biomedical studies.

INERT GAS EXCHANGE AND BUBBLE FORMATION

In evaluating the tendency for bubbles to form, the tissue dissolved gas tension must be known during decompression. Traditionally, it is assumed that inert gas exchange between capillaries and tissues is limited by blood perfusion and that diffusion is so rapid as to be negligible. This leads to a simple model where a step change in inspired gas pressure or composition results in an exponential gas exchange in each tissue at a rate determined by perfusion and gas solubility, and characterized by the tissue time constant or half-time, which for humans ranges from a few minutes to hundreds of minutes. There is evidence, however, that diffusion in cells may be from 10^2 to 10^4 times slower than in extracellular fluid, in which case at least three time constants may be needed to describe a single tissue type [3].

Bubble formation in tissue depends on the extent of supersaturation in that tissue, commonly measured by the supersaturation ratio, $\gamma = P_i/P_a$, and pressure difference, $\Delta P = P_i - P_a$ where P_i is the inert gas tension in a tissue, and P_a is the ambient hydrostatic pressure. The mechanism for bubble formation is still not clear, but research [4] seems to confirm an old theory that bubble formation is related at least in part to preexisting micronuclei. Recent work also suggests that not only inert gas tension, but the tensions of all dissolved gases, including oxygen, play a role in bubble formation and evolution. Nevertheless, practice dictates that bubbles form when γ or ΔP reach critical values which vary with tissue and dive profile.

In the traditional supersaturation approach, optimum decompression is achieved by maintaining γ or ΔP for each limiting tissue just below the critical threshold. In the "phase equilibration" approach [3], on the other hand, gas is assumed to separate immediately at low supersaturations and then be eliminated due to an "inherent unsaturation" of tissues relative to formed bubbles, largely caused by metabolic conversion of oxygen in tissues into highly soluble CO_2. Ultrasonic observations suggest that the truth lies between these two views, since for short dives bubbles appear only at relatively high values of γ (e.g. $\gamma = 2$) while for long saturation dives they indeed appear at very low supersaturations.

For animal studies an effective dive-ascent profile is a rapid increase to bottom pressure which is held for a time T and then followed by a linear return to original ambient pressure in a further time T. This selectively stresses tissues of time constant approximately equal to T, and permits study of specific tissues by controlling pressure and bottom time [5]. For such step-ramp dives, P_i, γ, and ΔP can be calculated for tissues of given time constants using the traditional gas exchange theory and presented in the form of computer plotted graphs such as shown in Figure 1.

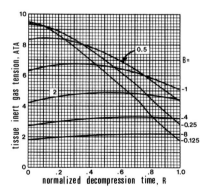

Figure 1. Computer plot of tissue inert gas tension, P_i, for a step-ramp dive, bottom time T, equal to the linear decompression time. Initial and final pressure 1 ATA, bottom pressure $P_b = 10$ ATA. R is the actual decompression time divided by T. Each curve is for tissue of normalized time constant B, equal to the tissue time constant divided by T. Gas mixtures: initially air; compression and decompression until 3.5 ATA, on 95% N_2 5% O_2; decompression below 3.5 ATA, air. The change in gas mixtures, to avoid oxygen toxicity, gives slight inflections in the curves.

ULTRASONIC BUBBLE DETECTION

Quantitative studies of the role of bubbles in decompression require in vivo knowledge of real-time size and location, and minimum detectable size of bubbles. This section explores some ultrasonic methods for resolving these questions.

A bubble in a sound field of given frequency reflects a signal whose amplitude decreases approximately linearly with decreasing bubble diameter until the bubble resonant diameter is reached, and then decreases as the cube of the diameter [6]. This general trend is interrupted in two regions by perturbations in the response. The first causes fluctuations in response when bubble size is comparable to the wavelength of sound. The second causes a peak in response when the size corresponds to the bubble resonant frequency, which in water at 1 ATA is given approximately by $d = 6.4/f$, where d is the diameter in microns, and f the frequency in MHz. The resonant frequency of a given diameter bubble varies directly with the square root of the pressure inside the bubble. In the scattering region, where the signal falls off as the cube of diameter, the signal is approximately 6400 times larger than from a rigid sphere of same diameter [7], which shows how effectively bubbles reflect sound waves, and why they are excellent contrast agents in decompression studies.

The above described variation in received, reflected signal voltage with diameter permits size estimation from measurements of signal voltage under standardized conditions. However, because of fluctuations and perturbations in response, a measured voltage may correspond to several bubble diameters [8], and the diameter is not always a single-valued function of voltage. Under proper conditions this ambiguity may be reduced substantially for three reasons. At high frequencies resonant bubble diameters are about 1 μm; such small bubbles collapse very rapidly due to surface tension, and are thus not likely to be present for any appreciable time during measurements. Secondly, in blood at 1 ATA the resonant peak is greatly attenuated (due to blood viscosity), although at higher pressures the attenuation is less and the ambiguity may reappear. Finally, in pulsed ultrasonic systems the resonant peak and flucatuations are considerably "smoothed" because the transmitted sound wave comprises a wide spectrum of frequencies and the bubble no longer reacts to a single frequency excitation [5].

The measured response of a pulsed imaging system in water [5] operating at 7.5 MHz is shown in Figure 2. Bubble 'targets' for these tests were observed with a microscope, and included free electrolytically generated bubbles, as well as collapsing bubbles restrained by an acoustically transparent piece of gelatin with a small depression into which the bubble floated. In vitro tests of CW Doppler devices [9] have shown nearly linear variation of reflected signal amplitude with bubble diameter.

Bubble size measurement with external Doppler systems usually gives only relative size indications because of uncertainties in orientation, bubble location, and transient nature of signal. Better measurements should be possible with in vivo reference [10], or with transducers implanted around veins or arteries.

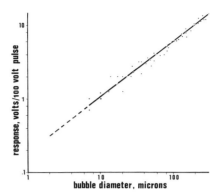

Figure 2. Normalized measured response of an ultrasonic scanner system to a small bubble in water. The response is the peak received echo amplitude at the amplifier output, using maximum 95 dB gain and a 7.5 MHz crystal transducer with 100 V pulse excitation. The noise at the output is about 0.2 V peak and is nearly independent of the transmitted pulse amplitude.

With careful calibration, an imaging system yields good size estimation [5] if the effect of all acoustic structures intervening between transducer and bubble is taken into account. Deflection modulation of the sector scan with scan lines spaced to prevent image fusion allows accurate measurement of echo amplitude, given by echo deflection height. The scan also gives the exact bubble distance from the transducer and thickness of intervening tissues. After correction of the echo amplitude for bubble distance, attenuation from tissue and other structures, excitation pulse height, receiver gain, and transducer temperature, a standardized plot such as Figure 2, gives the bubble size within limits of fluctuations in the plot.

Size determination based on variation of bubble resonant frequency with diameter has been much discussed and some promising results [11, 12] have been obtained. At atmospheric pressure, however, the resonant peak is sufficiently damped in blood, to make this technique difficult.

To measure bubble size with a sector-scan imaging system the bubble must be centered with respect to the thickness of the sector-scan slice. Clearly, an echo from such a centered bubble could also come from a larger off-center bubble (above or below the plane of scan). This ambiguity can be removed by either centering the scan plane to maximize a given echo, or by scanning three adjacent planes. Slowly varying bubble signals can be evaluated unambiguously by momentary recentering of the scan plane, but this is generally impossible with rapidly changing bubbles where an ambiguity may remain unless a three-plane scan is used. The probability that a given echo corresponds to a given bubble size depends on the azimuthal resolution of the scanner and on the bubble size distribution. Figure 3 shows a typical azimuthal resolution curve of a scanner together with the computed magnification factor of bubbles that are off-center relative to centered bubbles.

Bubbles are best located in vivo with imaging systems. The location accuracy improves with higher frequencies and low transducer "f-number," but this degrades

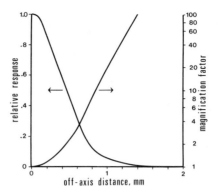

Figure 3. Azimuthal resolution of a 14.1 mm diameter, 7.5 MHz lithium sulfate transducer at the 7.1 cm focal point, with the corresponding computed magnification factor of bubbles that are off-center, to give the same response as an on-center unit bubble. Example: an echo from a centered 5 μm diameter bubble could also be produced by a 20 × 5 = 100 μm bubble, 1 mm above the center of the scan plane.

the ability to visualize deeper below the skin, so that a compromise must usually be made between resolution and penetration.

If sound velocity and refraction errors in tissues are compensated, a typical 7.5 MHz system focused at 7.1 cm can locate a tiny bubble to an accuracy of about 0.2–0.7 mm [5], depending on echo height and background echoes. Overlapping of adjacent bubble echoes makes it difficult for such a system to separate bubbles closer together than about 0.7 mm in range and 1.5 mm in azimuth.

A most promising method of real-time bubble detection and location uses imaging with a "phased array" in which the scanning probe is stationary and comprises an array of tiny transducers synchronized to scan electronically. Such units are currently under intensive commercial development. Figure 4 shows a column of tiny bubbles imaged by a 2.25 MHz phased array comprising 64 transducers on a 1 inch square probe, scanning thirty images per second [13]. The resolution is appropriate to the overall array size, but the subdivision of the transducer can cause phantom images to appear in directions other than that of momentary aim (as in a diffraction grating), which must be considered in design and use of such a system. Such a system can look through an intercostal space at bubbles that have drained into the right heart.

In vivo measurements of vascular bubble velocity is possible with CW Doppler detectors with known orientation to a blood vessel, though in practice this is difficult. A high speed scanner, such as the phased array described above, can also give bubble velocity.

The minimum bubble size detectable by ultrasound depends on the frequency, background noise surrounding the bubble, and scan depth, assuming optimum transducer and electronics design. An approximate limit to detectable size is probably set by the bubble resonant diameter. Based on an extrapolation of the curve in Figure 2, the smallest bubble detectable [5] in water with such a 7.5 MHz pulsed system is about 0.5 μm in diameter, just below the resonant diameter. Although

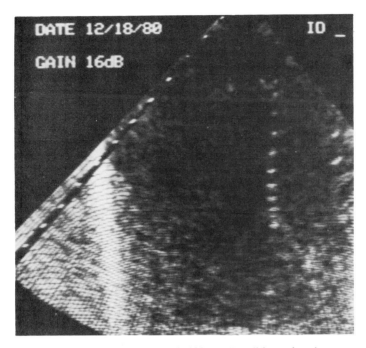

Figure 4. Real-time image of a column of tiny bubbles as "seen" by a phased-array system with a stationary probe. The two images at the far right are artifacts, and the column of light dots along the left margin of the sector scan is a set of range markers.

extremely unstable, such a bubble would be measured with a signal-to-noise ratio of about 9 dB, using 600 V excitation pulses. In practice no bubbles smaller than 7 μm in diameter were measured because smaller bubbles collapsed almost instantly in water. The 7.5 MHz system would resolve a 2 μm diameter bubble, 1 cm deep in guinea pig tissue in vivo, with a S/N ratio of about 5 dB, taking into account the 4.7 dB round trip attenuation (in excess of water attenuation) of guinea pig muscle tissue, and that background noise for 600 V pulses, 1 cm deep in muscle tissue, is about 0.6 V. Using different B-scan equipment operating at 8 MHz [8], a minimum detectable bubble size of 10 μm was reported.

The minimum size bubble detectable by Doppler is considerably larger than that using imaging, because of the increased background noise due to blood flow. Doppler observation of the thoracic caudal vena cava in Hanford miniature swine, following injection of glass microspheres, showed that 40 μm spheres are not detectable individually [14] while 80 μm spheres are detectable individually. Bubbles, however, should be better reflectors than rigid microspheres.

BUBBLE STABILITY

Small bubbles in solution are inherently unstable and will grow or decay depending upon the differences in gas tensions inside and outside the bubble, and upon surface tension. In water 10 μm bubbles collapse in some seconds and a 5 μm diameter bubble collapses in about 1 s. Thus, unless very small bubbles are stabilized, as has been suggested, by platelets or by a surface layer of fibrinogen, it is unlikely that they will exist and be visualized for more than a few seconds.

A bubble of initial radius R_0 will grow by a factor E, in a liquid of supersaturation ratio γ, in a time t, in seconds, given by [15], (R_0 in microns),

$$t = \frac{R_0^2}{80(\gamma - 1)} (E^2 - 1) \tag{1}$$

where surface tension has ben neglected, as has been verified experimentally. This enables estimating either bubble size, R_0, or γ in vivo. To measure R_0, a bubble is imaged ultrasonically and the hydrostatic pressure is adjusted to a value H_0, so that the bubble neither grows nor decays. The pressure is then decreased slightly by an increment h (to give a known $\gamma = 1 + h/H_0$) and the time is measured for the bubble size ratio to change a given amount. For bubbles larger than 10 μm in diameter, the surface tension can be neglected and equation (1) is used to calculate R_0. Alternatively, by measuring the time for a given bubble to grow by a given ratio, γ may be estimated for the tissue surrounding the bubble – a very useful technique.

DECOMPRESSION STUDIES

The original suggestion that ultrasonic imaging could show decompression bubbles in vivo, was confirmed in a decompressed rat observed with 15 MHz ultrasound [16]. Subsequently extensive experimental work has exploited imaging, Doppler, transmission, absorption, and resonance in decompression studies [1, 5, 17, 18, 19]. Some highlights of this work are reviewed below, starting with studies by the authors and then presenting other imaging and Doppler studies.

Studies with guinea pigs, hamsters, and human divers were made using a high performance B-scan imaging system, operating with a 7.5 MHz, 14.1 mm diameter lithium sulfate transducer, focused at 7.1 mm and excited by pulses adjustable from 100 to 1200 V at 1 kHz pulse rate. The average intensity for 200 V pulses was 0.61 mW/cm^2. Single bubbles could be located to about 0.5 mm, and adjacent bubbles or echoes separated at about 1.5 mm. Deflection modulation of the display was added to the conventional intensity modulation to permit accurate measurements of echo heights, and the real time display was photographed on Polaroid or movie film.

The guinea pig is a convenient animal for such studies because its relatively small size permits a variety of tissue types to be observed at typical depths below the skin of only 1 cm. This means that high frequencies may be used for higher bubble resolution without excessive signal loss from tissue attenuation, as would be the case if much deeper tissues were studied. The hind leg was scanned just below the knee, giving data on skin, muscle, fat, bone, nerve, connective and vascular tissue. Techniques were developed [5, 18] for immobilizing the leg in a perfectly non-constricting manner and for observing the animal ultrasonically and visually within a pressure chamber.

To facilitate locating elusive tiny bubble echoes against a background cluttered with various tissue echoes, a Polaroid oscilloscope camera-viewer was modified to include an optical comparator which could superimpose a reference Polaroid image on the real-time display. During decompression the reference image would be turned up whenever any doubt existed whether an echo was a new bubble echo or background. For long decompressions different reference photos were inserted depending upon needs. The background could be suppressed by superimposing a negative image of proper luminosity making newly appearing echoes stand out on a black background, but in practice this method was only moderately effective.

Figure 5 shows selected scans of a step-ramp dive to 10 ATA for 40 min together with a matching sketch of presumed anatomical features of the guinea pig leg. The area scanned was concurrently sampled with a 7.5 MHz high sensitivity external Doppler device viewing a volume about 4×10 mm in cross section over depths ranging from 1 to 2 cm. This device could detect from 5 to 10 μm moving bubbles in water.

Once bubble echoes appeared the decompression rate in Figure 5 was "bubble-controlled" to maintain imaged bubble echo heights at low to moderate levels. In the scan photos the sound beam is from the left and time in hundredths of minutes is shown at the right. Reference scan (a) taken well before bubble detection, shows skin at front and back of the leg, important triangular area of fat, some fascia below the fat (vertical triangular area of fat, some fascia below the fat (vertical lines), and the fibula and part of the tibia. The bones, being absorbent, cast ultrasonic "shadows." The first bubbles were imaged just before 71 min with no signs of guinea pig distress and no Doppler echoes detected. Bubbles appear in the fat in (b, c) and disappear after recompression at 71.7 min (d, e). Subsequent ascent maintained echoes at a moderate level shown in (f), corresponding to bubbles of about 20 μm diameter average. Bubbles first appeared at 3.5 ATA and were found to be stable when the pressure was increased to 5.5 ATA. This means that the inert gas tension at time of bubble appearance was about 5.5 ATA (neglecting surface tension) and that $\gamma = 5.5/3.5 = 1.6$. This is a powerful technique for measuring inert gas exchange in vivo at a determined site, in this case, fat. The time constant of this tissue can be estimated from Figure 1, at R = 0.72, as either 10 or 70 min (there are two curves corresponding to the same value of R = 0.72 and P_i = 5.5 ATA). Other data[5]; suggesting that the longest time constant in guinea pigs is 25–36 min, implies that the limiting tissue in this experiment had the 10 min time constant.

In scans (f, g, h, i) a sudden pressure drop from 2.75 to 2.50 ATA ($\gamma = 1$ changes to $\gamma = 1.1$) at 235.50 min, causes some initially stable bubbles to double their diameters in 30 s. From equation (1) the initial bubble diameter should thus be approximately 18 μm in close agreement with the 20 μm diameter determined from the echo height.

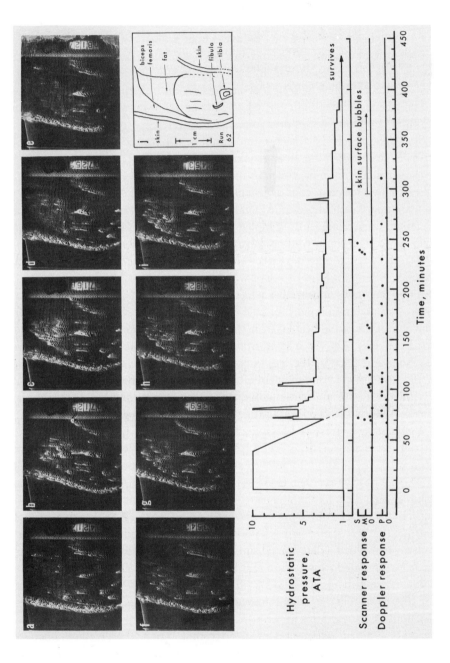

Figure 5. Bubble imaging during a "bubble-controlled" decompression of a guinea pig.

The repeatable reduction or disappearance of echoes with recompression confirms that real bubbles and not various aggregates were observed.

Another example of decompression bubbles is seen in Figure 6, in a step-ramp dive to 10 ATA for 60 min, where each scan image (occurring at 8 frames/s was photographed on movie film and then carefully analyzed for moving bubbles. In (a) the bubble echoes are just appearing (faint bars to the left of large echo near the number "71"). Developing bubbles fluctuate and migrate conspicuously over intervals of 5–20 s, as is even apparent in (c, d) taken only 0.5 s apart, until consolidation in the angular mass of bubbles (f, g) probably in the fat. In (f,g) echoes are so strong that they shade and mask everything behind them (as seen by the scanner).

These guinea pig experiments showed that: 1) bubble echoes represent true bubbles and not cellular or plasma aggregates; 2) over a wide range of decompression times bubbles form mostly in the blood or fatty tissue, and to a much lesser extent in muscle, fascia, etc. (except in short severe dives); 3) bubbles can appear

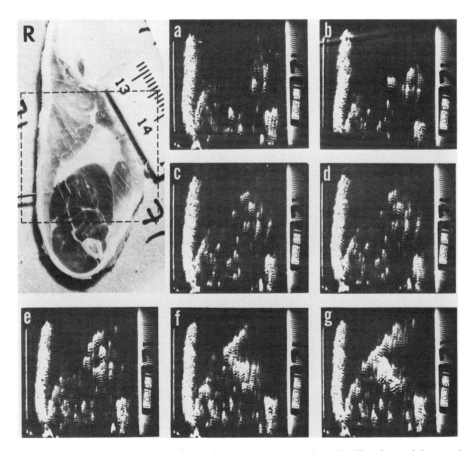

Figure 6. Transient bubbles imaged during decompression in a guinea pig. The photo of the actual frozen cross section of the leg is to the same scale as the scans – the white mass in the center is fat, and the black dots are blood vessels.

before symptoms of DS; 4) sometimes recompression produced "bubble showers" due to liberation of bubbles trapped in capillary beds; 5) bubbles occur in symptom-free long dives; 6) severe bends symptoms appeared when detected bubble diameters were approximately 40 μm; 7) bubble-controlled decompression worked; 8) important gas exchange parameters could be measured in vivo at a particular site; 9) a time lag of about 2 min appeared to exist from the time a critical decompression threshold was passed until bubbles formed.

In human studies conducted with divers in Hawaii, preliminary results showed probable bubble echoes at the site of pain in two cases of divers experiencing mild bends in the knee. Possible silent bubbles were observed in one very well controlled dive, and it was shown conclusively that no bubbles in the 50–200 μm range occurred in the areas scanned during and after decompression. Unforeseen environmental difficulties limited detection here to bubbles larger than 20 μm. Figure 7 shows scanning of a diver's knee in progress in a submersible habitat during a 400 ft helium dive. Monitoring equipment was locked in during the last 50 ft of the dive.

In other studies bubble development in goldfish (*Carassius auratus*) was observed by B-scan imaging [5, 7] and showed repeated survival following extensive bubbles in white muscle, gut, fins, ovaries, and along bones, resulting from ascent after 4 h at 8 ATA.

The above work has been elaborated and continued in studies [20, 21] with anesthetized guinea pigs using a modified commercial B-scan device operating at 8 MHz, 2.3 mW/cm^2 intensity, with sensitivity resolving approximately 10 μm diameter bubbles. Early-appearing bubbles were of varying and transient character, evolving to dynamic, which is suggestive of vascular bubbles. Further evolution led to stationary bubbles. The most active areas were blood vessels in fatty tissue at interfaces (e.g., blood vessels crossing the surface of the tibia at the junction of the tibia cranialis). EKG monitoring of DS was used but early clinical signs could not be observed because of anesthesia. The scanner output was stored in a computer [21] as a reference, permitting integration of pulses received in a region and then suppressing the background. A phased-array system is projected to work with this computer.

Decompression bubbles in hamsters have been successfully imaged using a novel acoustic-optical converter [22]. The method lacked resolution because the ratio of laser to ultrasonic wavelength was very small, but was able to image large volumes which could facilitate finding where bubbles originate.

Simplicity of design, lower cost, and relative ease of use have made Doppler bubble monitoring during decompression widespread, even though it is limited to the detection of moving bubbles. Such bubbles were first detected by Doppler [23] in the vena cava of a sheep during decompression from a 200 ft, 60 min dive and in the descending aorta upon surfacing. After considerable work during which Doppler bubbles were detected in humans an efficient precordial Doppler detector was designed and tested [24] using two 5 MHz half-inch square crystals separated by 2 cm to focus on the pulmonary artery 3-7 cm retrosternally. Extensive use of this technique has led to the evolution of a number of schemes for grading the level or

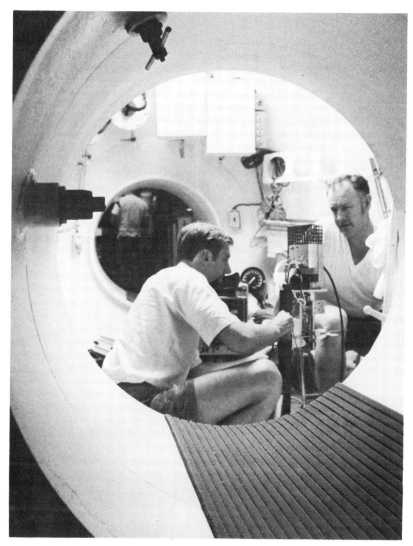

Figure 7. **B-scan monitoring of a diver's knee during a 400 ft helium dive in a submersible habitat. The** transducer is coupled to the leg through a thin water-filled balloon and acoustic gel; the scanner is accurately positioned with respect to the knee by a set of rods, a foot outline, measured coordinates, and standardized seating. Several divers were monitored.

intensity of Doppler bubble signals by comparing the number and level of audible signals with the heart and blood flow background sound [1].

A correlation in human divers of Doppler bubble grade [25] with some DS symptoms has been made. Prediction of dive outcome based on bubble grade was deemed possible, but not yet reliable, because bubbles monitored in the pulmonary artery are a long way removed from sites of bubble formation, and sometimes formed bubbles are not released into the circulation and hence undetected by

Doppler. The advantage of imaging methods, which can detect both stationary and moving bubbles, is apparent in this respect. Another extensive study [26] has found that DS symptom severity generally follows increase in bubble grade and that very minor DS symptoms, such as itches, have been recorded even when no Doppler bubbles were detected.

An interesting application of Doppler technique [27] has been the determination of maximum decrease in pressure, ΔP, from a saturation pressure, P_s, in rats and dogs, to produce no bubbles, some bubbles, and finally symptoms of DS. Significantly, it was found that the no-bubble threshold was the same for rats and dogs over a range of P_s from 3 to 10 ATA. Bubbles appeared before DS symptoms.

Of considerable interest to decompression studies is continuing work [28] on isobaric counterdiffusion where bubbles are produced at a fixed pressure by a change in breathing gases. Thus, it has been shown in goats and in miniature swine that a change to 4.7 ATA helium 0.3 ATA O_2, after saturation with 4.7 ATA nitrogen 0.3 ATA O_2, produced Doppler bubbles detected in the inferior vena cava after 1 h (goats) and 3.5 h (swine). The latter echoes persisted for over 48 h, suggesting that echoes may have arisen from circulating platelet aggregates or stabilized bubbles. This technique holds promise for future studies and contrast production for ultrasonic observations.

REFERENCES

1. Pearson R (ed): Early diagnosis of decompression sickness. Undersea Med Soc, Bethesda, MD, 1977.
2. Schilling CW, MF Werts: Physical methods of bubble detection in blood and tissues. Undersea Med Soc, Bethesda, MD, 1977.
3. Hills BA: Thermodynamic decompression: an approach based upon the concept of phase equilibration in tissue. In: Bennet PB, DH Elliot (eds) The physiology and medicine of diving, p 319–356, Bailliere Tindall and Cassell, London, 1975.
4a. Vann RD, J Grimstad, CH Nielsen: Evidence for gas nuclei in decompressed rats. Undersea Biomed Res 7(2):107–112, 1980.
4b. Yount DE: Skins of varying permeability: a stabilization mechanism for gas cavitation nuclei. J Acoust Soc Am 65(6):1429, 1979.
4c. Kunkle TD, EL Beckman, DE Yount: Non-haldanian decompression schedules. Session XX, Inert Gas Exchange and Decompression 7th Symp Underwater Physiol, Athens, July 1980.
4d. Lehto VP, I Kantola, T Tervo, LA Laitinen: Ruthenium red staining of blood–bubble interface in acute decompression sickness in rat. Undersea Biomed Res 8:101–111, 1981.
5. Rubissow GJ: A study of decompression sickness using ultrasonic imaging of bubbles. PhD thesis, University of California, Berkeley, 1973.
6. Nishi RY: Problem areas in the ultrasonic detection of decompression bubbles. In ref. [1] above, 1977.
7. Mackay RS, GJ Rubissow: Decompression studies using ultrasonic imaging of bubbles. IEEE Trans Biomed Eng BME-25(6):537–544, 1978.
8. Beck TW, S Daniels, WDM Paton, EB Smith: Detection of bubbles in decompression sickness. Nature 276:173–174, 1978.

9. Monjaret JL, R Guillerm, G Masurel: Detector of bubbles moving through blood vessels with Doppler signal, Colloq Int Capteurs Bio Med, Paris, 1975.
10. Nishy RY: Ultrasonic detection of bubbles with doppler flow transducers. Ultrasonics 10 (4):173–179, 1972.
11. Horton JW, CH Wells: Resonance ultrasonic measurements of microscopic gas bubbles. Aviat Space Environ Med 47:777–781, 1976.
12. Fairbank WM, MO Scully: A new noninvasive technique for cardiac pressure measurement: resonant scattering of ultrasound from bubbles. IEEE Trans Biomed Eng BME-24(2):107–110, 1977.
13. Mackay RS: Personal communication.
14. Gillis MF: Evaluation of swine as a hyperbaric analog to man and detection of emboli by use of ultrasonic Doppler flowmeter. Final Rep to ONR (AD 724 765), Battelle Mem Inst, Richland, Wash. 1971.
15. Epstein PS, MS Plesset: On the stability of gas bubbles in liquid-gas solutions. J Chem Phys 18:1505–1509, 1950.
16. Mackay RS: Proc Second Symp on Underwater Physiol, National Academy of Sciences/ National Research Council Publ 1181, p 41, 1963.
17. Mackay RS, GJ Rubissow: Detection of bubbles in tissues and blood. Fourth Symp on Underwater Physiol, Philadelphia 1969, In: Lambertsen C (ed) Underwater Physiology, pp 151–160. Academic Press, New York, 1971.
18. Rubissow GJ, RS Mackay: Ultrasonic imaging of in vivo bubbles in decompression sickness. Ultrasonics 9:225–234, 1971.
19. Smith KH, MP Spencer: Doppler indices of decompression sickness: their evaluation and use. Aerospace Med 41(12):1396–1400, 1970.
20. Daniels S, WDM Paton, EB Smith: Ultrasonic imaging system for the study of decompression-induced gas bubbles. Undersea Biomed Res 6(2):197–207, 1979.
21. Daniels S, JM Davies, WDM Paton, EB Smith: Monitoring bubble formation with an integrating pulse-echo ultrasonic method. Session XX, Inert Gas Exchange and Decompression 7th Symp Underwater Physiol Athens, July, 1980.
22. Buckles RS, C Knox: In vivo bubble detection by acoustic-optical imaging techniques. Nature 222:771–772, 1969.
23. Spencer MP, SD Campbell: Development of bubbles in venous and arterial blood during hyperbaric decompression. Bull Mason Clinic 22:26–32, 1968.
24. Spencer MP, N Simmons, HF Clarke: A precordial transcutaneous cardiac output and aeroembolism monitor. Fed Proc 30:703, 1971.
25. Powell MR: Physiological significance of doppler-detected bubbles in decompression sickness. In ref [1] above, 1977.
26. Nashimoto I, Y Gotah: Ultrasonic doppler detection of blood bubbles in caisson work. In ref [1] above, 1977.
27. Lin YS: Species independent maximum no-bubble decompression from saturation dive. Session XX, Inert Gas Exchange and Decompression 7th Symp Underwater Physiol, Athens, July 1980.
28. D'Aoust BG: Theoretical and practical review of concepts of ascent criteria. In ref [1] above, 1977.

B. CLINICAL APPLICATIONS

6. METHODOLOGY IN CONTRAST ECHOCARDIOGRAPHY

NELSON B. SCHILLER and JAMES A. GOLDSTEIN

The intravenous saline contrast technique has become standard and widely employed as it facilitates the detection of intracardiac shunts, enhances chamber identification by cavity opacification and definition of endocardial surfaces, and facilitates the detection of tricuspid insufficiency. A major limitation of this technique has been its inability to reproduce a sufficiently intense contrast effect [1, 2]. This limitation is of clinical importance because it is often necessary to perform a series of contrast maneuvers on the same patient. In our early experience with this technique, up to 75% of all injections were judged technically inadequate. However, we have evolved a technique which has circumvented the problem of reproducibility. There are several key elements which contribute to the success of this technique. Principal among these elements are the choice of intravenous catheter, the preparation of the contrast solution, and the selection of venous access. Minor considerations which contribute to the successful performance of the contrast technique are syringe size, the use of a three-way stopcock, and the performance of complimentary maneuvers such as upper arm massage and the Valsalva maneuver.

INTRAVENOUS CATHETER

A major limiting feature of our early attempts to achieve reproducible contrast studies was infiltration at the vena puncture site. This particular problem resulted from forceful delivery of contrast from the syringe, which is critical in achieving the contrast effect. Unfortunately, high velocity fluid delivery often resulted in extravasation of fluid and occasionally hematoma. We therefore abandoned the use of scalp vein infusion sets and adopted the use of a 20-gauge, $1\frac{1}{4}$ in. teflon catheter (Deseret Angiocath R). Once we had adopted the use of this equipment, the extravasation of fluid ceased to be a problem. (Figure 1).

PREPARATION OF THE SOLUTION

In our laboratory, we use saline solution because of its ready availability. We have not attempted to use any other type of contrast agent, although some centers report success with glucose and saline mixture, lactated Ringer's solution, or the patient's

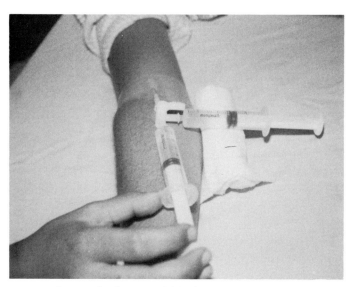

Figure 1. Appearance of preparation for contrast injection.

own blood. We feel that the contrast effect depends on an increase in the amount of dissolved or suspended air delivered. In order to achieve optimal aeration of the solution to be injected, we employ 30 ml multiple dose vials of bacteriostatic sodium chloride for injection. A 19-gauge needle attached to a 6 ml syringe (Figure 2) is introduced into the vial and the solution is rapidly injected in and out of the vial so as to aerate the contents. As shown in the photograph, the production of a cloudy gray appearance indicates adequate aeration. Just prior to injection, 4 cm^3 of this solution is rapidly withdrawn into the syringe and quickly delivered into the in-

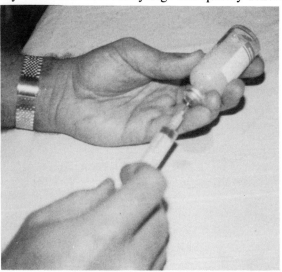

Figure 2. Aeration technique for preparation of saline contrast. Note cloudy gray appearance of fluid.

dwelling teflon catheter. The rapid delivery of aerated fluid consistently produces optimal contrast effect.

SELECTION OF VENOUS ACCESS SITE

The medial antecubital vein provides the most direct peripheral access to the central circulation allowing rapid delivery of a square wave contrast bolus to the right heart. Such a square wave delivery can be critical in locating the site of intracardiac shunting.

MINOR CONSIDERATIONS

The use of a three-way stopcock contributes to the success of the contrast technique by enabling rapid access to the intravenous line. Such rapid access is essential because the agitated saline retains the suspended air for only a short period of time. The choice of a 6 ml syringe has proved to be handy both in allowing rapid delivery of fluid and in its stability when attached to the stopcock.

Massage of the upper arm and the performance of the Valsalva maneuver are additional maneuvers which contribute to the success of the contrast technique.

MASSAGE OF THE UPPER ARM

After the injection of saline and visualization of a satisfactory contrast effect, another contrast effect can often be attained by raising the arm over the patient's head and massaging or milking the inner aspect of the upper arm toward the central circulation. This will, in most cases, produce a second contrast bolus almost equal in intensity to the first. This effect is achieved presumably by the release of residual contrast agent within the peripheral venous circulation.

THE VALSALVA MANEUVER

In order to temporarily reverse the usual diastolic pressure relationship between the right and left heart, the Valsalva maneuver can be employed. In preparation for this maneuver, we instruct the patient to exhale against a closed epiglottis. This particular instruction can be rendered comprehensible to the patient by explaining that the feeling is identical to that of straining at the stool. We have found that the best effect usually occurs on the first attempt at the Valsalva maneuver. Therefore, we instruct the patient not to undertake this maneuver until an actual recording is underway. We obtain most of our contrast studies with the Valsalva maneuver from the apical four-chamber view. Once a satisfactory four-chamber view is obtained, the saline bolus is given and the patient is instructed to "bear down". The arrival of the contrast in the right atrium, which is usually very rapid in a normal circulation, is often delayed by the elevation of intrathoracic pressure associated with this maneuver. Nonetheless, in 5–7 s contrast enters the right atrium. At that moment, the patient is instructed to release the strain. At the moment of release there is a sudden rise in right-sided filling pressure which may temporarily exceed left-sided filling pressure. Thus, in patients with an atrial septal defect or with a patent foramen ovale, this maneuver can often be effective in inducing a momentary right-to-left shunt. Such a shunt is confirmed when contrast material is seen to enter the left heart. If an M-mode beam is simultaneously passed through the left ventricle and left atrium during the release of the strain phase of the Valsalva maneuver, an atrial origin of the left-to-right shunt can be verified by observing that the contrast first appears in the left atrium, traverses the open mitral valve, and then enters the left ventricle. This pattern suggests either an atrial septal defect or patent foramen ovale. If the initial appearance of contrast is on the ventricular side of the mitral valve, a shunt at the ventricular level is suggested. When a large right-to-left shunt is suspected, it is best to limit the number of contrast injections given. While undue effects of contrast administration are very rare, a few reported instances of central nervous system symptomatology have occurred in the setting of a large right-to-left shunt. In all cases, signs and symptoms were reversible, but such experiences should introduce caution when such shunts are suspected.

In summary, we have presented a simple method for reproducible performance of saline contrast studies employing readily available materials and skills common to most physicians.

ACKNOWLEDGMENT

The authors wish to thank Dr. Joan E. Schiller, Laura E. Schiller, Emily W. Schiller and Steven J. Younger for their assistance.

REFERENCES

1. Bommer WJ, DT Mason, AN DeMaria: Studies in contrast echocardiography: development of new agents with superior reproducibility and transmission through the lungs. Circulation (Suppl II) 60:53, 1979 (abstract).
2. Meltzer RS, EG Tickner, TP Sahines, RL Popp: The source of ultrasonic contrast effect. J Clin Ultrasound 8:121–127, 1980.

7. STRUCTURE IDENTIFICATION BY CONTRAST ECHOCARDIOGRAPHY

RICHARD L. POPP and CHARLES R. TUCKER

The exciting technique of structure identification by contrast echocardiography has many developing applications and is now especially useful in defining cardiac chambers and in the recognition of congenital heart defects, as well as of complications of the abnormal flow resulting from such defects. But, if we are trying to define a given chamber, or the time sequence of flow of contrast moving from one chamber to another, the basic identity of each structure is the most important information we must begin with. Most people doing echocardiography now believe they understand cardiac anatomy very well, and in fact they do. But as the equipment has allowed us to see more and more details of the cardiac anatomy, and we are presented a more comprehensive view of the heart than has been possible in the past, the subtle details of anatomic features that were not visible or not important before become crucial to our diagnosis.

We must come to ask ourselves, "Do I understand the internal anatomy of the right atrium in enough detail to visualize it in three dimensions?", "Do I understand the attachments of the pericardium around the heart and great vessels sufficiently to know all of the potential spaces for pericardial fluid collection?" This type of detailed information is the source of diagnosis or, alternatively, the source of frustration when dealing with imaged structures that are not commonly seen. A firm basis in anatomy is the prime need of echocardiographers. Contrast echocardiography is an excellent tool for clarifying distortions of the heart due to disease superimposed on a normally formed heart, as well as for clarifying the pathophysiology of congenital defects. For example, there is a reflection of the pericardium around the right atrium in most people and, in the presence of pericardial effusion, this can give rise to some very confusing patterns. Figure 1 shows a structure which is possibly within the right atrium of a patient in whom a right atrial mass could have clinical significance. The patient also had pericardial effusion and, after injection of contrast material into the venous system, the extent of the right atrium was defined. The apparent "structure" within the right atrium was actually the posterior atrial wall, with an accumulation of pericardial effusion posterior to the atrial wall.

Further, one can inject a small amount of contrast into a needle introduced for pericardiocentesis in order to have the contrast agent circulate in the

52

space marked by the end of the needle so one can tell if the tip of the needle is in the heart, the pericardium or the pleural space. In the usual contrast study, the contrast agent is introduced into a peripheral vein. The common defect of a persistent left superior vena cava emptying via the coronary sinus into the right atrium is well defined using injection into the left arm. The large circular space in the posterior atrioventricular groove that is present on parasternal long-axis views of the heart fills with contrast material prior to flow of the contrast agent into the right heart [1].

Structure identification by contrast echocardiography within the heart is limited by and defined by the flow patterns in a given patient. Recently several groups have primarily introduced contrast agents for echocardiogra-

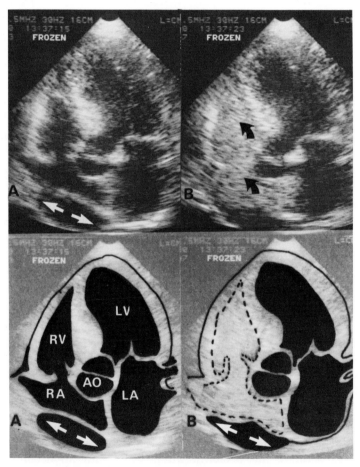

Figure 1. Apical four-chamber view prior to (panel A) and during (panel B) contrast injection. The space (white arrows), apparently part of the right atrium (RA), does not fill with contrast (black arrows) and is extracardiac. This is pericardial effusion posterior to the RA. Other abbreviations are standard.

phy by means of catheters in the left heart. However, if we do not use the newly developed technique for introducing contrast agents into the left heart via the pulmonary circulation, we should primarily concern ourselves with right heart flow. We will discuss structure identification roughly in the sequence of flow after venous injection.

The normal pattern of flow from the vena cavae to the right atrium can be well visualized in the majority of cases where adequate contrast is introduced intravenously. Reflux of contrast material into the inferior cava, after introduction of the material via the superior cava, occurs in some normal situations and several pathologic conditions. Many investigators have found M-mode records, taken through the inferior cava or hepatic veins, to be useful in precisely timing the appearance of the contrast material in the infradiaphragmatic vessels [2]. It is not at all unusual to see contrast material arrive in the inferior cava after venous injection and before ventricular systole in the presence of a relatively non-compliant right ventricle. This does not mean the patient has tricuspid regurgitation, since the contrast is refluxing into the venous system prior to ventricular systole. With a comprehensive view of the atrial-caval junction, such as is seen with subcostal views, one can get a good idea of the sequence of flow and of the timing of this flow. Nevertheless, the average observer cannot keep track of the electrocardiogram and the two-dimensional image at one time and so it is necessary to use M-mode recording or an audible signal, such as a signal joined to the QRS complex, if one wishes to adequately assess the timing of flow using contrast agents. Flow within the right atrium is generally viewed as a reference for flow targets passing into the left atrium or some other structure. When trying to track this flow, or when looking for negative contrast effects of flow from the left atrium to the right, we must be aware of the right atrial anatomy. The ostium of the coronary sinus, the valve of the inferior cava, the Chiari network, and the potential flow from the thebesian veins may lead to confusion in interpreting right atrial flow. When analyzing the echocardiogram for possible defects in the interatrial septum, one should be very clear on the anatomy of the septum primum and septum secundum. Figure 2 is a diagrammatic representation of the anatomy of the interatrial septum pertinent to the views used with most two-dimensional systems. This figure shows some of the anatomic features of the atrium and indicates the usual sites of ostium secundum, ostium primum, and sinus venous atrial septal defects.

Right atrial anatomy is generally termed "complex" or "variable" and can be properly described by both of these terms. However, the amount of trabeculation within the right ventricle, the general form of the right ventricle, and the anatomic definition of the tricuspid valve and the pulmonic valve within the normal right ventricle are rather uniform. The anatomy of the great vessels is extremely consistent in most adults, but may

54

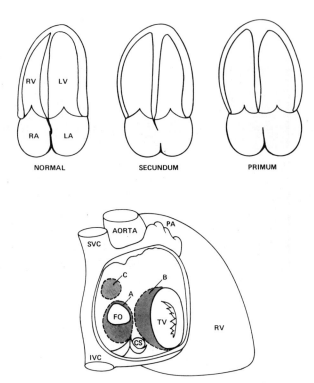

Figure 2. Diagrams of atrial septal defects as viewed by echocardiography (above) and right atrial anatomy (below). The locations of (A) ostium secundum, (B) ostium primum and (C) sinus venosus defects are indicated.

CS = coronary sinus, FO = fossa ovalis, IVC = inferior vena cava, SVC = superior vena cava, TV = tricuspid valve, RV = right ventricle.

be arranged along a full spectrum of interrelationships in patients with congenital malformations. Because the current limitations of display give us only black, white and gray pictures of the structures, it is not possible to consistently record a given chamber in a contrasting color for consistent identification. If we could do this it would not be necessary to standardize our examination techniques. Actually this is just the reason that forces us to use standardized examination techniques for transducer placement and manipulation [3]. Once the anatomy is firmly visualized and the examiner has a clear idea of the three-dimensional anatomy involved, innovative examination techniques can be used. Methods to visualize the right ventricular inflow tract, the junction of the right ventricular outflow and the pulmonary artery, and the extent of the pulmonary artery and its bifurcation, are available (Figure 3).

Transducer positions at the cardiac apex are most consistently useful for evaluation of intracardiac flow when the question of shunt is being explored. From this apical position, the four-chamber view can be used to interrogate

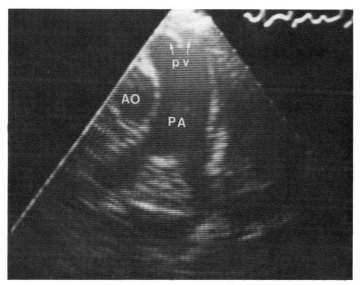

Figure 3. Echo image of the main pulmonary artery and its branches.
AO = aorta, PA = pulmonary artery, pv = pulmonary valve.

the volume which includes virtually all of the heart. Choosing the appropriate level for imaging, one can then observe the timing of the contrast
echocardiographic target's appearance in the various chambers and structures. In the presence of a post-infarction ventricular septal defect, for
example, one may choose parasternal or other views to further localize and
define the nature of the defect once the four-chamber views have clarified
the general level of the defect. As in most shunt lesions, there is some
bidirectional flow across such ventricular septal defects as shown in
Figure 4.

We have commented little on the identification of left heart structures
since generally one needs to have a catheter introduced into the left heart in
order to visualize these structures. In the presence of a large volume
right-to-left shunt the identification of left heart structures has more perti-
nence. When injecting contrast agents into the left heart by catheter, the
velocity of flow in the left heart often presents a problem for structure
identification since there is very rapid washout of contrast material from the
left heart. Also there may be considerable streaming of blood within the left
heart.

Some very exciting studies have recently been performed with catheters
placed in the coronary vessels and special contrast agents introduced
selectively into the coronary arteries in animals [4]. In these studies there is
considerable enhancement of reflectance of the myocardium after contrast
injection. Sub-selective coronary artery injections show the distribution of
coronary flow by segmental myocardial contrast enhancement and, with

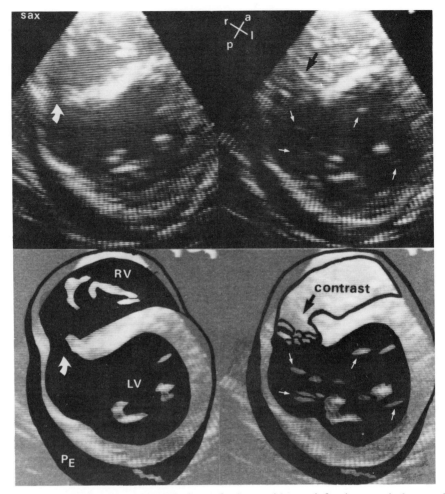

Figure 4. Short-axis (sax) parasternal views of a heart with post-infarction ventricular septal defect (large arrow). After peripheral contrast injection (right panel) contrast echoes are seen in the left ventricle (LV) (small arrows).

PE = pericardial effusion, a = anterior, p = posterior, r = right, l = left, RV = right ventricle.

some agents, slow egress of contrast agent appears to occur, indicating the level of flow present. This is an exciting area for the future.

LIMITATIONS

Structure identification by contrast echocardiography is limited by several factors. First among these is the introduction of contrast material into the venous system and its adequate transmission into the right heart. We will not go into this in detail here but, when very slow venous flow is occurring, there will obviously be an effect on transmission of the contrast agent to the right heart. Also, if the patient is in the left lateral decubitus position and the left arm is used for injection, there is sometimes an apparent compression of the left venous vessels with ineffectual contrast introduction. In general, the more proximal the injection site, the more reproducible and adequate will be the contrast visualization. Of course if one uses artificial targets or commercially produced contrast material, the reproducibility of contrast delivery is improved. Any contrast agent may be introduced into the heart and be virtually invisible if the imaging system is so noisy that a great amount of random signal is occurring and obscuring the transit of contrast through the heart. Conversely, if the system is either so insensitive or the gains are reduced to such an extent that the contrast signals are not made visible by the instrument, no structure identification can take place. It is important to note that the signal distal to a chamber highly filled with gaseous contrast material may not be well visualized. This is because a great deal of the sound transmitted into the chamber containing contrast is scattered or absorbed, with little remaining sound to be transmitted to the subsequent potential sound reflectors [5].

A different type of physical limitation relates to the volume of resolution of ultrasonic imaging systems. While we commonly speak of the axial resolution of an ultrasound system, this measurement seldom comes into consideration with contrast echocardiography. We are not trying to resolve two sides of the contrast target but we are only asking the instrument to present a single interface (the leading edge of the target) defining the location of the contrast agent. The lateral spread of such highly reflective structures may lead to apparent spread of the signal into a chamber where the contrast is not truly present. This is not usually a problem when dealing with lateral resolution in the plane of scan. In this case one can tell if the signals are being spread in both lateral directions from a location representing the true reflector site. If there is spread of the signal into a neighboring chamber, the observer can generally perceive this. There is more of a problem when we consider resolution out of the plane of scan. Resolution in this third dimension is usually worse than in either of the other two directions because of transducer construction. At least this has been true in studies done at Stanford by our group. If a signal appears in the chamber because of highly reflective targets being "behind" or "in front of" the visualized scan-plane, the observer has virtually no way of knowing that these echoes are spuriously presented. The recognition of this phenomenon goes some way toward avoiding improper diagnoses resulting from this error. As instrument sensitivity improves, this problem could become more prevalent, but as the equipment is improved with regard to transducer design, the volumetric resolution should be better and the problem just described should be reduced. It is important for each person working with contrast echocardiography to understand the physical limitations of the equipment in order to avoid problems now while the equipment is being improved beyond our current levels.

REFERENCES

1. Snider RA, TA Ports, NH Silverman: Venous anomalies of the coronary sinus: Detection by M-mode, two-dimensional and contrast echocardiography. Circulation 60:721–727, 1979.
2. Wise NK, S Myers, JA Stewart, R Waugh, T Fraker, J Kisslo: Echo inferior venacavography: A technique for the study of right sided heart disease. Circulation (Suppl II) 59 and 60:II–202, 1979.
3. Henry WL, A DeMaria, R Gramiak, DL King, JA Kisslo, RL Popp, DJ Sahn, NB Schiller, A Tajik, LE Teichholz, AE Weyman: Report of the American Society of Echocardiography Committee on Nomenclature and Standards in Two-dimensional Echocardiography. Circulation 62:212–217, 1980.
4. DeMaria AN, WJ Bommer, K Riggs, A Dajee, M Keown, OL Kwan, DT Mason: Echocardiographic visualization of myocardial perfusion by left heart and intracoronary injections of echo contrast agents. Circulation (Suppl III) 62:III–143, 1980.
5. Meltzer RS, EG Tickner, RL Popp: Why do the lungs clear ultrasonic contrast? Ultrasound Med Biol 6:263–269, 1980.

8. SPONTANEOUS LEFT VENTRICULAR MICROBUBBLES IN PATIENTS WITH METALLIC MITRAL PROSTHETIC VALVES

Randolph P. Martin and Lehman K. Preis, Jr.

INTRODUCTION

Small intracavitary echoes are often visualized in the right atrium and right ventricle following the intravenous injection of various agents such as saline, dextrose in water, or indocyanine green dye. Occasionally, these microbubbles can be seen within the left atrium or left ventricle when there is a right-to-left shunt at the atrial or ventricular level. The etiology of these echoes has been attributed to visualization of microcavitation or microbubbles formed from dissolved gasses in the intravenous solution [1–3]. However, spontaneous microbubbles are rarely seen in the left heart. One theory of the genesis of these spontaneous left ventricular microbubbles is the release of gasses from red blood cells during hemolysis [4].

Two-dimensional echocardiography, while useful in the evaluation of patients with mitral bioprosthetic valves, has not been shown to play a key role in the valvular evaluation of patients with metallic mitral prosthetic valves. During two-dimensional echocardiographic evaluation of patients with Beall mitral prostheses, we noted unusual spontaneous echoes in the left ventricle which were similar to microbubbles visualized in the right heart after intravenous injection of various agents. Because dysfunction of the Beall prosthesis is associated with significant hemolysis [5–9], we initiated this study to determine the role of the two-dimensional echo in assessing metallic prosthetic function and to determine if spontaneous left ventricular microbubbles represent hemolysis of red cells secondary to possible subclinical valvular dysfunction. Accordingly, the microbubbles might identify a subset of patients with metallic prosthetic valve dysfunction who warrant close follow-up.

METHODS

From February 1972 until April 1975, 105 patients underwent Beall valve (model 103, model 104) implantation at the University of Virginia Hospital. As part of a follow-up evaluation, 33 patients with Beall prostheses (with a mean insertion duration of 68 months) were evaluated for prosthetic function by single and two-dimensional echocardiography over a six month period (from March until October 1979). Of the 33 patients, 22 had isolated mitral Beall prostheses, eight had combined mitral Beall and aortic Starr-Edwards prostheses, two had combined mitral and tricuspid Beall prostheses, and one had an isolated tricuspid Beall prosthesis. Patients underwent full cardiologic evaluation and had two-dimensional echoes and M-mode echoes combined with phonocardiograms. Laboratory evaluation included hemoglobin, hematocrit, red blood cell count, mean corpuscular volume, mean corpuscular hemoglobin, hemoglobin concentration, platelet and reticulocyte count, serum glutamic oxaloacetic transaminase (SGOT), serum glutamic pyruvic transminase (SGPT), lactic dehydrogenase (LDH), and serum bilirubin. The serum LDH levels were used to determine the presence of hemolysis [10–13]. The M-mode echocardiograms were obtained using a Smith-Kline Ekoline 20A with a 2.25 MHz transducer. Returning signals were recorded on a paper strip chart at 50 and 100 mm/s, using an Irex 101 strip chart recorder. Lead two of the ECG and a phonocardiogram at the lower left sternal border using a 120 Hz–50 Hz band pass filter were recorded simultaneously with the M-mode echocardiograms. The M-mode echoes were recorded so that the prosthetic valve was magnified and the time compensation gain ramp set to approximate the anterior cage of the prosthesis. Accordingly, the majority of echoes anteriorly to the cage were attenuated.

The two-dimensional echocardiograms were performed with either a commercially available wide angle phased-array ultrasongraph (Varian 3000R) using a 2.25 MHz transducer, or a mechanical sector scanner (ATL Mark III-850A) using a 3.0 MHz transducer. Conventional two-dimensional echocardiographic imaging was performed from both the parasternal and apical windows.

While all studies were read initially as part of the patients' clinical evaluation, the two-dimensional echocardiograms were later reread in a blinded fashion by observers without knowledge of the patients' clinical or laboratory findings to assess echocardiographic quality (good, fair, poor) and evidence of microbubbles (none, rare, moderate, gross). The microbubbles seen by two-dimensional echocardiography were small, echo dense circular structures that moved within the left ventricle in a somewhat chaotic manner in diastole and, occasionally, in systole (Figure 1). These were best appreciated in real time. None of the patients had intravenous needles or solutions in place at the time the echocardiographic exams were performed. The M-mode and phonocardiograms were read to determine the interval between the aortic valve closure and the opening click of the mitral prosthesis (A2–OC interval). The A2–OC interval for the normal mitral Beall prosthesis varies between 0.09 and 0.12s [14–17]. Beat-to-beat variation of this interval greater than 30 ms in patients in atrial fibrillation or greater than 20 ms in patients in normal sinus rhythm is considered abnormal. Additionally, the M-mode echocardiograms were read to determine the presence or absence of linear streaks anterior to the mitral prosthesis, a potential sign of microbubbles (Figure 2).

Similar evaluations, including two-dimensional echocardiographic and single-dimensional echo-phono evaluations, and laboratory evaluations were performed on a control group of 31 patients who had either mitral non-Beall prosthetic valves or significant mitral regurgitation. This group was composed of 31 patients, 13 of

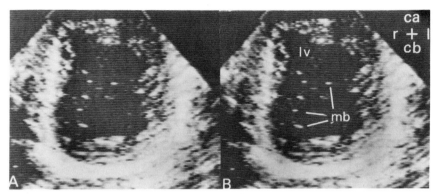

Figure 1. A stop-frame photograph of the left ventricular cavity. The two figures are identical, with panel B being labeled. The numerous microbubbles (mb) can be seen floating within the left ventricular cavity (lv). A small portion of the Beall struts can be seen as the bright echoes below the label mb. The orientation is shown in the upper right had corner of panel B. ca = cardiac apex; cb = cardiac base; l = left; lv = left ventricular cavity; mb = microbubbles; and r = right.

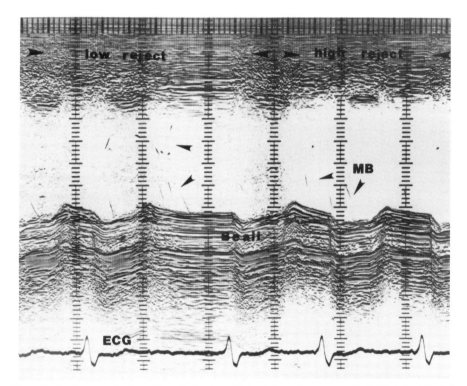

Figure 2. A photograph of an M-mode tracing obtained from the same patient. The characteristic M-mode of the Beall valve can be seen (labeled Beall). This figure illustrates the effect of instrument setting or reject on the appearance of the microbubbles, which appear as linear streaks (labeled mb). In the left half of the figure, low instrument reject was used and the linear streaks are much more apparent than in the right side of the figure where high instrument reject was used. Utilizing the high reject, the linear streaks are nearly removed from the tracing, a finding which may explain their relative absence on many previous M-mode studies of the Beall valve.

whom had mitral prosthetic valves (five Kay-Shiley mitral prostheses, five mitral porcine heterografts, and three mitral Starr-Edwards prostheses) and 18 patients who had stable, but significant mitral regurgitation. None of the control patients had active bacterial endocarditis.

RESULTS

While all two-dimensional echocardiographic examinations were performed from multiple transducer positions, the apical four-chamber view was the view most often used to attempt to elucidate mitral Beall function. In none of the 33 patients was there evidence of the prosthetic disc sticking or rocking and in none of the patients was there obvious foreign material visualized on the ventricular side of the struts. The apical four-chamber view proved to be the best view for detecting microbubbles.

Figure 3 graphically represents the relationship of the two-dimensional echocardiographic detection of microbubbles with the serum LDH levels according to the position and number of metallic prosthetic valves. As can be seen, 16 of the 22 patients with isolated mitral Beall prostheses (73%) had evidence of left ventricular microbubbles and a mean LDH of 1643 ± 628 IU. The remaining six patients with isolated mitral Beall prostheses who failed to show microbubbles on their two-dimensional studies had a mean LDH of 1200 ± 254 IU. Of the eight patients with mitral Beall prostheses and Starr-Edwards aortic prostheses, four or 50% had evidence of left ventricular microbubbles on their two-dimensional studies.

These patients had a much higher mean LDH level than the remaining four patients without two-dimensional echocardiographic evidence of microbubbles (2257 ± 1492 IU versus 1678 ± 271 IU, respectively). The two patients with mitral and tricuspid Beall prostheses both had evidence of microbubbles on their two-dimensional echo study, but these only occurred in the left ventricular cavity. The single patient with an isolated tricuspid Beall prosthesis had no evidence of right or left ventricular microbubbles and had a normal LDH level (289 IU). While no statistical significance was found between the level of the LDH and the presence of microbubbles, a trend did appear to exist between the laboratory evidence of hemolysis (increasing LDH levels and decreasing hematocrit) and the presence of left ventricular microbubbles on the two-dimensional study. For purposes of further discussion, only the 22 patients with isolated mitral Beall prostheses will be considered.

Figure 4 illustrates that those patients with isolated mitral Beall prostheses who showed marked signs of hemolysis (as indicated by LDH levels of greater than 1600 IU) were commonly found to have left ventricular microbubbles on their two-dimensional echocardiographic examinations. Similarly, four out of five of these patients, or 80%, without microbubbles on their two-dimensional echo, had hematocrits greater than 38%, whereas 14 of 16 patients (88%) with two-dimensional

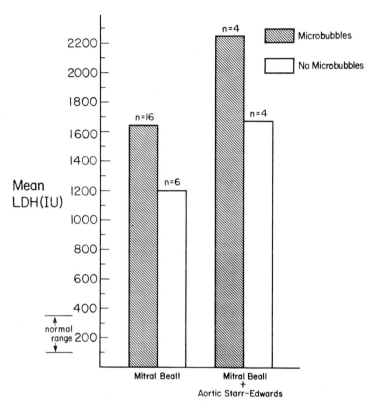

Figure 3. A bar graph showing the relationship between the two-dimensional echocardiographic appearance or absence of microbubbles and the mean lactic dehydrogenase level for patients with isolated mitral Beall valves and patients with combined mitral Beall and aortic Starr-Edwards valves. Those patients with microbubbles on their two-dimensional echo studies consistently had a higher mean LDH level than those patients without the echocardiographic appearance of microbubbles.

echocardiographic findings of microbubbles had hematocrits of less than 38% (Figure 5). Those patients who had numerous microbubbles on their two-dimensional echocardiographic studies also had LDH levels of greater than 1600 IU and hematocrits much less than 38%. None of the control group patients (patients with non-Beall prosthetic valves, or stable significant mitral regurgitation) had echocardiographic evidence of microbubbles or laboratory evidence of significant hemolysis. The mean LDH level was 383 ± 107 IU in the control patients with other forms of mitral prosthetic valves, and 308 ± 126 IU in the nonprosthetic mitral regurgitation patients.

The frequency of finding microbubbles by the two-dimensional echocardiographic technique in the patients with isolated mitral Beall prostheses appeared to vary according to the instrument used. As will be discussed shortly, this may have been secondary to either echocardiographic technique or lack of recognition to the

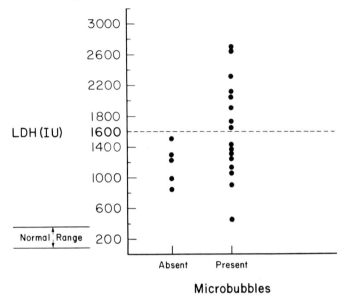

Relationship of LDH and 2-D Echo Microbubbles in Patients with Isolated Mitral Beall Valves

Figure 4. A graph representing the relationship of the LDH level and the echocardiographic appearance of microbubbles in those patients with isolated mitral Beall valves. As can be seen, all patients who had a mean LDH level of greater than 1600 IU had the obvious appearance of microbubbles on their two-dimensional echocardiographic study.

potential presence of microbubbles as the phased-array 2.25 MHz instrument was used initially, and then, the mechanical 3.0 MHz system subsequently. With the 2.25 MHz transducer of the phased-array system, nine of 14 (64%) of the patients with isolated mitral Beall prosthese demonstrated microbubbles. Utilizing the 3.0 MHz transducer of the mechanical system, all five patients studied showed left ventricular microbubbles. When both instruments were used on the remaining three patients, there was complete agreement as to the presence or absence of microbubbles.

Not all patients who had microbubbles detected by their two-dimensional echocardiographic studies had M-mode findings which were judged to be diagnostic of the presence of microbubbles on their M-mode tracings. Again, this may have been secondary to technique as many of the initial M-mode echocardiograms were performed with all echoes anterior to the cage of the prosthesis (when imaged from an apical transducer position) damped. While 16 of the 22 patients with isolated mitral Beall prosthesis had two-dimensional evidence of microbubbles within the left ventricular cavity, only 11 of the 16 showed M-mode findings of microbubbles.

The correlation between the phonocardiographic detection of potential prosthetic dysfunction with the two-dimensional echocardiographic recognition of microbubbles is shown in Figure 6. Fifteen of the 22 patients with isolated mitral Beall prosthesis had phonocardiograms and two-dimensional echoes performed.

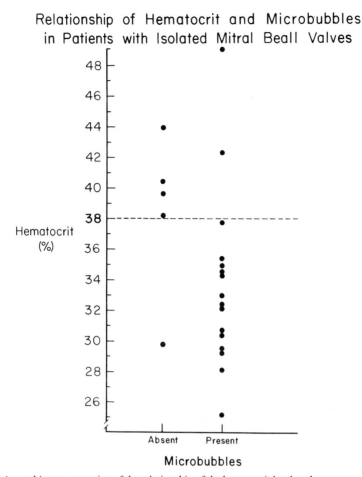

Figure 5. A graphic representation of the relationship of the hematocrit level to the presence or absence of microbubbles in patients with isolated mitral Beall valves.

As can be seen, five of the 15 (33%) had a markedly abnormal A2 opening click interval. This group had a significantly lower hematocrit and a significantly higher mean LDH level than the ten remaining patients with a normal A2 opening click interval. While all five patients with an abnormal A2 opening click interval exhibited two-dimensional echocardiographic findings of microbubbles, seven of the ten patients with normal A2 opening click intervals also had two-dimensional echocardiographic findings of microbubbles. Therefore, no significance could be attributed to the two-dimensional echocardiographic findings of microbubbles as it relates to the A2 opening click interval, but the finding of an abnormal A2 opening click interval and microbubbles appeared to represent real prosthetic dysfunction.

Four of the 22 patients with isolated mitral Beall prostheses underwent cardiac catheterization for suspected prosthetic dysfunction. All had significant hemolytic anemias requiring multiple transfusions. All demonstrated marked two-dimen-

66

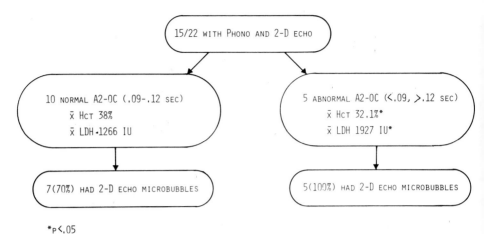

*p<.05

Figure 6. A graphic illustration of the relationship between the A2 opening click interval as obtained on the phono and the two-dimensional echocardiographic presence or absence of microbubbles in those patients who had both exams performed. As can be seen, the echocardiographic appearance of micro-bubbles did not necessarily correlate with an abnormal A2 opening click interval. However, those patients who had both an abnormal A2 opening click interval and microbubbles on their echocardio-graphic exam showed a significantly lower hematocrit and higher mean LDH level than those patients who had a normal A2 opening click interval.

sional echocardiographic evidence of left ventricular microbubbles. Three of the four patients underwent replacement of their prosthesis secondary to marked val-vular dysfunction (significant mitral regurgitation or combined regurigitation and obstruction). At surgery, all three valves demonstrated the classical finding of marked notching of the disc about its margin and associated wear of the metal struts [18].

DISCUSSION

Exogenously induced bright echoes, described as microcavitations or microbub-bles, have been routinely employed to diagnose the direction of intracardiac shunts and the presence of significant tricuspid regurgitation by both the M-mode and two-dimensional echocardiographic technique. The etiology of these small echoes has been attributed to visualization of microcavitations formed from dissolved gasses secondary to a drop in pressure in the intravenous solution [1–3].

Rare cases of spontaneous microbubbles seen within the left ventricular cavity within the M-mode technique have been reported in mitral regurgitation [4] or in disseminated intravascular coagulation [19]. One theory of the genesis of these spontaneous microbubbles, as seen by the M-mode technique, has been the release of gasses from red blood cells during hemolysis [4]. In an experimental model, Gramiak and Waag utilized a hemolyzing agent to induce the release of gasses from red blood cells and simultaneously recorded, with the M-mode technique, the small microbubbles that floated upward in a column toward the transducer. These authors concluded that the gaseous release from the hemolyzed red cells had produced the echo signal [4]. Other authors have described microbubble-like echoes in patients with Starr-Edwards mitral prostheses and have attributed them to fibrin clots or sewing ring cloth degeneration of the prosthetic valve [19]. There have been few, if any, descriptions of spontaneous, left ventricular microbubbles detected by the two-dimensional echocardiographic technique.

While routinely imaging our patients with mitral Beall prosthetic valves as a method for evaluating prosthetic function, we were struck by the appearance of spontaneous microbubbles in the left ventricle in patients who often showed marked signs of hemolysis. Therefore, we undertook this study to determine if the detection of left ventricular microbubbles in patients with metallic prosthetic valves might not be a new role for the two-dimensional echocardiographic technique. Additionally, we had hoped to determine whether or not there might be a correlation between the echocardiographic presence of microbubbles and signs of significant hemolysis, a fact which would lend credence to the theory that microbubbles may represent hemolysis of red blood cells. Among our patient population with isolated mitral Beall prosthesis, 73% had evidence of microbubbles. While the presence of the microbubbles was often associated with marked laboratory and clinical findings of ongoing hemolysis, no statistical significance was found between the presence of microbubbles and the serum level of LDH. Despite this fact, Figures 4 and 5 graphically demonstrate that microbubbles were present in 100% of our patients with an LDH level greater than 1600 IU and 98% of our patients with a hematocrit of less than 38%. Our control population group, with rheumatic mitral regurgitation, mitral valve prolapse, and various other prosthetic mitral valves (Starr-Edwards, porcine, and Kay-Shiley valves) had minimal or no laboratory evidence of hemolysis and no two-dimensional echocardiographic evidence of microbubbles. Subsequent to this study, these authors have seen rare isolated microbubbles in the left ventricle of patients with active mitral and aortic bacterial endocarditis. Again, this is the setting in which ongoing hemolysis is known to occur. While not all patients with two-dimensional echocardiographic evidence of microbubbles had substantiation of significant Beall prosthetic dysfunction, those patients with large number of spontaneous left ventricular microbubbles more often had severe clinical and laboratory evidence of marked hemolysis. From this group with marked presence of microbubbles on the two-dimensional echocardiographic examination, three patients who underwent surgical replacement of the mitral Beall prosthesis (for clinical and catheterization proved indications), all had significant wear of the disc and struts. The authors feel that the presence of a significant amount of left ventricular microbubbles in patients with Beall and potentially other types of prosthetic valves, may indicate a subset of patients with prosthetic other types of prosthetic valves, may indicate a subset of patients with prosthetic valves who warrant close follow-up evaluation. The authors also feel that these spontaneous diastolic microbubbles most likely represent spontaneous hemolysis of red blood cells secondary to subclinical or clinically apparent valvular dysfunction.

The fact that some of our patients with laboratory evidence of hemolysis did not exhibit microbubbles on their two-dimensional echocardiographic studies may be explained by: 1) echocardiographic technique, 2) instrumentation, and 3) associated multiple valvular prostheses. Conventional M-mode echocardiographic evaluation of patients with metallic mitral prosthesis has employed an apical transducer position, magnification of the prosthetic valve, and high reject settings in order to further delineate fine valvular detail. Initially, we utilized the apical transducer position with our two-dimensional echocardiographic examination in our patients with mitral Beall prosthesis. We also attempted to decrease extraneous echoes, which commonly are seen on the two-dimensional echo exam of mitral metallic prostheses, by altering the gain or reject setting so that only bright echo targets were present. Utilizing this method, the left ventricular cavity often became quite "silent" and there was a loss of subtle echoes. It was easy to understand that this way of investigating metallic mitral prosthesis might "reject" out subtle fine echoes such as the microbubbles. Once we did begin to detect microbubbles on routine clinical examinations, strict attention was paid to revising this method of studying the mitral prosthesis and attempts were made to bring out subtle small echo targets. Hence, the delineation of a better "gray-scale" was attempted so that small echo targets could be better visualized. Other factors relating to instrumentation may also determine the ability of the two-dimensional echo technique to image microbubbles. All patients studied with the mechanical sector alone (which utilized a higher frequency transducer) were positive for the presence of microbubbles, whereas those patients imaged with the acoustically focused phased-array system, with the lower frequency transducer, yielded a lesser number of patients showing microbubbles. While it is tempting to attribute these differences to sensitivity of instrumentation alone, or to the ability of higher frequency transducers to detect these small targets, other factors may have been equally important. The phased-array system was singularly employed early in our experience, while the mechanical system was used almost exclusively in patients studied later. Our ability to maximize detection of microbubbles by using appropriate reject and damping settings may have improved simultaneously with the adoption of the use of the mechanical system. While the fine echoes, such as the microbubbles, most likely could be better detected by a higher frequency transducer, other factors, such as attention on the part of the user of the instrument, may have been involved.

Finally, the failure of the two-dimensional echocardiographic technique to detect microbubbles in patients with laboratory evidence of hemolysis may be explained by patients who have other prosthetic valves in addition to the mitral Beall valves. The eight patients who had mitral Beall and aortic Starr-Edwards valves had the highest level of LDH (Figure 3). Among the eight patients with combined mitral Beall and aortic Starr-Edwards valves, the group with left ventricular microbubbles had a significantly higher level of LDH than did those without microbubbles on their two-dimensional echo studies. However, the four patients without left ventricular microbubbles had an LDH level which was similar to the 16 patients with isolated mitral Beall valve prosthesis and two-dimensional echocardiographic findings of microbubbles. While our study indicates that the presence of microbubbles in patients with isolated mitral Beall prosthesis, especially if they are very prominent and plentiful on the two-dimensional echocardiographic study, may be well associated with significant laboratory signs of hemolysis, the converse is not necessarily true. Patients who have mitral Beall prosthesis and another left sided metallic prosthetic valve will often have elevated LDH levels, but may not have the two-dimensional echocardiographic findings of left ventricular microbubbles present. It is still the authors' belief that those patients who have marked two-dimensional echocardiographic findings of microbubbles, whether they do or do not have associated aortic metallic prosthesis, should be carefully evaluated for potential or subclinical prosthetic dysfunction.

The ability to detect microbubbles on the M-mode echo exam as fine linear streaks anterior to the struts of the prosthetic valve may also be directly influenced by the echocardiographic technique. The routine way of evaluating mitral metallic prostheses may often reject or damp out the fine linear echoes as can be easily seen in Figure 2. When simultaneous or derived M-modes are generated from the two-dimensional echocardiographic exam microbubbles are more often visualized (if they were present on the two-dimensional exam).

Of interest is the fact that the A2 opening click interval has frequently been employed as an indicator of prosthetic valve dysfunction [14, 15, 20, 21]. In our patients with isolated mitral Beall prostheses, an abnormal A2–OC interval was significantly associated with laboratory evidence of hemolysis and the two-dimensional echocardiographic presence of microbubbles. This finding tends to support the concept that an abnormal A2 opening click interval may be a valuable indicator of prosthetic valve dysfunction. However, the fact that some patients with a normal A2 opening click interval have numerous microbubbles may indicate that the A2 opening click interval, while valuable when abnormal, is relatively insensitive in detecting subclinical valvular dysfunction. Follow-up information on later overt mechanical malfunction is required, however, to determine the validity of this assumption.

The use of two-dimensional echocardiography in mitral and aortic bioprosthetic valves is recognized. However, the role of two-dimensional echocardiography in the mitral metallic prosthesis has yet to be proven. Problems with reverberations make identification of real versus artifactual echoes (especially on the atrial side of the prosthesis) most difficult. Additionally, problems with lateral and axial resolution make the detection of fine intraprosthetic abnormalities most difficult. The two-dimensional echo technique, with its wide angle of view, allows for a much quicker localization of the best acoustic window for interrogating the heart. Similarly, the apical four-chamber view allows for multiple sources of information to be rapidly obtained in the patients with metallic mitral prosthetic valves. Qualitative, if not quantitative, information about left ventricular size and function, and mitral prosthetic dehiscence can be rapidly obtained. We believe that the ability to detect spontaneous microbubbles within the left ventricle of patients with metallic mitral prosthesis, especially the Beall prosthesis, may represent a new or different use of the two-dimensional echo technique. These patients may well represent a subset of patients with prosthetic valves who deserve close clinical evaluation and follow-up for potential or real prosthetic dysfunction. We also believe that spontaneous endogenous microbubbles most likely do represent hemolysis of red blood cells as Gramiak and Waag had earlier indicated [4]. The relationship between other cardiologic abnormalities associated with hemolysis, such as bacterial endocarditis, and the presence and number of microbubbles offer stimulating avenues for futher investigation.

REFERENCES

1. Bove AA, DF Adams, AE Hugh, PR Lynch: Cavitation at catheter tips – a possible cause of air embolus. Invest Radiol 3:159, 1968.
2. Bove AA, MC Ziskin, WL Mulchin: Ultrasonic detection of in vivo cavitation and pressure effects of high-speed injections through catheters. Invest Radiol 4:236, 1969.
3. Kremkau FW, R Gramiak, EL Carstensen, PM Shah, DH Kramer: Ultrasonic detection of cavitations at catheter tips. Am J Roentgenol 110:177, 1970.
4. Gramiak R, RC Waag (eds): Cardiac Ultrasound, p 30–33. CV Mosby, St. Louis, 1975.
5. Williams JC Jr., CR Vernon, GR Daicoff, TD Bartley, MW Wheat Jr., HW Ramsey: Hemolysis following mitral valve replacement with the Beall valve prosthesis. J Thorac Cardiovasc Surg 61:393, 1971.
6. Henderson BJ, As Mitha, BT le Roux, Gotsman: Haemolysis related to mitral valve replacement with Beall valve prosthesis. Thorax 28:488, 1973.
7. Clark RE, FL Grubbs, RC McKnight, TB Ferguson, CL Roper, CS Weldon: Late clinical problems with Beall model 103 and 104 mitral valve prostheses: hemolysis and valve wear. Ann Thorac Surg 21:475, 1976.
8. Clark RE, TA Pavlovic, BE Knight, JH Joist, SD Burrows, RC McKnight, EG Brown: Quantification of wear, hemolysis and coagulation deficits in patients with Beall mitral valves. Cardiovasc Surg (Suppl II) 56:II–138, 1977.
9. Silver MD, GJ Wilson: The pathology of wear with Beall model 104 heart valve prosthesis. Circulation 4:617, 1977.
10. Walsh JR, A Starr, LW Ritzman: Intravascular hemolysis in patients with prosthetic valves and valvular heart disease. Circulation (Suppl I) 39:I–135, 1969.
11. Myhre E, K Rasmussen: Mechanical hemolysis in aortic valvular disease and aortic ball-valve prosthesis. Acta Med Scand 186:543, 1969.
12. Myhre E, K Rasmussen: Serum lactic dehydrogenase activity and intravascular haemolysis. Lancet 1:355, 1970.
13. Myhre E, K Rasmussen, A Anderson: Serum lactic dehydrogenase activity in patients with prosthetic heart valves: a parameter of intravascular hemolysis. Am Heart J 80:463, 1970.
14. Benchimol A, CL Harris, KB Desser: Alteration of the mitral opening click time in a patient with the Beall mitral valve prosthesis. Chest 64:343, 1973.
15. Karwai N, BL Segal, JW Linhart: Delayed opening of Beall mitral prosthetic valve detected by echocardiography. Chest 67:239, 1975.

16. Smith RA, RE Kerber, JW Snyder: Noninvasive diagnostic evaluation of the normal Beall mitral prosthesis. Cath Cardiovasc Diag 2:289, 1976.
17. Benchimol A: Noninvasive diagnostic techniques in cardiology. Williams & Wilkins, Baltimore, 1977.
18. Silver MD, GJ Wilson: The pathology of wear in the Beall model 104 heart valve prosthesis. Circulation 56:617, 1977.
19. Schuchman H, H Feigenbaum, JC Dillon, S Chang: Intracavitary echoes in patients with mitral prosthetic valves. J Clin Ultrasound 3:107, 1975.
20. Brodie BR, W Grossman, L McLaurin, PJK Starek, E Craige: Diagnosis of prosthetic mitral valve malfunction with combined echo-phonocardiography. Circulation 53:93, 1976.
21. Berndt TB, DJ Goodman, RL Popp: Echocardiographic and phonocardiographic confirmation of suspected caged mitral valve malfunction. Chest 70:221, 1976.

9. CONTRAST ECHOCARDIOGRAPHY OF THE LEFT VENTRICLE

J. ROELANDT, R.S. MELTZER, and P.W. SERRUYS

INTRODUCTION

Rapid injection of biologically compatible solutions produces a "cloud of echoes" in the blood which is otherwise echo free. The source of this echocardiographic contrast is microbubbles of air introduced during injection [1, 2].

Left ventricular catheter injections have been employed to identify left side structures from M-mode echocardiograms [3, 4] and to validate cardiac views imaged by two-dimensional echocardiography [5, 6]. The method has also been found to be accurate and sensitive for the demonstration of small, intracardiac, left-to-right shunts and of minimal degrees of aortic and mitral valve regurgitation [7, 8, 9].

Injection of echo contrast material into the left ventricle, however, requires cardiac catheterization, making it an invasive procedure. This probably explains why left ventricular contrast echocardiography has not gained widespread clinical application.

Recently the possibility of transmitting echo contrast material across the capillary bed of the lungs to the left heart with pulmonary wedge injections [10, 11, 12] or with peripheral venous injections using experimental contrast agents [13, 16] has been demonstrated. These possibilities show great promise and may stimulate an increasing interest in ultrasonic left heart opacification. This chapter aims to review some methodological and clinical aspects of left ventricular contrast echocardiography. Most of this area is still investigational.

METHODOLOGIC ASPECTS OF LEFT VENTRICULAR CONTRAST ECHOCARDIOGRAPHY

At present, echocardiographic contrast studies of the left ventricle are performed in the catheterization laboratory. M-mode or two-dimensional techniques can be employed, each having its specific advantages and limitations for clinical problem-solving and research.

Two-dimensional echocardiographic views employed

Our experience with left ventricular echo contrast has been mainly with two-dimensional echocardiography, using a dynamically focused linear-array instrument (Fociscan, Organon Teknika) or a phased-array sector-scanner (Toshiba SSH-10A). The long-axis and short-axis views from the parasternal transducer position as well as the four-chamber and long-axis views from apical transducer position are routinely recorded [6, 14]. The apical views are especially useful for quantitative left ventricular studies, since the entire left ventricle from apex to base can often be recorded.

Left ventricular injection of echocardiographic contrast material

The rapid injection through a catheter of any biologically compatible fluid into the left ventricle causes echocardiographic contrast. We routinely use a manual flush of 5 to 10 ml of 5% dextrose in water.

Indocyanine green dye may yield a better contrast effect because of its surfactant properties, which keep the microbubbles of air, resulting from the vigorous shaking during preparation, stabilized in the solution [2]. One milliliter of indocyanine green solution (5 mg/ml for adults) is injected into the catheter and manually flushed with 5 to 10 ml of physiologic saline or 5% dextrose [7]. We have never observed any adverse patient reaction to direct left ventricular injections during echocardiographic contrast studies [15].

Pulmonary wedge injection of echocardiographic contrast material

Bommer et al. [10] reported in 1979 that catheter injections in the pulmonary wedge position in dogs cause echocardiographic contrast on the left side of the heart. Reale et al. [11] studied 43 patients with acquired or congenital heart disease and injected different echo-producing substances (indocyanine green dye, saline and carbon dioxide) via a balloon-tipped catheter in the pulmonary wedge position. Echocardiographic contrast was seen in the left ventricle in all patients studied. No complications or side effects were observed. We have studied 41 patients, using a Cournand 7F catheter alone in 27, a Swan-Ganz 7F catheter alone in 3 and both catheters in 11, for pulmonary wedge injections. Left ventricular echocardiographic contrast was seen in 3 out of 14 patients with the Swan-Ganz catheter and in 30 out of 38 patients when the Cournand catheter was used (Figure 1). We found that injection pressure proximal to the catheter had to be more than 40 kPa (300 mmHg) in order to obtain left side echocardiographic contrast.

Angiocardiographic studies with injections of Amipaque® further demon-

74

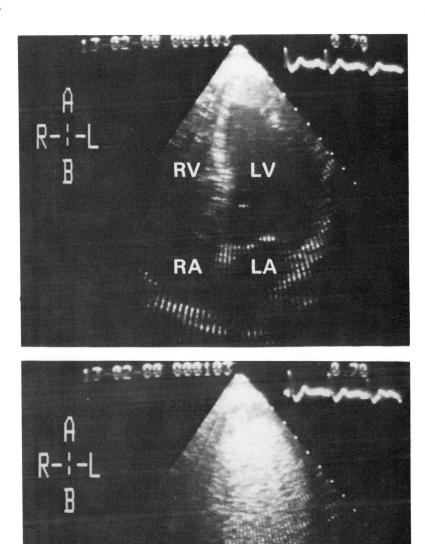

Figure 1. Stop-frame, apical four-chamber views obtained from a patient with a normal left ventricle immediately before (upper panel) and after pulmonary wedge injection of echocardiographic contrast (lower panel). The echo contrast fills both the left atrium (LA) and left ventricle (LV), of which the cavity contour becomes clearly delineated.

A = apical; B = basal; L = left; R = right; RA = right atrium and RV = right ventricle.

strated that a complete occlusive wedge position of the catheter must be achieved. The latter finding probably explains the higher success rate with a Cournand catheter: its higher stiffness allows more complete occlusion. It is conceivable that the pressure applied during occlusive injections may allow deformation of the air bubbles into a "dumbbell" shape resulting in their intact passage, rather than being retained by the "sieve" action of the capillary bed [16]. Apart from coughing, none of our patients had symptoms or worsening of their cardiopulmonary status related to the pulmonary wedge injections. Nonetheless, the method must still be considered as an experimental procedure until its safety has been finally established [12, 16].

Transmission of peripherally injected contrast through the lungs

Microbubbles of gas larger than the capillary diameter (approximately 8 microns) are stopped by the "sieve" action of the pulmonary capillary bed. On the other hand, microbubbles small enough to pass the pulmonary capillaries have an internal pressure which is significantly higher than the ambient blood pressure. Gas inside the microbubble therefore dissolves down its concentration gradient into the surrounding blood. The duration of this process is shorter than the pulmonary transit time and explains why the commonly employed contrast materials for peripheral venous injection are removed from the circulation before they reach the left side cavities [17].

We have created left side echocardiographic contrast in pigs by the injection of diethyl ether and hydrogen peroxide in the right heart or proximal pulmonary artery. Our studies demonstrated, however, that these agents are potentially dangerous [16]. Recently, transmission of echocardiographic contrast through the pulmonary capillary bed following peripheral venous injection has been demonstrated in dogs by Bommer et al. [10] using 2 to 10 micron diameter microballoons. Human application must await toxicity studies.

Opacification of the left ventricle following peripheral venous injection is thus a valid research goal. A better understanding of physical characteristics and physiological behaviour of microbubbles will probably permit successful attainment of this goal in the not too distant future.

CLINICAL APPLICATIONS OF LEFT VENTRICULAR CONTRAST ECHOCARDIOGRAPHY

Demonstration of valvular insufficiency

Sytolic regurgation of echo contrast material injected into the left ventricle to the left atrium is indicative of mitral regurgitation. The method is sensitive and minimal

amounts or regurgitation are readily detected [9, 18]. In moderate to severe degrees of mitral incompetence, the clearance time of the echo contrast from both the left atrium and left ventricle is considerably prolonged. Normally, echo contrast material remains from 4 to 10 cycles in the left ventricle and from 4 to 6 cycles in the left atrium. Uchiyama et al. [19] were able to determine the site or regurgitation in two patients with mitral valve prolapse syndrome using the echo contrast technique. Aortic regurgitation is demonstrated with a high degree of sensitivity by injecting echo contrast material in the aortic root and detecting its appearance in the left ventricle during diastole. The clearance time of the echo contrast from the left ventricle is much prolonged (15 to 50 cycles). In some instances, the regurgitant pattern of echo contrast may be observed as a "shower of echoes" hitting the anterior mitral valve or interventricular septum. Clearance time cannot be used to quantify mitral or aortic regurgitation reliably. It may serve, however, to confirm or exclude its presence in patients in whom roentgenographic contrast studies are contraindicated due to pregnancy [20] or angiographic dye allergy.

Demonstration of left-to-right shunts

Echo contrast flow patterns after left ventricular injection are helpful in identifying ventricular septal defects with left-to-right shunting and are at least as sensitive as indicator-dilution studies. Appearance of the echo contrast in the right ventricle or right ventricular outflow tract may be simultaneous with injection or be delayed by one cycle. The appearance time is dependent upon the timing of injection during the cardiac cycle and the position of the catheter in the left ventricle. A left-to-right shunt as small as 5 % of the pulmonary flow may be detected [8]. We have experience with two patients in whom a ventricular septal defect was missed by oximetry and diagnosed by left ventricular contrast echocardiography (Figure 2). The method is useful for the demonstration of a left ventricular to right atrial shunt and the localization of small defects in the trabecular septum using the apical four-chamber view. Recently, Reale et al. [11] have demonstrated the possibility of using pulmonary wedge injections (see paragraph 2.3) for direct visualization of a left-to-right shunt at atrial or ventricular level, thus obviating left heart catheterization. They rightly concluded that the method could be used as a simple screening procedure during right heart catheterization to avoid invasion of the left heart in some patients. The toxicity of pulmonary wedge injections and the sensitivity of this approach as compared to oximetry and indicator dilution techniques need further evaluation.

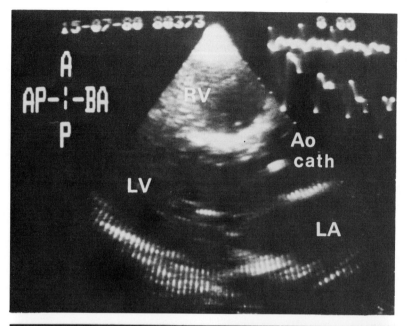

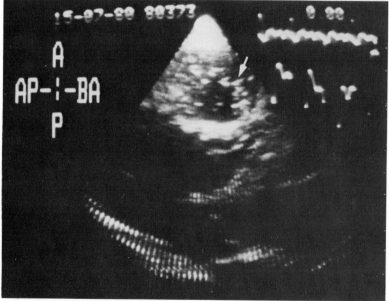

Figure 2. Parasternal long-axis views of a patient with a small ventricular septal defect before (upper panel) and after (lower panel) catheter injection of echo contrast in the left ventricular outflow tract. Echoes appear in the right ventricular outflow tract (arrow) proving the existence of a small left-to-right shunt.

A = anterior; AP = apical; BA = basal; P = posterior; Ao = aorta; cath = catheter; LA = left atrium; LV = left ventricle; RV = right ventricle.

Delineation of the left ventricular cavity

Feigenbaum et al. [4] utilized left ventricular injections of indocyanine green dye to identify the endocardium from other echoes within its cavity. Even when using newer equipment, non-structural echoes often obscure the endocardial boundaries and make proper delineation of the left ventricular cavity difficult or even impossible [21]. It is conceivable that opacification of the left ventricular cavity with echocardiographic contrast would improve border recognition and increase the accuracy of left ventricular volume determination from two-dimensional images (Figure 3). We therefore made recordings of the left ventricle in four views (parasternal long-axis view and short-axis view, at mitral level; apical four-chamber view and long-axis view) before and after left ventricular or pulmonary wedge injections of 5% dextrose in water in 13 patients (Figure 4). Long-axis length and surface area within the endocardial contours were measured from stop-frame images, independently from recordings with and without contrast, using a light pen system and a digital computer. The measurements were repeated by the same investigator one month later. Long-axis length was longer and the surface area larger with contrast than without contrast and this was significant (P >0.001). To our surprise, measurements on contrast images showed a higher intra-observer variability. In another series of 18 patients we compared left ventricular volumes determined by angiocardiography with these measured from two-dimensional echocardiographic views (apical four-chamber view and apical long-axis view) before and after injections of echocardiographic contrast. The use of contrast did not improve the correlation between echocardiographic and angiocardiographic volumes. Our studies, although preliminary, indicate that contrast echocardiography improves on the systematic error (it largely corrects for the known systematic underestimation of left ventricular volumes by two-dimensional echocardiography) but does not improve the random error or reproducibility.

3.4. Study of blood flow patterns

The non-contrast blood flowing from the left atrium into the left ventricle after its opacification with echo contrast allows us to observe transmitral blood flow. The negative contrast shadow delineates the functional mitral valve orifice. This is demonstrated in Figure 5, obtained from a patient with mitral valve stenosis. The anatomical dimension of the valve is visualized during the baseline study in the parasternal long-axis view (Figure 5, upper panel). The functional dimension is visualized by the echo-free blood entering the left ventricle after its opacification and appears smaller in the same cross-section (Figure 5, middle panel). Intracavitary flow patterns

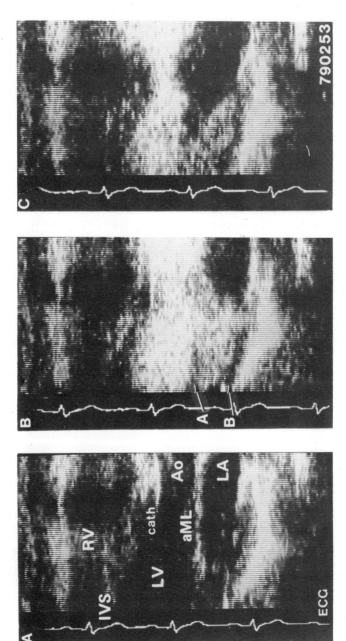

Figure 3. Left ventricular cavity opacification by direct catheter injection of echocardiographic contrast in a patient with right ventricular volume overload. Panel A: before injection. Panel B shows a systolic frame with echocontrast outlining the left ventricular cavity. Arrow A indicates the papillary muscle. Arrow B indicates the myocardium of which the endocardial surface is delineated by the posterior limitation of the echocardiographic contrast. The transmitral blood flow is visualized in panel C by the negative shadow resulting from noncontrast blood entering the left ventricle from the left atrium during diastole. Ao = aorta; aML = anterior mitral valve leaflet; cath = injecting catheter; ECG = electrocardiogram; IVS = interventricular septum; LA = left atrium; LV = left ventricle; RV = right ventricle.

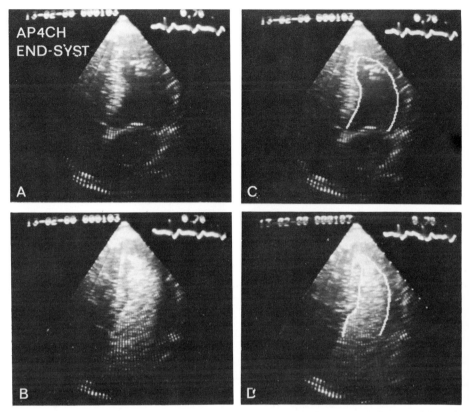

Figure 4. End-systolic stop-frame images of apical four-chamber views obtained before (panel A) and after (panel B) pulmonary wedge injection of echo contrast to opacify the left ventricular cavity. The apical area is poorly defined on the basal study and is better delineated after echo contrast. Contouring of the cavjty before and after opacification will give different results (panels C and D).

produced by a mitral valve prosthesis can be followed after pulmonary wedge injections. Occasionally one may observe a vortex of echo contrast circulating within an ischemic aneurysm in patients with coronary artery disease (Figure 6). Left ventricular contrast echocardiography thus allows a new type of study on local flow, turbulence and stasis, which promises to become more useful in the future if transpulmonary echo contrast transmission becomes available.

Densitometric dilution curves of echocardiographic contrast

Bommer et al. [22] described in 1978 a method of obtaining dilution curves of echocardiographic contrast by videodensitometry. They focused an analog photometer upon the screen of the videomonitor over the middle of the right ventricular cavity during two-dimensional echocardiographic contrast stu-

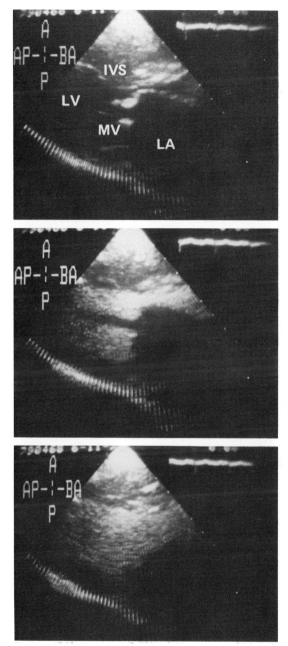

Figure 5. Stop-frame photographs of parasternal long-axis views of a patient with mitral valve stenosis before (upper panel) and after injection of echo contrast via a catheter in the left ventricle. The middle panel shows a frame recorded during diastole. The negative shadow caused by the non contrast blood flowing from the left atrium into the ventricle visualizes the transmitral blood flow pattern. During systole (lower panel), the echo contrast does not pass into the left atrium, excluding mitral incompetence.

A = anterior; AP = apical; BA = basal; P = posterior; IVS = interventricular septum; LA = left atrium; LV = left ventricle; MV = mitral valve.

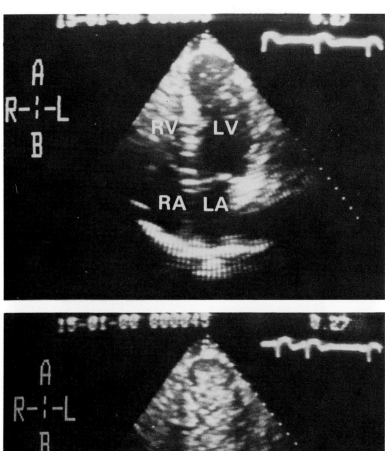

Figure 6. Apical four-chamber views before (upper panel) and after (lower panel) left ventricular opacification by echo contrast via a pulmonary wedge injection in a patient with an apical aneurysm. Wash-out of echo contrast from within the aneurysm was delayed.

A = apical; B = basal; L = left; R = right; LA = left atrium; LV = left ventricle; RA = right atrium; RV = right ventricle.

dies. The dilution curves were reproducible on multiple echocardiographic contrast injections to an accuracy of 15%. The time course of decay made it possible to separate patients with normal from those with low cardiac output and/or tricuspid regurgitation. Echo-contrast indicator dilution curves of the left ventricle were subsequently performed in dogs using injections of 10 ml of a 1:100,000 concentration by volume of 30 micron diameter microballoons. Good correlations with cardiac output measurements were found [23]. We have used an image-processing computer to analyze video recordings of contrast injections in order to follow the decay of density after left ventricular and pulmonary wedge injections in 17 patients. A meaningful calculation of the area under the curve could not be made because of limitations due to video "overload" immediately after injection. In consequence, contrary to the studies by DeMaria et al. [23], it seems that cardiac output measurements cannot be estimated reliably using routine contrast dilution techniques. The decay phase was found to be exponential and has characteristics of indicator-dilution curves, as predicted theoretically. Preliminary data indicate that R-wave gating may allow estimation of ejection fraction [24].

Hagler et al. [25] used computer-based videodensitometric techniques to analyze video recordings of left ventricular contrast echocardiograms to quantitate left-to-right shunts. Time-density histograms were generated from the right and left ventricular cavities after injection of echo contrast in the left ventricle in 7 patients with a ventricular septal defect. Their results indicate the possibility of quantitating shunts with these techniques.

ACKNOWLEDGMENT

The authors wish to thank Willem Gorissen, Jackie McGhie and Wim Vletter for technical assistance and Machtelt Brussé for help in manuscript preparation.

REFERENCES

1. Gramiak R, PM Shah: Echocardiography of the aortic root. Invest Radiol 3:356, 1968.
2. Meltzer RS, EG Tickner, TP Sahines, RL Popp: The source of ultrasonic contrast effect. J Clin Ultrasound 8:121, 1980.
3. Gramiak R, PM Shah, DH Kramer: Ultrasound cardiography: contrast studies in anatomy and function. Radiology 92:939, 1969.
4. Feigenbaum H, JM Stone, DA Lee, WK Nasser, S Chang: Identification of ultrasound echoes from the left ventricle by use of intracardiac injections of Indocyanine green. Circulation 41:614, 1970.

84

5. Sahn DJ, DE Williams, S Shackelton, WF Friedman: The validity of structure identification for cross-sectional echocardiography. J Clin Ultrasound 2:201, 1975.
6. Tajik AJ, JB Seward, DJ Hagler, DD Mair, JT Lie: Two-dimensional real-time ultrasonic imaging of the heart and great vessels: technique, image orientation, structure identification and validation. Mayo Clin Proc 53:281, 1978.
7. Seward JB, AJ Tajik, JG Spangler, DE Ritter: Echocardiographic contrast studies. Mayo Clin Proc 50:163, 1975.
8. Pieroni DR, J Varghese, RM Freedom, RD Rowe: The sensitivity of contrast echocardiography in detecting intracardiac shunts. Cathet Cardiovasc Diagn 5:19, 1979.
9. Kerber RE, JM Kioschos, RM Lauer: Use of ultrasonic contrast method in the diagnosis of valvular regurgitation and intracardiac shunts. Am J Cardiol 34:722, 1974.
10. Bommer WJ, DT Mason, AN DeMaria: Studies in contrast echocardiography: development of new agents with superior reproducibility and transmission through lungs. Circulation 59 and 60 (Suppl II):II–17, 1979 (abstract).
11. Reale A, F Pizzuto, PA Giaffré, A Nigri, F Romeo, E Martuscelli, E Mangier, G Scibilia: Contrast echocardiography: transmission of echoes to the left heart across the pulmonary vascular bed. Europ Heart J 1:101, 1980.
12. Meltzer RS, PW Serruys, J McGhie, N Verbaan, J Roelandt: Pulmonary wedge injections yielding left-sided echocardiographic contrast. Brit Heart J 44:390, 1980.
13. Bommer WJ, EG Tickner, J Rasor, T Grehl, DT Mason, AN DeMaria: Development of a new echocardiographic contrast agent capable of pulmonary transmission and left heart opacification following peripheral venous injection. Circulation 62 (Suppl III):III–34, 1980 (abstract).
14. Meltzer RS, C Meltzer, J Roelandt: Sector Scanning views in echocardiography: a systematic approach. Europ Heart J 1:379, 1980.
15. Serruys PW, F Hagemeijer, J Roelandt: Echocardiological contrast studies with dynamically focussed multiscan. Acta Cardiol 34:283, 1979.
16. Meltzer RS, OEH Sartorius, CT Lancée, PW Serruys, PD Verdouw, CE Essed, J Roelandt: Transmission of ultrasonic contrast through the lungs. Ultrasound in Med & Biol 7:377, 1981.
17. Meltzer RS, EG Tickner, RL Popp: Why do the lungs clear ultrasonic contrast. Ultrasound in Med & Biol 6:263, 1980.
18. Amano K, T Sakamoto, Y Hada, T Yamaguchi, T Ishimitsu, H Adachi: Contrast echocardiography: application for valvular incompetence. J Cardiography 9:697–716, 1979.
19. Uchiyama I, T Isshiki, K Koizumi, Y Ohuchi, K Kuwako, T Umeda, K Machii, S Furuta: Detection of the site and severity of mitral valve prolapse by real-time cross-sectional echocardiography with contrast technique. J Cardiography 9:689–696, 1979.
20. Meltzer RS, PW Serruys, J McGhie, PG Hugenholtz, J Roelandt: Cardiac catheterization under echocardiographic control in a pregnant woman. Amer J Med 71:481, 1981.
21. Roelandt J, WG van Dorp, N Bom, PG Hugenholtz: Resolution problems in echocardiology, a source of interpretation errors. Amer J Cardiol 37:256, 1976.
22. Bommer W, J Neef, A Neumann, L Weinert, G Lee, DT Mason, AN DeMaria: Indicator-dilution curves obtained by photometric analysis of two-dimension echo-contrast studies. Amer J Cardiol 41:370, 1978 (abstract).

23. DeMaria AN, W Bommer, K Riggs, A Dajee, L Miller, DT Mason: In vivo correlation of cardiac output and densitometric dilution curves obtained by contrast two-dimensional echocardiography. Circulation (III–101) 1980 (abstract).

24. Bastiaans OL, J Roelandt, L Piérard, RS Meltzer: Ejection fraction from contrast echocardiographic videodensity curves. Clin Res 29:176A, 1981 (abstract).

25. Hagler DJ, AJ Tajik, JB Seward, DD Mair, DG Ritter, EL Ritman: Videodensitometric quantitation of left-to-right shunts with contrast sector echocardiography. Circulation 57 and 58 (Suppl II), II–70, 1978 (abstract).

10. PULMONARY WEDGE INJECTIONS FOR THE EVALUATION OF LEFT-TO-RIGHT SHUNTS

ATTILIO REALE and FRANCESCO PIZZUTO

Contrast echocardiography or echoangiography has gained wide acceptance in many echo and cardiac catheterization laboratories (see Chapter 9). The method is applied in the verification of cardiac structures and in the demonstration of flow patterns through the recording of echoes produced by injecting into the blood stream substances such as indocyanine green, saline, blood and dextrose [1–13]. These agents are characterized by the fact that their echo-producing quality is lost during passage through the pulmonary or systemic capillary beds [2, 9, 13, 14]. Thus, when the contrast material is injected into a peripheral vein or a right heart cavity, the echoes appear only as far as the pulmonary arteries, and direct visualization of intracardiac septal defects and aortopulmonary communications are obtainable only in the presence of a right-to-left shunt. In order to demonstrate the passage of echoes from left to right it has been necessary to inject the agent directly into the left heart cavities [3, 13–16].

Recently a new agent was developed consisting of gas-containing microballoons in liquid suspension capable of pulmonary transmission and left heart opacification following peripheral venous injection. This, however, was a preliminary report of studies performed on three dogs [17]. Until now pulmonary transmission of echographic contrast in humans has been achieved only by means of pulmonary wedge injections of conventional echo-producing agents.

This chapter deals with the above mentioned technique, which was developed in our laboratory [18–22]. Results obtained with a similar technique were reported by other researchers on dogs [23] and on humans [24] (see Chapter 11).

The working rationale was based upon the hypothesis that echoes might be preserved across to the left heart by attaining concentrations upstream from the pulmonary capillaries higher than can be obtained by peripheral venous or right heart injections, and by introducing the echo-producing agent closer to the pulmonary capillary bed.

In preliminary trials various substances were injected into a larger peripheral pulmonary arterial branch without success. We then reasoned that still higher concentrations would be possible by means of forceful injection through an end-hole catheter in a pulmonary wedge position. However, transmission of echoes to the left heart did not occur in the first two patients in whom Cournand catheters were used. The technique was thus further modified to insure rapid delivery of the contrast in as much a bolus form as possible, and the following procedure was standardized and used throughout this study.

METHOD

A balloon-tipped catheter (Fast USCI No. 5–7 F) is wedged under fluoroscopic control in a right or left pulmonary arterial branch, usually in the lower lung fields. An echocardiographic display is then obtained. When screening for a left-to-right shunt, M-mode imaging of aorta, pulmonary artery, and left atrium by the suprasternal approach, is selected. Subsequently, if echoes appear in the pulmonary artery, other M-mode and two-dimensional displays are used to identify the site of the shunt. Recordings were obtained with an Aloka model SSD-110S mechanical sector scanner. As soon as a satisfactory echo picture is seen, the balloon is inflated and an echo-producing substance is rapidly injected. Toward the end of the injection, the balloon is deflated and the catheter is flushed with saline.

Previous studies in our laboratory [25] have shown that CO_2 bubbles produce very dense echoes in comparison to other agents. This was the substance used in the first patients of our series. This gas was selected on the basis of the reported safe use of injection of CO_2 bubbles directly into the coronary arteries for the purpose of coronary blood flow measurement [26]. It later became apparent that good pulmonary transmission of echoes could also be obtained with indocyanine green and saline, and we now reserve CO_2 for the cases yielding unsatisfactory echoes with other agents. Thus, CO_2 (0.5 ml) was used in 16 patients, saline (5 ml) in eight, and indocyanine green (5 ml) in 44.

RESULTS

Observations were performed during diagnostic cardiac catheterization in 68 patients, 39 males and 29 females, aged from 2 to 69 years (mean age 22).

Group I consisted of 26 patients with acquired valvular ischemic or congenital heart disease without oxymetric and/or angiographic evidence of septal defects or aortopulmonary communications.

Group II consisted of 42 patients; 17 with atrial septal defect, 16 with ventricular septal defect and nine with persistent ductus arteriosus, and a left-to-right shunt of variable magnitude. Calculated q_p/q_s ratios ranged from 1/1 to 4.3/1 (mean 1.8/1). Q_p/Q_s was 1.5/1 or less in 20 patients. In seven of these there was no O_2 saturation step-up and the left-to-right shunt was documented by selective left heart cineangiography.

Pulmonary transmission of echoes with subsequent visualization of the left heart chambers and aorta was obtained in 64 patients (24 in Group I and 40 in Group II). In the absence of a left-to-right shunt, the transmitted echoes were confined to the left atrium, left ventricle and aorta (Figures 1–3). When a left-to-right shunt was present, the right heart chamber or pulmonary artery receiving the shunt was shown to fill with echoes (Figures 4–7). CO_2 usually produced denser echoes than indocyanine green and saline. In two of the 64 successful cases, left heart echoes could be

88

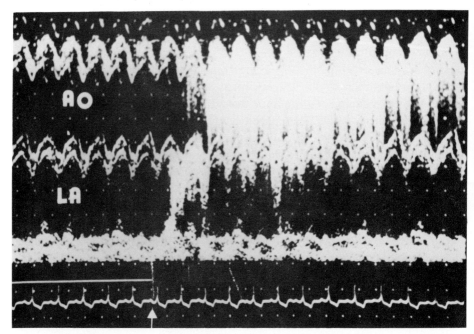

Figure 1. M-mode echocardiogram after pulmonary wedge injection of indocyanine green (arrow) in a patient with aortic insufficiency, showing echoes in left atrium (LA) and aorta (AO).

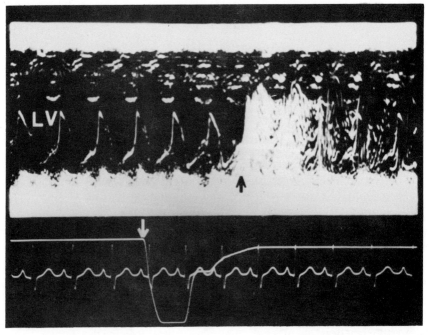

Figure 2. M-mode echocardiogram after pulmonary wedge injection of CO_2 (white arrow) in a patient with a functional systolic murmur, showing echoes in left ventricle (LV) appearing first posterior and subsequently anterior to the mitral valve.

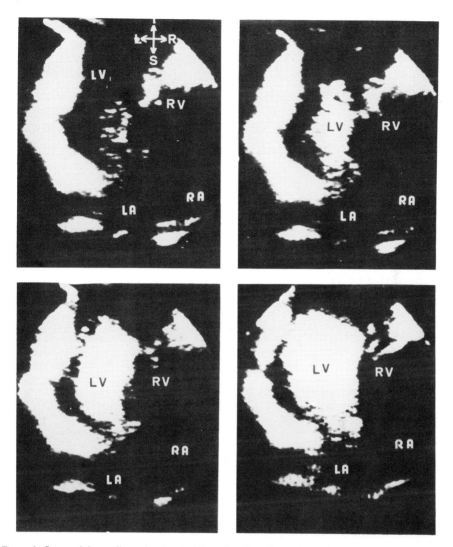

Figure 3. Sequential two-dimensional apical four-chamber views after pulmonary wedge injection of indocyanine green in a patient with aortic coarctation, showing progressive visualization of left ventricle (LV).

obtained only with CO_2, after the other two agents had failed to appear on the left side.

In four of the 68 patients, two in each group, pulmonary transmission could not be obtained, in spite of repeated injections in different wedge positions.

No clinical complications or side effects were noted in any of the patients, some of whom received up to 15 wedge injections. In most instances the actual injection was not perceived by the patient, while occasionally it produced short bursts of coughing.

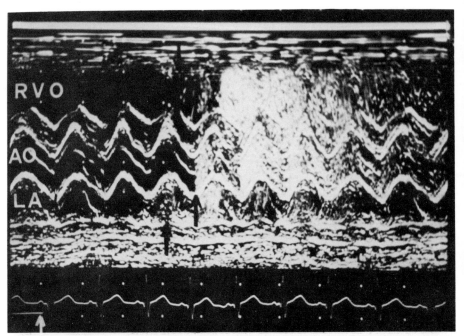

Figure 4. M-mode echocardiogram after pulmonary wedge injection of saline (white arrow) in a patient with atrial septal defect, showing echoes appearing sequentially in left atrium (LA), right ventricular outflow (RVO) and aorta (AO).

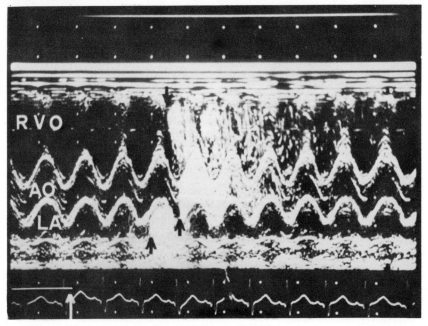

Figure 5. Same patient as in Figure 4, after injection of saline into a pulmonary vein (white arrow). The picture demonstrates the similarity in sequence of appearance and density of echoes as with pulmonary wedge injection.

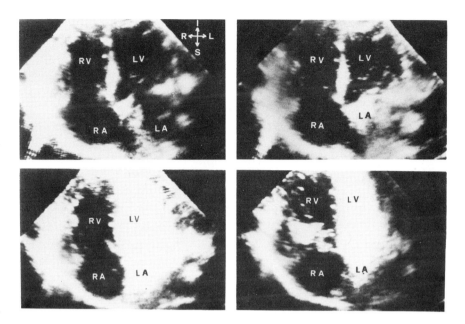

Figure 6. Sequential two-dimensional apical four-chamber views after pulmonary wedge injection of indocyanine green in a patient with ventricular septal defect. The right ventricle (RV) receives echoes from the left ventricle (LV) below the tricuspid valve. The right atrium (RA) remains echo-free.

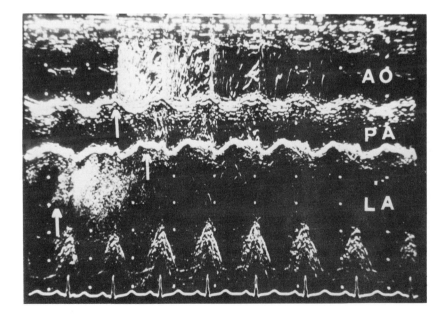

Figure 7. M-mode suprasternal view after pulmonary wedge injection of indocyanine green in a patient with persistent ductus arteriosus, showing sequential appearance of echoes in left atrium (LA), aorta (AO) and pulmonary artery (PA).

DISCUSSION

This and other studies demonstrate that transmission of echoes across the pulmonary capillaries is possible in the great majority of patients when the echo-producing agent is injected in a pulmonary wedge position. The exact mechanism, however, is not clear. There are several possible explanations:

a. The echoes produced at the catheter tip, being introduced into a smaller volume of blood than when injected in a peripheral vein or right heart cavity, achieve a much higher concentration, thus preventing total disappearance of the echo phenomenon along the pulmonary capillaries.

b. The short transit time of the agent injected nearer to the pulmonary capillaries reduces the dissolving effect of surface tension upon the echo-producing microbubbles.

c. The pulmonary capillaries are distended by the rapid and forceful injection, the larger caliber thus obtained allows the passage of unaltered microbubbles.

In our experience visualization of the left heart was usually quite intense. There was no apparent correlation between echo density and factors such as age and sex of patients, underlying cardiac disease, pulmonary arterial and venous pressures, systemic arterial oxygen saturation, and respiratory function.

There was no recognizable reason for the failure of the four patients in our series in whom pulmonary transmission could not be obtained. Two had ischemic heart disease, one had a ventricular septal defect (Q_p/Q_s 1.7/1), and one an atrial septal defect (Q_p/Q_s 3.3/1). All had normal pulmonary arterial and venous pressures and normal systemic arterial oxygen saturation. It should be noted that in one of these unsuccessful cases even peripheral vein injection produced only very poor echoes.

The site of pulmonary wedge injection seems to be important in some cases: in a few patients, left heart echoes were obtained only after changing the position from right to left lung or from lower to upper lobes or vice versa.

A comparison with the only other published observations on humans [24] yields significant differences in methodology which are rather difficult to interpret. The quoted authors obtained consistently better results with the use of the Cournand catheter (11/15 positive) than with the Swan-Ganz catheter (1/8 positive). They also state that in preliminary unpublished studies they were unable to obtain pulmonary transmission of echoes with the Swan-Ganz catheter when the balloon was inflated during the wedge injection. In our study, the use of the Cournand catheter was abandoned after the first unsuccessful trials and thereafter the balloon of the Fast catheter was always inflated during injection. We have the impression that it is important to deflate the balloon immediately at the end of injection. This maneuver, together with rapid flushing, probably provides a further "kick" to the bolus of echo-producing agent. It is difficult to judge whether this difference in methodology can explain the lower incidence of unsuccessful pulmonary transmission in our series (5.8%) in comparison to that of the other observations (23%) [24].

The sensitivity of the method is high: in each of the patients with successful pulmonary transmission and a left-to-right shunt, the latter was demonstrated by the appearance of right heart echoes; even in the seven patients who had shunts small enough not to cause oxygen saturation step-up in the right heart chambers of pulmonary artery (Figure 8). In these subjects visualization of the shunt would have required left heart angiography or echoangiography.

It is well known that septal defects can be demonstrated by peripheral venous contrast echocardiography [27–30]. This occurs either because of some right-to-left shunting, which is frequent in atrial septal defects, rare in ventricular septal defects, and patent ductus arteriosus in the absence of right ventricular and pulmonary hypertension, or as echo-free areas along the septal margins at the site of a left-to-right shunt ("negative contrast" effect). In our series, venous echoangiography was performed in a few cases at the time of cardiac catheterization prior to wedge injection. The fact was evidenced by a small right-to-left shunt in six out of 12 patients, by echo-free aspect in three out of 12 patients with an atrial septal defect; three out of eight patients with a ventricular septal defect showed a right-to-left shunt (right ventricular pressure respectively 58, 60 and 70 mm Hg); none showed echo-free zones.

Serious complications such as pulmonary hemorrhage and hemoptysis have been

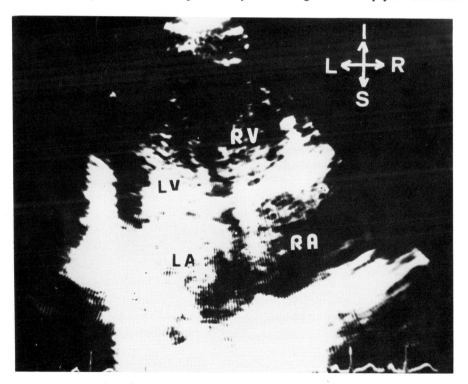

Figure 8. Two-dimensional apical four-chamber view after pulmonary wedge injection of indocyanine green in a patient with atrial septal defect and no oxymetric evidence of a left-to-right shunt. The picture shows echoes filling the right atrium (RA) from the left atrium (LA).

reported from the use of the flow-directed balloon-tipped catheter [31, 32]. They seem to occur when the catheter is inserted blindly, or when there are prolonged periods of flow occlusion in the pulmonary wedge position. Our method requires manipulation of the catheter under fluoroscopic control and a short time of wedging and balloon inflation. These precautions are essential as a safeguard against the above mentioned complications. The injection of foreign materials into the pulmonary capillaries is a potential cause of embolization to the systemic circulation. None of our cases nor of Meltzer's had any clinical evidence of such complication. Prolonged wedging may cause pulmonary infarction, but this never occurred in any patient studied until now. All of our patients had postcatheterization chest films, five had complete pulmonary function tests, four had lung scans in the anterior and left lateral position, before and within 24 to 48 hours after the procedure. In three patients cineangiography of the pulmonary arterial district selected for wedge injection was performed before the procedure and at the end of cardiac catheterization. In eight patients LDH determinations were carried out on blood samples drawn immediately before and 2, 4, 6, 12, 24 and 48 hours after wedge injection. None of these tests showed variations postcatheterization in any of the patients thus studied. Similar observations with regard to chest films and lung scans have been reported [24]. Therefore, the method of pulmonary transmission of echoes by wedge injection appears to be safe procedure for humans, in our experience and in that of others [24].

It is a simple and sensitive method which can be used during right heart catheterization for demonstration of left-to-right shunts at the atrial, ventricular, and pulmonary arterial sites. It seems to be particularly useful when the shunt is small and unrevealed by oxygen saturation differences. In the patients in whom good transmission of echoes to the left heart is obtained, there is no passage to right heart and pulmonary artery, the absence of left-to-right shunts through septal defects and aortopulmonary communications can be assumed with certainty. Thus, if no other specific indications exist for left heart invasion, this can be avoided. If the test reveals left-to-right shunting, cineangiographic visualization of the defect, if necessary according to the individual clinical situation and the diagnostic and therapeutic surgical needs, will be more easily programmed and the number of radiopaque contrast injections possibly reduced.

It is obvious that the ultimate goal of echoangiography is to obtain an echoproducing agent which would pass the pulmonary capillaries with peripheral venous injection. Experimental studies with new indicators are underway [17, 33], but until they are proved to be applicable to human use the method of pulmonary transmission of echoes by wedge injection remains the only available procedure.

REFERENCES

1. Gramiak R, PM Shah: Echocardiography of the aortic root. Invest Radiol 3:356–366, 1968.
2. Gramiak R, PM Shah, DH Kramer: Ultrasound cardiography: contrast studies in anatomy and function. Radiology 92:939–948, 1969.
3. Feigenbaum H, JM Stone, DA Lee, WK Nasser, S Chang: Identification of ultrasound echoes from the left ventricle by use of intracardiac injections of indocyanine green. Circulation 41:615–621, 1970.
4. Pieroni Dr, PJ Varghese, RD Rowe: Echocardiography to detect shunt and valvular incompetence in infants and children. Circulation (Suppl IV) 48:81, 1973 (abstract).
5. Kerber RE, JM Kioschos, RM Lauer: Use of an ultrasonic contrast method in the diagnosis of valvular regurgitation and intracardiac shunts. Am J Cardiol 34:722–727, 1974.
6. Seward JB, AJ Tajik, JG Spangler, DG Ritter: Echocardiographic contrast studies: initial experience. Mayo Clin Proc 50:163–192, 1975.
7. Valdes-Cruz LM, DR Pieroni, JM Roland, PJ Varghese: Echocardiographic detection of intracardiac right-to-left shunts following peripheral vein injections. Circulation 54: 558–562, 1976.
8. Duff DF, HP Gutgesell: The use of saline for ultrasonic detection of right-to-left shunt in post-operative period. Am J Cardiol 37:132, 1976 (abstract).
9. Seward JB, AJ Tajik, DJ Hagler, BG Ritter: Peripheral venous contrast echocardiography. Am J Cardiol 39:202–212, 1976.
10. Valdes-Cruz LM, DR Pieroni, JM Roland, PJ Varghese: Recognition of residual post-operative shunts by contrast echocardiography techniques. Circulation 55:148–152, 1977.
11. Assad-Morell JL, JB Seward, AJ Tajik, DJ Hagler, ER Giuliani, DG Ritter: Echo-phonocardiographic and contrast studies in conditions with systemic arterial trunk overriding the ventricular septum. Circulation 53:663–673, 1976.
12. Seward JB, AJ Tajik, DJ Hagler, ER Giuliani, GT Gau, DG Ritter: Echocardiogram in common (single) ventricle: angiographic-anatomic correlation. Am J Cardiol 39: 217–225, 1977.
13. Tajik AJ, JB Seward: Contrast echocardiography. In: Kotler MN, BL Segal (eds) Clinical Echocardiography, p 317–341. F.A. Davis, Philadelphia, 1978.
14. Pieroni DR, PJ Varghese, RM Freedom, RD Rowe: The sensitivity of contrast echo-cardiography in detecting intracardiac shunts. Cathet Cardiovasc Diagn 5:19–29, 1979.
15. Tajik AJ, JB Seward, DJ Hagler, DD Mair, JT Lie: Two-dimensional real-time ultra-sonic imaging of the heart and great vessels. Mayo Clin Proc 53: 271–303, 1978.
16. Hagler DJ, AJ Tajik, JB Seward, DD Mair, DG Ritter: Real-time wide-angle sector echocardiography: atrioventricular canal defects. Circulation 59: 140–150, 1979.
17. Bommer WJ, EG Tickner, J Rasor, T Grehl, DT Mason, AN DeMaria: Development of a new echocardiographic contrast agent capable of pulmonary transmission and left heart opacification following peripheral venous injection. Circulation (Suppl III) 62:34, 1980 (abstract).
18. Reale A: Visualizzazione ecocontrastografica delle sezioni sinistre del cuore mediante iniezione di anidride carbonica in arteria polmonare. Policlin Sez Prat 86:216–219, 1979.
19. Reale A: Contrast echocardiography: Transmission of echoes to the left heart across the pulmonary vascular bed. Am J Cardiol 45:401, 1980 (abstract).
20. Reale A, F Pizzuto, E Martuscelli, E Mangieri, PA Gioffrè: Echoangiographic visualization of left-to-right shunts by venous cardiac catheterization. World Congress on Paediatric Cardiology, London, June 1980:170 (abstract).

21. Reale A, F Pizzuto, F Romeo, A Nigri, G Scibilia: Venous echoangiography of the left heart. European Congress of Cardiology, Paris, June 1980:31 (abstract).
22. Reale A, F Pizzuto, PA Gioffrè, A Nigri, F Romeo, E Martuscelli, E Mangieri, G Scibilia: Contrast echocardiography: transmission of echoes to the left heart across the pulmonary vascular bed. Eur Heart J 1:101–106, 1980.
23. Bommer WJ, DT Mason, AN DeMaria: Studies in contrast echocardiography: development of new agents with superior reproducibility and transmission through lungs. Circulation (Suppl II) 59, 60:17, 1979.
24. Meltzer RS, PW Serruys, J McGhie, N Verbaan, J Roelandt: Pulmonary wedge injections yielding left-sided echocardiographic contrast. Br Heart J 44:390–394, 1980.
25. Gioffrè PA, F Pizzuto, F Romeo, E Martuscelli, G Scibilia, A Reale: Ecoangiografia con anidride carbonica. Atti Congr Ital Cardiol, Bari, June 1979:123 (abstract).
26. Tambe A, WR McLaughlin, HA Zimmerman: Double contrast medium technique for coronary blood flow studies. Am J Cardiol 21:117, 1968 (abstract).
27. Rasmussen K, S Simonsen, O Storstein: Quantitative aspects of right-to-left shunting in uncomplicating atrial septal defect. Br Heart J 35:894–897, 1973.
28. Kronik G, I Slany, H Moesslacher: Contrast M-mode echocardiography in diagnosis of atrial septal defect in acyanotic patients. Circulation 59:372–378, 1979.
29. Fraker TD, PJ Harris, VS Behar, JA Kisslo: Detection and exclusion of interatrial shunts by two-dimensional echocardiography and peripheral venous injection. Circulation 59:379–384, 1979.
30. Weyman AE, LS Wann, RL Caldwell, RA Hurwitz, JC Dillon, H Feigenbaum: Negative contrast echocardiography: a new method for detecting left-to-right shunts. Circulation 59:498–505, 1979.
31. Pape, LA, CI Haffajee, JE Markis, et al: Fatal pulmonary hemorrhage after use of the flow-directed balloon-tipped catheter. Ann Intern Med 90:344–347, 1979.
32. Haapaniemi J, R Gadowski, M Naini, H Green, D Mackenzie, M Rubenfire: Massive hemoptysis secondary to flow-directed thermodilution catheters. Cathet Cardiovasc Diagn 5:151–157, 1979.
33. Reale A: Unpublished observation reported at International Symposium on Ultrasound in Cardiology, Madrid, February 27–28, 1981.

11. FACTORS AFFECTING THE SUCCESS OF ATTAINING LEFT HEART ECHO CONTRAST AFTER PULMONARY WEDGE INJECTIONS

PATRICK W. SERRUYS, RICHARD S. MELTZER, JACKIE MCGHIE, and JOS ROELANDT

INTRODUCTION

Peripheral venous contrast echocardiography has become an important diagnostic method and finds increasing application for the detection of intracardiac right-to-left shunts [1–21] and tricuspid insufficiency [22, 23]. It has been established that microbubbles of air injected into the blood stream are responsible for the echocardiographic contrast effect [24, 25]. The pulmonary capillary bed acts as a filter for these microbubbles [26]. Thus, after a peripheral venous or right heart injection, the appearance of ultrasonic contrast in the left heart cavities proves the existence of an intracardiac of extracardiac right-to-left shunt.

We, and others, have demonstrated the feasibility and safety of ultrasonic contrast injections in the aorta or left ventricle. The clinical utility of the procedure has been limited to a relatively small number of special cases [18, 27]. Nonetheless, acoustic opacification of the left heart cavities and the imaging of blood flow patterns in these cavities without invasion of the left heart, are attractive concepts to the "semi-invasive echocardiographer". For these reasons, we attempted transpulmonary transmission of echocardiographic contrast as early as 1976 (unpublished data). We employed a Swan-Ganz catheter in the wedge position, and all of our initial efforts to achieve left heart echo contrast met with failure. Recently, Bommer et al. demonstrated the feasibility of achieving transpulmonary transmission of echocardiographic contrast by wedge injections in dogs [28]. Several types of catheter were tested, and the authors underlined the importance of the type of catheter used. This animal study prompted us to reevaluate the possibility of transpulmonary transmission of echocardiographic contrast after wedge injections in our patients.

We thus designed a study in order to answer the following questions:
a. Is it possible to detect echocardiographic contrast in the left heart after injection of a biologically compatible solution in the pulmonary capillary wedge position?
b. Do pulmonary wedge injections damage the pulmonary parenchyma?
c. What is the route and mechanism of transmission through the pulmonary capillary bed?
d. What is the success rate of this procedure and what factors influence this success rate (type of catheter, pulmonary vascular pressures, site of injection, pressure of injection, etc.)?
e. What could be the clinical utility of this investigation?

PATIENTS STUDIED AND METHODS

Our study population consists of 41 patients who were studied consecutively using pulmonary wedge injections. All of these patients underwent diagnostic right and left heart catheterization for routine clinical indications. Their cardiac diagnosis and hemodynamic parameters, which could influence a positive test result, are summarized in Table 1.

The patients were divided into two groups according to the type of catheter used for the wedge injections: Group I patients had a Cournand catheter alone, and Group II patients had a Swan-Ganz catheter, with or without an additional Cournand catheter.

Group I

Twenty-seven patients underwent right heart catheterization with a 7 French Cournand catheter. After measuring the wedge pressure, 5–6 vigorous manual injections were performed in the same position, using 8 ml of either a saline or a 5% dextrose solution. Patients were in a slight left lateral decubitus position. Simultaneous echocardiography was performed during each injection to monitor for the appearance of left heart echocardiographic contrast. After each wedge injection, the wedge pressure was measured. No attempt was made to aspirate blood back through the system.

The echocardiographic instrument used to monitor left heart contrast during these studies was a Toshiba SSH-10A phased-array sector scanner. The following two-dimensional echocardiographic views were recorded: apical four-chamber, apical long-axis, and parasternal long- and short-axis views [29]. In order to study the toxicity of pulmonary wedge injections, three different tests were performed on subgroups of the study population:

a. Perfusion lung scans using macro-aggregated albumen complexed with technetium (11 patients)
b. Two follow-up chest X-rays: these were obtained the evening after catheterization and the following morning and compared to the precatheterization chest X-ray (ten patients)
c. Lactic dehydrogenase (LDH) isoenzyme determinations from 8 to 12 h after the pulmonary capillary injections (14 patients).

The lung scan and the three chest films were examined by two experienced observers blinded to the site of wedge injection. A record of the injection site was made after each series of injections in the catheterization laboratory by brief cineangiocardiography of the position of the Cournand catheter.

In order to identify the anatomic pathway followed by the ultrasonic contrast on its passage through the pulmonary parenchyma, special cineangiography (50 frames/s) was performed immediately after the echocardiographic study in ten patients, via the Cournand catheter in the same wedge position. The angiographic contrast agent was Amipaque[R] (Nyegaard & Co. AS, Oslo, Norway), a new nonionic agent, which is hypotonic and which has a viscosity approximately equal to that of blood. These ten patients did not have a lung scan and LDH isoenzyme determinations were not made. They were reserved for those patients with pulmonary wedge injections of 5% dextrose alone. In five out of the ten patients, who later had Amipaque injections, the precatheter pressure in the injection system was measured during hand injection of 5% dextrose. In order to accomplish this, two different pressure transducers were interposed by means of 3-way stopcocks and short lengths of tubing between the injecting syringe and Cournand catheter.

Group II

Fourteen patients underwent catheterization with a 7 French Swan-Ganz thermo-dilution catheter to attempt transpulmonary echocardiographic contrast transmission. In all of these patients the catheter was advanced to the wedge position, so that the wedge pressure could be obtained without balloon inflation. Injections were performed from this position. In 11 of these patients, after either successful or unsuccessful attempts at creating left heart ultrasonic opacification, the Swan-Ganz catheter was replaced by a 7 French Cournand catheter, which was carefully positioned using biplane fluoroscopy in the same position as the original Swan-Ganz catheter. This protocol thus attempted to compare, within a given patient, the effect of a catheter with a large or small lumen on the success of transpulmonary echo contrast transmission.

RESULTS

Transmission of ultrasonic contrast through the lungs

In 27 of the 41 study patients the injections were only performed through a Cournand catheter, in three patients only through a 7 French Swan-Ganz catheter, and in 11 patients through both catheters. Of the 41 study patients, 31 had contrast observed ultrasonically in the left heart after wedge injections. The overall success rate for left heart opacification through a Cournand catheter (31/38, or 82%) was higher than that through a Swan-Ganz catheter (3/14, or 21%). In the 11 patients with injections through both catheters in the identical wedge position, the frequency of successful left heart ultrasonic opacification was twice as high with the Cournand catheter (6/11) compared to the Swan-Ganz catheter (3/11).

In an attempt to semiquantitatively analyze the success of transpulmonary echocardiographic transmission, we employed a 0 to + + + scale for the intensity of left ventricular ultrasonic opacification on two-dimensional echocardiography after wedge injection. If the left ventricular cavity was totally opacified with a clear demarcation of endocardium throughout the cardiac cycle, we called the opacifi-

Table 1.

Patient	Age/Sex	Diagnosis	Catheter	Localization	Mean wedge pressure	Oxygen saturation in the pulmonary artery	Mean pulmonary artery pressure	LHEC	Chest film	Lung scan	LDH (I.U.)	Iso enzyme 1, 2, 3, 4, 5
Group I												
1	55/m	aortic stenosis and regurgitation	Cournand 7F	RLL	13	73	23	+++	unchanged	normal	444	1, 2 ++ 3, 4 +
2	45/m	CAD	Cournand 7F	RLL	6	–	–	+++	unchanged	RLL defect	244	nl
3	38/m	CAD	Cournand 7F	RLL	13	–	–	+++	unchanged	normal	344	1, 2 +
4	21/f	atrial septal defect	Cournand 7F	RLL	8	93	19	–	unchanged	–	276	nl
5	49/m	fixed subvalvular aortic stenosis	Cournand 7F	RLL	6	80	13	+++	unchanged	normal	238	nl
6	60/m	CAD	Cournand 7F	RLL	12	–	–	+++	unchanged	normal	290	1, 2 +
7	43/m	mitral regurgitation	Cournand 7F	RLL	5	80	13	+	unchanged	normal	270	nl
8	68/m	aortic stenosis and regurgitation, mitral regurgitation	Cournand 7F	RLL	14	73	20	++	unchanged	normal	270	1, 2 +
9	34/m	aortic and mitral regurgitation	Cournand 7F	RLL	15	–	–	+	unchanged	–	344	nl
10	20/m	aneurysm of the interventricular septum	Cournand 7F	RLL	10	92	17	+++	unchanged	RLL defect	321	nl

11	22/f	open foramen ovale	Cournand 7F	RLL	6	79	8	+++	unchanged	nl	236	1, 2, 3
12	39/m	subvalvular aortic stenosis	Cournand 7F	RLL	6	83	14	+++	unchanged	nl	329	1, 2, 3
13	61/f	aortic aneurysm with aortic regurgitation	Cournand 7F	RLL	6	71	18	+++	unchanged	RLL defect	–	–
14	37/m	aortic regurgitation	Cournand 7F	RLL	8	81	14	+++	–	–	286	nl
15	55/m	mitral valve prolaps	Cournand 7F	RLL	9	72	18	++	measurement of the pressure of injection			
16	45/m	impending infarction	Cournand 7F	LLL	15	–	–	++	measurement of the pressure of injection			
17	36/f	CAD	Cournand 7F	RLL	13	77	28	+++	measurement of the pressure of injection			
18	66/f	CAD	Cournand 7F	RLL	16	78	29	+++	measurement of the pressure of injection			
19	54/m	CAD	Cournand 7F	RLL	6	–	–	+++	cine of pulmonary wedge injection			
20	26/m	ventricular septum defect	Cournand 7F	LLL	6	87	28	++	measurement of the pressure of injection / cine of pulmonary wedge injection			
21	62/m	CAD	Cournand 7F	RLL	13	–	–	+++	cine of pulmonary wedge injection			
22	43/m	CAD	Cournand 7F	RLL	6	–	–	–	cine of pulmonary wedge injection			
23	38/f	mitral stenosis and regurgitation	Cournand 7F	RLL	14	77	23	+++	cine of pulmonary wedge injection			
24	47/m	aortic stenosis and regurgitation	Cournand 7F	RLL	14	79	27	+++	cine of pulmonary wedge injection			
25	31/m	subvalvular aortic stenosis	Cournand 7F	RLL	12	–	–	+	cine of pulmonary wedge injection			
26	58/m	mitral stenosis	Cournand 7F	RLL	–	–	–	++	cine of pulmonary wedge injection			
27	44/m	CAD	Cournand 7F	RLL	5	76	–	+++	cine of pulmonary wedge injection			

Table 1. (continued)

Patient	Age/Sex	Diagnosis	Catheter	Localization	Mean wedge pressure	Oxygen saturation in the pulmonary artery	Mean pulmonary artery pressure	LHEC	Chest film	Lung scan	LDH (I.U.)	Iso enzyme 1, 2, 3, 4, 5
Group II												
28	48/m	CAD	Swan Ganz 7F	RLL	10	79	12	+++	cine of pulmonary wedge injection			
			Cournand 7F	RLL	10	79	12	+++				
29	65/f	aortic and mitral stenosis	Swan Ganz 7F	RLL	14	72	24	–				
			Cournand 7F	RLL	16	72	24	–				
		CAD	Cournand 7F	LLL	16	72	24	–				
30	20/m	aortic re-gurgitation	Swan Ganz 7F	RUL	14	85	17	–				
			Cournand 7F	RLL	14	85	17	–				
		mitral valve prolaps	Cournand 7F	RML	14	85	17	–				
31	50/m	Löffler's syndrome	Swan Ganz 7F	RLL	24	–	35	–				
			Cournand 7F	RLL	24	–	35	+++				
32	55/m	CAD	Swan Ganz 7F	RLL	5	73	12	+				
			Cournand 7F	RLL	5	73	12	+				
33	61/m	CAD	Swan Ganz 7F	RLL	–	–	–	–				

No.	Age/sex	Diagnosis	Catheter	Location							
34	38/m	ventricular septum defect	Cournand 7F	RLL	—	—	—	+			
			Swan Ganz 7F	RLL	14	87	29	—			
35	50/f	mitral stenosis and regurgitation	Cournand 7F	RLL	14	87	29	—			
			Swan Ganz 7F	RLL	31	77	55	—			
36	42/m	CAD	Cournand 7F	RLL	31	77	55	—			
			Swan Ganz 7F	RLL	15	77	20	—			
37	59/f	mitral stenosis and regurgitation. aortic regurgitation. tricuspid regurgitation. pulmonary hypertension. CAD	Cournand 7F	RLL	15	77	20	+++			
			Swan Ganz 7F	RML	27	67	54	+++			
			Cournand 7F	RML	27	67	54	+++			
38	22/m	coarctation of the aorta	Cournand 7F	LLL	7	80	12	—	unchanged	246	1, 2 +
			Swan Ganz 7F	RLL							
39	49/m	CAD	Swan Ganz 7F	LLL	14	75	21	—			
40	52/m	aortic stenosis and regurgitation	Swan Ganz 7F	RLL	15	87	34	—			
41	51/m	CAD	Swan Ganz 7F	RLL	7	74	13	—			

cation + + + (Figure 1A). If there was good left ventricular opacification, but the entire endocardial contour was not well delineated throughout the cardiac cycle, we graded the opacification as + + (Figure 1B). If only a few microbubbles were imaged, with poor definition of the ventricular cavity, we called the opacification + (Figure 1C). Of the 31 positive studies, 21 were judged + + +, 5 + +, and 5 +.

Hemodynamic studies showed a wide range of mean wedge pressures (6–31 mm HG) and mean pulmonary aterial pressures (8–55 mm Hg). Two of the three patients with a mean wedge pressure above 22 mm Hg had + + + opacification of the left ventricle. There was no relationship between either wedge pressure of

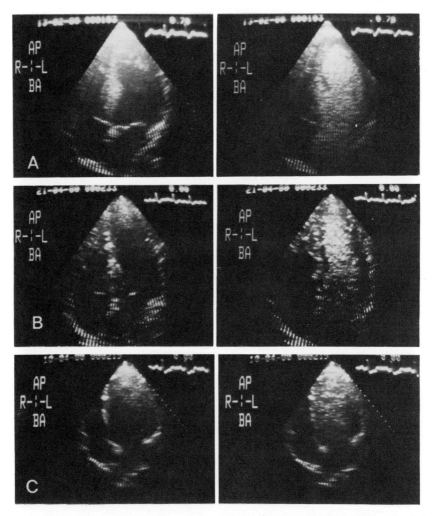

Figure 1. Still frames from two-dimensional echocardiogram in the apical four-chamber view before (left) and after (right) wedge injections. A) Totally opacified left ventricle (LV), with clear demarcation of the endocardium. Opacification rated + + +. B) Good LV opacification, but endocardial contour not entirely delineated throughout cardiac cycle, rated + +. C) Poor opacification with only a few micro-bubbles imaged, rated +. Orientation: AP = apical, BA = basal, R = right, L = left.

pulmonary arterial pressure and the success of contrast transmission. In two patients with a ventricular septal defect the left-to-right shunt was directly visualized after wedge injections (Figure 2). Analysis of the precatheter pressures during injection showed that pressures above 0.4 atmospheres were needed in order to achieve left heart contrast. Usually our vigorous hand injections reached values of several atmospheres, the mean value of the peak pressures recorded during 25 injections being 2.9 atmospheres. Since the mean duration of these injections was 1.6 ± 1.4 s and the injected volume was 8 cm^3, the mean flow rate during injection was 6.9 ± 2.3 cm^3/s (Table 2).

Analysis of the cineangiocardiograms of the ten patients undergoing Amipaque wedge injections suggested that there was no network of vessels, such as pulmonary arteriovenous fistulas, that bypass the pulmonary capillary bed. In the eight patients with grade $+ +$ or $+ + +$ left heart echo opacification prior to Amipaque injection, there was a progress of Amipaque in an exclusively anterograde direction, with opacification first of the arteriolar network and capillary blush before pulmonary venous contrast appearance (Figure 3). However, the two patients with 0 or $+$ left heart echo opacification evidenced reflux of Amipaque along the injection catheter, with retrograde opacification of the pulmonary arteries. In other words, the catheter did not appear to remain firmly wedged during these injections.

Table 2. Duration, mean flow rate and maximal pressure of hand injections in wedge position.

Injections	Duration s	Mean flow ml/s	Pressure (atmospheres)
1	1.00	8.00	3.4
2	0.80	10.00	5.5
3	0.92	8.70	4.4
4	1.00	8.00	3.4
5	1.04	7.69	3.0
6	1.14	7.02	2.4
7	1.08	7.41	2.9
8	1.00	8.00	3.4
9	1.12	7.14	2.5
10	0.80	10.00	5.6
11	0.90	8.84	4.6
12	1.00	8.00	3.5
13	1.06	7.55	3.0
14	2.00	4.00	0.9
15	1.44	5.56	1.4
16	1.12	7.14	2.4
17	1.20	6.67	2.0
18	0.96	8.33	3.5
19	0.94	8.51	4.2
20	1.50	5.33	1.5
21	2.10	3.81	0.7
22	4.60	1.74	0.6
23	7.00	1.14	0.4
Mean ± 1 s.d.	1.55 ± 1.43	6.90 ± 2.33	2.83 ± 2.32

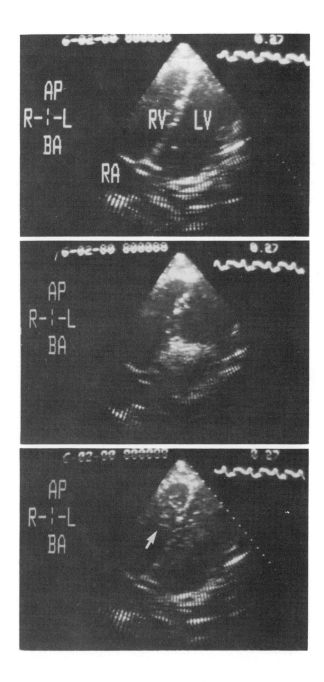

Figure 2. Still frames from two-dimensional echocardiogram, apical four-chamber view, of a patient with a ventricular septal defect. Upper panel: before wedge injection. Middle panel: shortly after appearance of contrast in the left ventricle (LV). Lower panel: several cardiac cycles later, with contrast still present in the LV and now also present in the right ventricle (RV). Throughout the study there was an absence of contrast in the right atrium (RA) as expected in a VSD. Orientation: AP = apical, BA = basal, R = right, L = left.

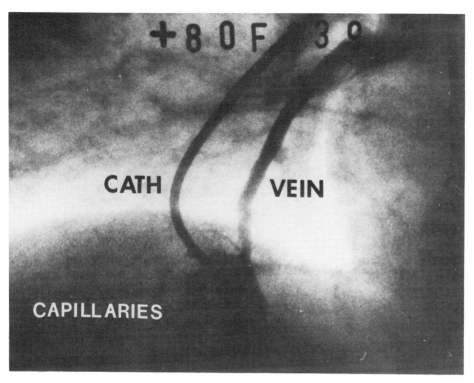

Figure 3. Frame from cineangiogram during injection of Amipaque in the pulmonary wedge position. Note capillary blush and pulmonary venous filling. In this patient there was no retrograde flow of contrast material around the catheter, indicating a firmly wedged position.

From the 50 frame/s cineangiocardiograms the pulmonary capillary to left atrial transit time was determined (Table 3). This entailed counting the number of frames between the appearance of contrast at the end of the catheter and its entry into the left atrium. This value was 254 ± 104 ms (mean ± 1 s.d.). The time from appearance at the catheter tip to satisfactory left atrial opacification was 536 ± 160 ms.

Toxicity of wedge injections

1. Clinical and hemodynamic: no patient complained of chest pain during the wedge injection or the 24 h immediately following catheterization. The wedge pressure was measured immediately after each wedge injection, and never changed significantly. Auscultation of the lungs after catheterization, paying particular attention to the lobe where the wedge injections were performed, was always normal.
2. Chest films (n = 10): there were no changes in the pre- and postcatheterization chest films.
3. Lung scans: of the 11 lung scans performed after catheterization, three showed segmental perfusion defects in the postero-inferior segment of the right lower lobe.

Table 3. Analysis of the cineangiograms performed in wedge position.

Pts no.	A (ms)	B (ms)
1	440	580
2	140	580
3 (2 injections)	160	420
	220	400
4	240	640
5	240	360
6	200	440
7 (2 injections)	280	540
	300	480
8	440	940
9	140	520
10	No opacification	
Mean ± s.d.	254 ± 106 ms	536 ± 160 ms

Column A: time from appearance of angiographic contrast material at the catheter tip to its entry into the left atrium.
Column B: time from appearance at the catheter tip to satisfactory left atrial opacification.

Late follow-up of all three patients revealed that their lung scans had normalized. 4. LDH isoenzyme levels: total LDH and its isoenzyme fractions were measured 8–12 h after catheterization in 12 of the study patients, as well as ten other patients undergoing diagnostic right and left heart catheterization without wedge injections. Total LDH in the study patients was 296 ± 57 U (normal 150–350 U) and in the control patients 336 ± 42 U. Only one study patients had an elevated total LDH level (444), and this was due to elevated isoenzyme 1 and 2. All three patients with segmental defects on their postcatheterization lung scans had normal total and isoenzyme fractions of LDH.

DISCUSSION

Mechanism

The results of this study cause us to pose the question: why can ultrasonic contrast reach the left heart after wedge injections, but not after peripheral venous injection? The pulmonary capillary diameter is approximately 8–10 μm [30]. One can conceive that smaller microbubbles would transit the pulmonary capillary "sieve" and reach the left heart. It is then necessary to know if microbubbles this small are still sufficient reflectors to be detectable by commercially available echocardiographic equipment. Using a solution of precision microbubbles, Meltzer et al. demonstrated that indeed bubbles this size yield contrast [26]. We must therefore conclude that microbubbles injected in the peripheral venous circulation never reach the left heart. This disappearance is due to diffusion of the gas contents of the microbubble into the ambient plasma, causing the bubble to shrink. Due to surface-tension factors in these extremely small bubbles, an unstable equilibrium results: the interior pressure is higher in this smaller bubble, accelerating the diffusion of gas down its concentration gradient into the ambient plasma, and thus accelerating the dissolution of the bubble. It has been calculated that a microbubble of air with an 8 μm diameter would dissolve completely in 190–550 ms, depending on the degree of saturation of the blood [26]. In humans the normal circulation time between the pulmonary capillaries and left atrium is above 2 s [31]. This explains why microbubbles are not ultrasonically imaged in left heart chambers after peripheral venous injections.

Thus, to explain the success of wedge injections in causing left heart ultrasonic opacification we need to invoke other mechanisms. A possible hypothesis is that the microbubbles can take a route through the lungs where the minimum diameter is greater than 8 μm, so that the capillary to left atrial circulation time is shorter than normal; and the total dissolution time of the microbubble is longer than that for an 8 μm bubble. This hypothesis implies the existence of anatomic arteriovenous communications opened during wedge injections, but not available after peripheral or right heart injections. We are unaware of studies establishing the existence of such channels and our Amipaque wedge cineangiograms did not suggest them. A viable hypothesis to explain the mechanism of transmission of microbubbles through the lungs would have to explain our observation that there seems to be a threshold pressure which must be attained in order to achieve left heart echo contrast.

Another important factor to take into consideration is the difference between the 7F Cournand and 7F Swan-Ganz catheters. The former has a larger internal lumen and thus a smaller resistance. It is also more rigid and allows a better "wedging" in the capillary position, with better transmission of injected pressures to the pulmonary capillary bed. One possibility is thus that the pulmonary capillary bed is distended by the injection to the point that it can allow passage of bubbles larger than 8 μm in diameter. Another possibility is that the bubbles themselves can be deformed by the pressures proximal to them, and in this way larger bubbles may pass the pulmonary capillary sieve (Figure 4). We estimate the pulmonary capillary to left atrium transit time from our Amipaque wedge injection cineangiograms, though realizing that conditions were not identical to those with aqueous solutions. The interval between contrast appearance at the catheter tip and initial entry into the left atrium was 254 ± 104 ms. Furthermore, the interval of 536 ± 160 ms between the appearance of Amipaque at the catheter tip and total left atrial opacification suggests that wedge injections decrease the capillary to left heart circulation time from normal.

Toxicity

The negative clinical and chest film findings and minor LDH elevations are relatively reassuring with respect to the possibility of toxicity in this technique. How-

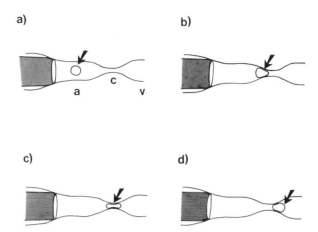

Figure 4. Diagrammatic representation of proposed mechanism by which microbubbles of gas larger than the pulmonary capillary diameter may pass through the lungs to yield left heart echo contrast. a) A bubble of gas (arrow) injected through a catheter (shaded) in the wedge position enters a pulmonary arteriole (a). b) Due to the hydrodynamic force applied to the local pulmonary circulation from an injection directly in the wedge position. The bubble is deformed and forced into a pulmonary capillary (c). c) The bubble elongates and may even fill a capillary entirely with gas. d) The bubble emerges on the venous (v) side of the pulmonary capillary bed. Reproduced with permission of Ultrasound in Medicine and Biology.

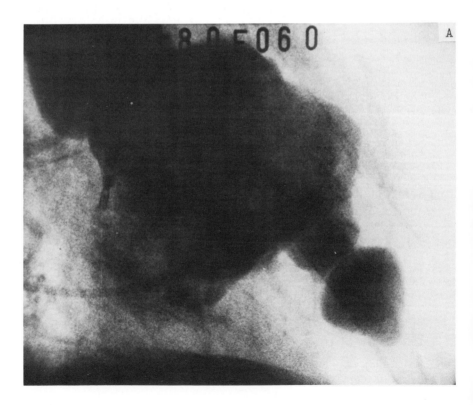

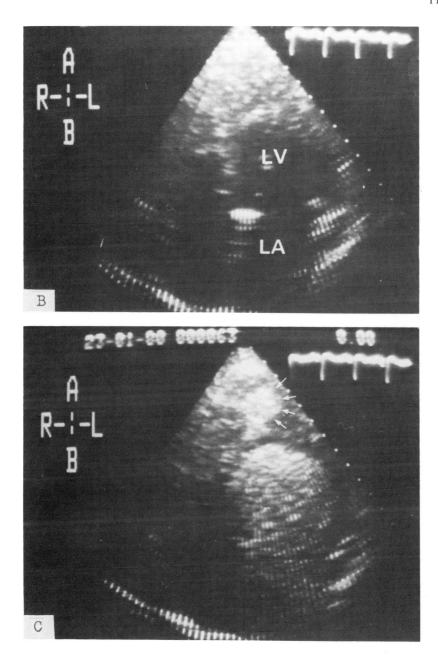

Figure 5. A) Frame from cineangiogram in the right anterior oblique position showing a small residual lumen to the left ventricle due to apical endocardial thickening in a patient with Löffler's eosinophilic endocarditis. B) Still frame from two-dimensional echocardiogram in the apical four-chamber view. Before wedge injection, no apical lumen is apparent. C) After wedge injection, the endocardial thickening is better defined, and the residual apical lumen is now seen (arrows). LA = left atrium, LV = left ventricle, A = apical, B = basal, R = right, L = left.

ever, the three segmental defects on lung scans after catheterization are disturbing. Certainly one can conceive that repeated wedge injections under pressure damaged arteriolar and capillary endothelium and thus caused the positive scans. It is important to remember that pulmonary infarction has been described as the sequel of leaving a catheter in the wedge position for an extended period of time [32]. Fatal exsanguination due to pulmonary artery rupture after Swan-Ganz balloon inflation has also been reported [33–35]. Aside from pulmonary toxicity, a major cause of concern for possible toxicity is systemic air embolus. In this context, it is important to realize that the routine flushing and angiography performed in the left heart during diagnostic catheterization usually contain microbubbles which are imaged as contrast by echocardiographic equipment. Indeed, this was how echocardiographic contrast was originally discovered. Furthermore, Reale et al. have recently published data on pulmonary wedge injections using an inflated Swan-Ganz catheter and $0.5–1.0\,cm^3$ of carbon dioxide, followed by 5% dextrose or saline solution [36, 37].

Since there are risks of both pulmonary and systemic toxicity, we feel that this procedure should be considered experimental until further data about toxicity is available.

Clinical implications

This procedure allows for the visualization of exclusively left-to-right intracardiac shunts only, necessitating the catheterization of the right heart. Abnormal flow patterns, such as turbulence and aortic or mitral regurgitation, may also be imaged. In half of our wedge injections we have attained + + + left ventricular opacification, which may aid in echocardiographic analysis of the left ventricle. Figure 5 illustrates this point. In this patient with Löffler's syndrome, the resting two-dimensional echocardiogram (Figure 5B) failed to bring out the apical deformation and thickening due to endocardial fibrosis that could be seen after transpulmonary left ventricular opacification (Figure 5C). However, all of these clinical problems are also amenable to solution by standard catheterization techniques and more work will be needed before wedge injections for transmission of echocardiographic contrast through the lungs becomes a clinical tool.

REFERENCES

1. Seward JB, AJ Tajik, JG Spangler, DG Ritter: Echocardiographic contrast studies: initial experience. Mayo Clin Proc 50:163–192, 1975.
2. Valdes-Cruz LM, DR Pieroni, JM Roland, PH Varghese: Echocardiographic detection of intracardiac right-to-left shunts following peripheral vein injections. Circulation 54: 558–562, 1976.
3. Duff DF, HP Gutgesell: The use of saline for ultrasonic detection of right-to-left shunt in post-operative period. Am J Cardiol 37:132, 1976 (abstract).
4. Seward JB, AJ Tajik, DJ Hagler, DG Ritter: Peripheral venous contrast echocardiography. Am J Cardiol 39:202–212, 1976.

5. Assad-Morell JL, JB Seward, AJ Tajik, DJ Hagler, ER Giuliana, DG Ritter: Echophonocardiographic and contrast studies in conditions with systemic arterial trunk overriding the ventricular septum. Circulation 53:663–673, 1976.

6. Hagemeijer F, PW Serruys, WG Van Dorp: Contrast echocardiology. In: N Bom (ed) Echocardiology. Martinus Nijhoff, The Hague, 1977.

7. Serruys PW, WB Vletter, F Hagemeijer, CM Ligtvoet: Bidimensional real-time echocardiological visualization of a ventricular right-to-left shunt following peripheral vein injection. Eur J Cardiol 6:117, 1977.

8. Serruys PW, CM Ligtvoet, F Hagemeijer, WB Vletter: Intracardiac shunts in adults studied with bidimensional ultrasonic contrast techniques after peripheral intravenous injections. Circulation (Suppl III) 26:55, 66, 1977.

9. Valdes-Cruz LM, DR Pieroni, JM Roland, PH Varghese: Recognition of residual postoperative shunts by contrast echocardiography techniques. Circulation 55:148–152, 1977.

10. Seward JB, AJ Tajik, DJ Hagler, ER Giuliani, GT Gau, DG Ritter: Echocardiogram in common (single) ventricle: angiographic—anatomic correlation. Am J Cardiol 39: 217–225, 1977.

11. Serruys PW, F Hagemeijer, CM Ligtvoet, J Roelandt: Echocardiologie de contraste en deux dimensions et en temps réel — I. Techniques ultrasoniques. Arch Mal Coeur 71:600, 1978.

12. Serruys PW, F Hagemeijer, AH Bom, J Roelandt: Echocardiologie de contraste en deux dimensions et en temps réel — II. Applications cliniques. Arch Mal Coeur 71: 611, 1978.

13. Tajik AJ, JB Seward, DJ Hagler, DD Mair, JT Lie: Two-dimensional real-time ultrasonic imaging of the heart and great vessels. Mayo Clin Proc 53:271–303, 1978.

14. Tajik AJ, JB Seward: Contrast echocardiography. In: Kotler MN, BL Segal (eds) Clinical Echocardiography, pp 317–341. FA Davis, Philadelphia, 1978.

15. Pieroni DR, PJ Varghese, RM Freedom, RD Rowe: The sensitivity of contrast echocardiography in detecting intracardiac shunts. Cathet Cardiovasc Diagn 5:19–29, 1979.

16. Hagler DJ, AJ Tajik, JB Seward, DD Mair, DG Ritter: Real time wide angle echocardiography: atrioventricular canal defects. Circulation 59:140–150, 1979.

17. Serruys PW, M Van den Brand, PG Hugenholtz, J Roelandt: Intracardiac right-to-left shunts demonstrated by two-dimensional echocardiography after peripheral vein injection. Br Heart J 42:429–437, 1979.

18. Serruys PW, F Hagemeijer, J Roelandt: Echocardiological contrast studies with dynamically focussed multiscan. Acta Cardiol 34:283, 1979.

19. Kronik G, I Slany, H Moesslacher: Contrast M-mode echocardiography in diagnosis of atrial septal defect in acyanotic patients. Circulation 59: 372–378, 1979.

20. Fraker TD, PJ Harris, VS Behar, JA Kisslo: Detection and exclusion of interatrial shunts by two-dimensional echocardiography and peripheral venous injection. Circulation 59: 379–384, 1979.

21. Weyman AE, LS Wann, RL Caldwell, RA Hurwitz, JC Dillon, F Feigenbaum: Negative contrast echocardiography: a new method for detecting left-to-right shunts. Circulation 59:498–505, 1979.

22. Lieppe W, VS Behar, R Scallion, JA Kisslo: Detection of tricuspid regurgitation with two-dimensional echocardiography and peripheral vein injection. Circulation 57:128, 1978.

23. Meltzer RS, DCA Van Hoogenhuyze, PW Serruys, M Haalebos, J Roelandt: Diagnosis of tricuspid regurgitation by contrast echocardiography. Circulation 63:1093–1099, 1981.

24. Barrera JG, PK Fulkerson, SE Rittgers, RM Nerem: The nature of contrast echocardiographic "targets". Circulation (Suppl II) 58:233, 1978 (abstract).

25. Meltzer RS, EG Thickner, TP Sahines, RL Popp: The source of ultrasound contrast

114

effect. J Clin Ultrasound 8:121, 1980.
26. Meltzer RS, EG Tickner, RL Popp: Why do the lungs clear ultrasonic contrast? Ultrasound Med Biol 6:263–269, 1980.
27. Kerber RE, JM Kioschos, RM Lauer: Use of an ultrasonic contrast method in the diagnosis of valvular regurgitation and intracardiac shunts. Am J Cardiol 34:722–727, 1974.
28. Bommer WJ, DT Mason, AN DeMaria: Studies in contrast echocardiography: development of new agents with superior reproducibility and transmission through lungs. Circulation (Suppl II) 59–60:11–17, 1979 (abstract).
29. Meltzer RS, C Meltzer, J Roelandt: Sector scanning views in echocardiology: a systematic approach. Eur Heart J 1:379–394, 1980.
30. Weibel ER, DM Gomez: Architecture of the human lung: use of quantitative methods establishes fundamental relations between size and number of lung structures. Science 137:577–585, 1962.
31. Hamilton WF (ed): Handbook Physiology: Circulation sec 2, vol 2, p 1709. Am Physiological Society, Washington DC, 1963.
32. Hagemeijer F, CJ Storm: Fan-shaped shadows due to pulmonary artery catheters: heparin prohylaxis. Br Med J 701:1124–1125, 1977.
33. Golden M, T Pinder, W Anderson, M Cheitlin: Fatal pulmonary hemorrhage complicating rupture of flow-directed balloon-tipped catheter in a patient receiving anticoagulant therapy. Am J Cardiol 32:865–867, 1973.
34. Pape LA, CI Haffajee, JE Markis et al.: Fatal pulmonary hemorrhage after use of the flow-directed balloon-tipped catheter. Ann Intern Med 90:344–347, 1979.
35. Haapaniemi J, R Gadowski, M Naini, H Green, D Mackenzie, M Rubenfire: Massive hemoptysis secondary to flow-directed thermodilution catheters. Cathet Cardiovasc Diagn 5:151–157, 1979.
36. Meltzer RS, OEH Sartorius, CT Lancée, PW Serruys, PD Verdouw, CE Essed, J Roelandt: Transmission of ultrasonic contrast through the lungs. Ultrasound Med Biol 7:377–384, 1981.
37. Reale A: Visualizzazione echocontrastografica delle sezioni sinitre del cuore mediante iniezione di anidride carbonica in arteria polmonare. Policlinico Sez Prat 86:216–219, 1979.
38. Reale A, F Pizzuto, PA Gioffrè, A Nigri, F Romeo, E Martuscelli, E Mangieri, G Scibilia: Contrast echocardiography: transmission of echoes to the left heart across the pulmonary vascular bed. Eur Heart J 44:101–106, 1980.

12. ECHO CONTRAST FOR THE DETECTION OF ATRIAL SEPTAL DEFECTS*

JOSEPH KISSLO

INTRODUCTION

Patients with atrial septal defects and other forms of right ventricular volume overload frequently manifest right ventricular enlargement and paradoxical septal motion on echocardiography [1–5]. Unfortunately, these findings are non-specific for atrial septal defects alone.

Two-dimensional echocardiography has been shown to provide spatial information concerning cardiac structures not readily available by conventional M-mode echocardiography and when combined with M-mode offers additional information for the ultrasonic evaluation of patients with atrial septal defects. Rarely, the atrial septal defect can be imaged. More commonly, the echocardiographer must resort to contrast methods to verify the presence of an atrial septal defect [6].

This chapter discusses the use of contrast two-dimensional echocardiography for detection of the right-to-left shunting present in all patients with atrial septal defects.

RATIONALE

Slight degrees of right-to-left shunt flow are present in atrial septal defects, even when the predominant shunt is left-to-right. Levin [7] demonstrated this by angiographic techniques in children with uncomplicated ostium secundum atrial septal defects. Further evidence substantiating this point was reported by Swan [8], who used indicator dilution methods. Alexander [9] created atrial septal defects in dogs and was able to measure directly the phasic shunt flow (including transient right-to-left shunting) during the cardiac cycle.

Some reports have demonstrated the use of contrast M-mode echocardiography in identifying and localizing significant right-to-left intracardiac shunts at the atrial level using peripherally injected contrast material [10, 11]. Seward has shown that small amounts of right-to-left shunting are not always detected by contrast M-mode echocardiography in patients with secundum atrial septal defect when there is predominant left-to-right shunt. This failure of M-mode presumably results

* Supported in part by USPHS Grants HL-12715, HL-14228, and HL-01613.

because of its narrow field of view.

As Fraker [6] has shown, however, two-dimensional echocardiography increases the probability of detecting right-to-left shunts at the atrial level, because it provides greater spatial information and allows simultaneous examination of the right atrium, left atrium, and interatrial septum. This wide field of view enhances the ability to visualize contrast as it crosses right-to-left.

METHODS

Preferences for contrast material vary with each laboratory. In this institution we prefer 8–10 cm^3 of saline rapidly injected into a peripheral vein. This solution produces excellent contrast targets with little risk of allergic reaction and none of the inconvenience of green dye. A bolus of 8–10 cm^3 of saline is then rapidly injected while recording appropriate views. It is important to remember that injections are made as rapidly as possible to ensure maximum turbulence and thus produce the greatest amount of contrast possible. Multiple injections in multiple views are usually required. Occasionally, 8–10 injections are needed.

It is always best to make injections during suspended respiration to avoid any artifact induced during the respiratory cycle. If possible, injections are always made into the left anticubital vein so that a coexistent aberrant left superior vena cava is not missed [12].

One maneuver which may be helpful in shunt detection when combined with contrast study is for the patient to perform a Valsalva with sudden release [13]. During the Valsalva maneuver venous return is impeded during the strain phase by the elevated intrathoracic pressure. When released, the peripheral veins rapidly empty into the right atrium, while the left atrium receives little blood from the pulmonary veins. Thus, small degrees of right-to-left shunt may be exaggerated during release and can be detected with the two-dimensional echocardiographic approach. This maneuver may be of real value when the clinician is confronted with the possible diagnosis of paradoxical emboli through a small atrial defect or patent foramen ovale [14].

RESULTS

Anatomic detection

Although rarely fruitful, the direct inspection of the atrial septum is accomplished by an apical four-chamber view. Because the atrial septum lies parallel to the interrogating beam, portions of the atrial septum "drop out" even in normal individuals. Thus, absence of portions of this structure should not be regarded as reliable criterion for atrial septal defect. A modified apical view where the trans-

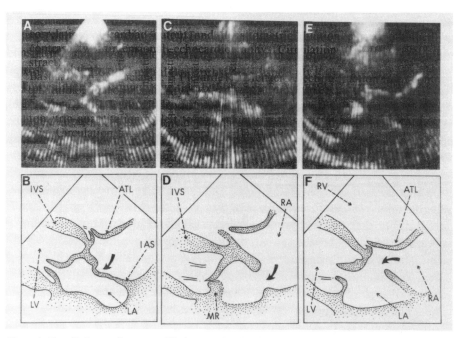

Figure 1. Systolic frames from a modified reversed apical four-chamber view. Panels A and B are from a normal subject. Solid arrows in B indicates the area of the foramen ovale. Panels C and D are from a patient with an ostium secundum atrial septal defect. Solid arrow in D indicates the area of the septal defect. ATL = anterior tricuspid leaflet; IAS = interatrial septum; IVS = interventricular septum; RA = right atrium; MR = mitral ring; RV = right ventricle.

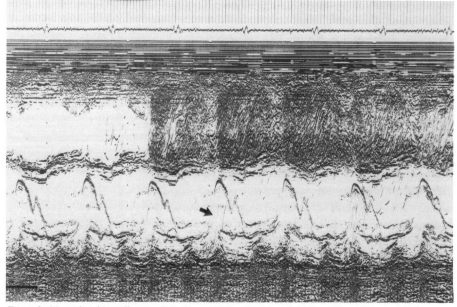

Figure 2. M-mode echocardiogram following peripheral contrast injection. The right ventricle is seen to fill with contrast followed by a lesser degree of contrast in the mitral valve orifice (arrow).

ducer is positioned more medially over the right ventricle sometimes eliminates this problem and is slightly more beneficial (Figure 1).

The entirety of the atrial septum is occasionally detected (Figure 1A and 1B) in normals and the foramen ovale is only rarely seen. Ostium secundum defects appear in the upper portions of the septum, but are sometimes difficult to differentiate from normals (Figure 1C and D) where "drop out" occurs. Ostium primum defects occur in the proximal portions of the septum and are more reliably detected (Figure 1E and F), particularly when a cleft mitral leaflet is seen on ventricular short-axis [15].

Contrast studies

When M-mode is used, contrast is usually best detected when the transducer is angled at the tips of the mitral valve (Figure 2). In this position the relative timing of appearance of the contrast in the mitral orifice before it enters the ventricle helps to identify an atrial septal defect.

Figure 3 shows a two-dimensional study with contrast transiting from the left atrium to the left ventricle through the open mitral valve in diastole. In this case, the patient had a rather large right-to-left component of atrial shunting.

More commonly, smaller degrees of right-to-left shunting are seen (Figure 4). The immediate appearance of one bubble in the left atrium is enough to confirm the presence of an atrial level shunt (Figure 5).

Although the initial data from this laboratory suggested that contrast echocardiography was both 100% specific and sensitive for detection of atrial septal defects [6], continued experience has tempered these results. In the past 114 patients with catheterized-proven atrial septal defect, there were only four false negatives for right-to-left shunting. As many as ten or more injections were occasionally required before confirmation was obtained. When contrast appeared in the left atrium within three beats after appearance in the right side, there were no false positives. Fraker [6] has shown that properly performed contrast echocardiography is more sensitive than indocyanine green dye curves or oximetry for shunt detection.

Another feature of contrast echocardiography is the negative contrast effect seen within the right atrium that results from the left-to-right component [16] (Figure 6). This criterion will be dealt with in more detail in the following chapter. Too inferior angulation of the transducer will, however, detect uncontrasted blood entering the right atrium from the inferior vena cava rendering a false positive result for left-to-right shunt. Bidirectional shunting is sometimes seen (Figure 7).

It has been reported that persistent left superior vena cava with drainage into the coronary sinus occurs in 0.5% of the general population and in 3–10% of patients with atrial septal defects [17–20]. When unsuspected, this entity may complicate cardiac catheterization and the establishment of cardiopulmonary bypass during open heart surgery.

Careful examination of abnormal targets in the posterior atrio-ventricular groove in the left ventricular long-axis with contrast techniques will usually re-

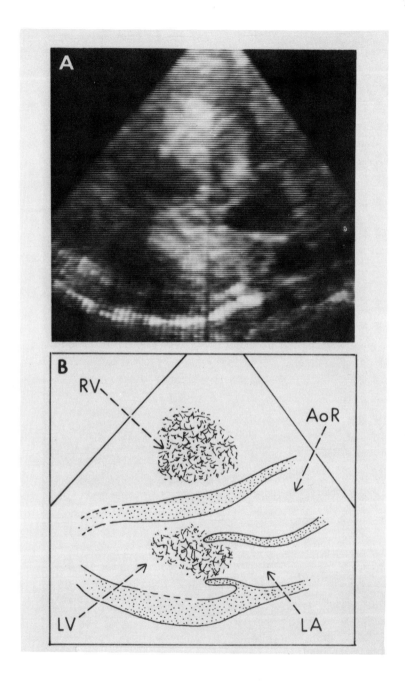

Figure 3. A large right-to-left shunt in the long-axis view of the left ventricle. Panel A and the accompanying schematic diagram in panel B show equal opacification of the left and right ventricles in this patient with an atrial septal defect and pulmonary hypertension. AoR = Aortic root; RV = right ventricle; LV = left ventricle; LA = left atrium.

120

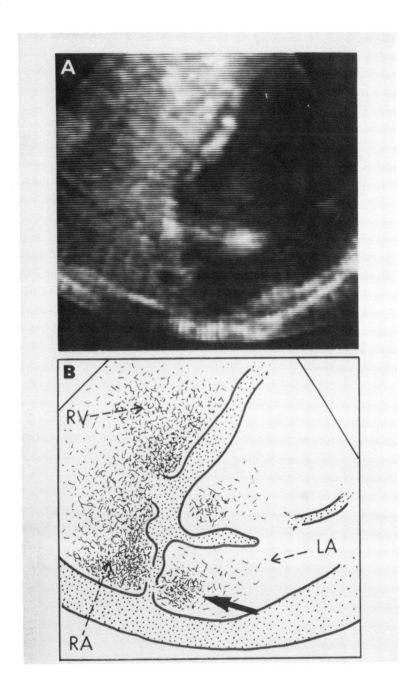

Figure 4. A moderate right-to-left atrial level shunt using the apical four-chamber view in a patient with an atrial septal defect. The solid arrow indicates a small, dense cloud of microcavitations just as they appear in the left atrium.

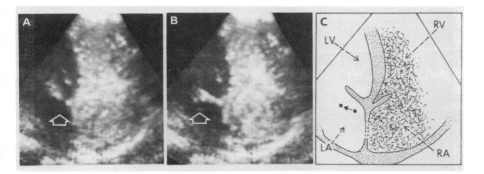

Figure 5. A small right-to-left atrial level shunt shown by sequential late diastolic stop-frame videotape images (panels A and B) and composite schematic diagram (panel C) in a reversed apical four-chamber view. Microcavitations are seen filling the right atrium and ventricle. The arrows in panels A and B indicate a single microcavitation as it moves from the atrial septum toward the mitral orifice (1/15th s time interval). Movement of the single microcavitation is illustrated in panel C.

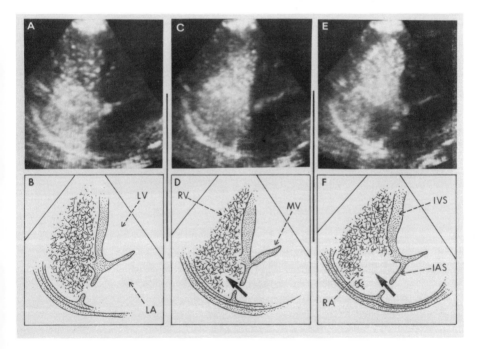

Figure 6. Sequential late diastolic stop-frame videotape images (panels A, C, and E) in the apical four-chamber view with accompanying schematic diagrams (panels B, D, and F) from a patient with an ostium secundum atrial septal defect. Blood without microcavitations (negative contrast) is seen to enter the right atrium (panels C and D) and to partially fill it (panels E and F). IVS = interventricular septum; IAS = interatrial septum; LV = left ventricle; RV = right ventricle; LA = left atrium; RA = right atrium; MV = mitral valve.

122

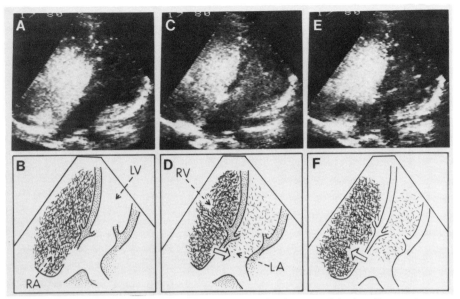

Figure 7. Bidirectional atrial septal defect proved by peripheral contrast injection. Contrast is seen to enter the right atrium (RA) and right ventricle (RV) in panels A and B. A moderate right to left shunt is seen in panels C and D. A negative contrast effect is seen in panels E and F. LA = left atrium; LV = left ventricle.

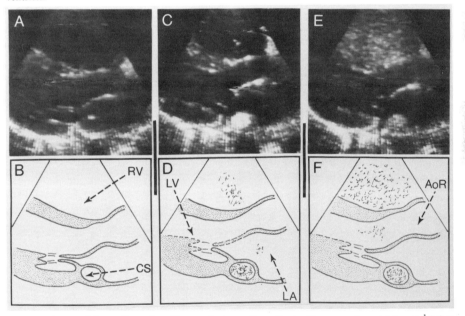

Figure 8. Sequential two-dimensional long-axis views of a patient with a secundum atrial septal defect and persistent left superior vena cava. Panel A illustrates the enlarged coronary sinus devoid of contrast. Following injection of contrast material in a peripheral left arm vein, the coronary sinus opacifies early (panel C), followed by opacification of the right ventricle (panel E). Note the appearance of a small amount of contrast material in the left atrium (panel C) and left ventricular outflow tract (panel E) demonstrating right-to-left shunting at the atrial level. RV = right ventricle; CS = coronary sinus; LV = left ventricle; LA = left atrium; AoR = aortic root.

veal this aberrant venous drainage [12]. Contrast fills the coronary sinus first, then right-sided structures and ultimately the left atrium when an atrial septal defect is present (Figure 8).

This phenomenon is only seen when the left arm is used for injection. Differential injections from both arms will confirm the venous drainage pattern (Figure 9).

Limitations

The echocardiographer should use this method prudently. Other cardiac abnormalities may be present in patients with atrial septal defects, necessitating cardiac catheterization. Some patients have poor sound transmission characteristics due to obstructive lung disease, obesity, or anterior chest wall abnormalities; so the diagnostic certainty of the ultrasonic information may, in itself, be questionable. Right-to-left atrial shunts may also be more difficult to demonstrate by contrast two-dimensional echo at faster heart rates, as is frequently the case in children.

Intrapulmonary shunting in patients without atrial septal defect may result in the appearance of bubbles within the left atrium. Usually this appearance is somewhat delayed taking eight or more beats following initial detection in the right heart.

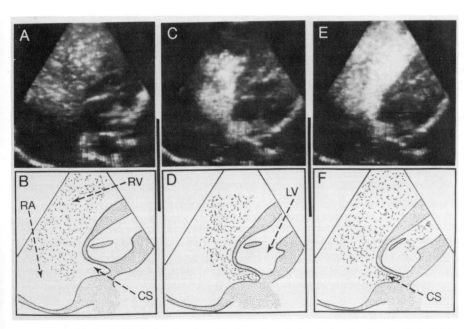

Figure 9. Modified apical four-chamber view. The beam is angled such that the plane is tilted slightly below the level of the left atrium and visualizes the area of entry of the coronary sinus into the right atrium. Panel A shows the distrubtion of contrast material following injection from a peripheral right arm vein. The right atrium and right ventricle opacify normally. Note the absence of contrast in the area of the coronary sinus. Panels C and E illustrate the distribution following injection of contrast material from a peripheral left arm vein. Note the complete opacification in the area of the coronary sinus and subsequent right ventricular filling. RA = right atrium; RV = right ventricle; CS = coronary sinus; LV = left ventricle.

When contrast appears within two beats, atrial septal defect is usually certain. Between these two extremes differentiation of atrial septal defect from intrapulmonary shunting is frequently difficult.

Spontaneous bubbles in the left heart occur rarely and are of unknown etiology. In these patients the results of contrast echocardiography are impossible to interpret with certainty.

Lastly, not all patients with contrast echo evidence for right-to-left shunting at the atrial level will have an anatomic atrial septal defect. In cases of pulmonary hypertension positive contrast echo results have been shown where only a patent foramen ovale was present. Fraker [6] has pointed out the clinical value of this approach for detecting a patent foramen ovale in patients with pulmonary hypertension, unexplained peripheral desaturation or paradoxical embolization.

REFERENCES

1. Diamond MA, JC Dillon, CL Haine, S Chang, H Feigenbaum: Echocardiographic features of atrial septal defect. Circulation 43:129, 1971.
2. Meyer RA, DC Schwartz, G Benzing, S Kaplan: Ventricular septum in right ventricular volume overload. Am J Cardiol 30:349, 1972.
3. Kerber RE, WF Dippel, FM Abboud: Abnormal motion of the interventricular septum in right ventricular volume overload. Circulation 48:86, 1973.
4. Hagan AD, GS Francis, DJ Sahn, JS Karliner, WF Friedman, RA O'Rourke: Ultrasound evaluation of systolic anterior septal motion in patients with and without right ventricular volume overload. Circulation 50:248, 1974.
5. Radtke WE, AJ Tajik, GT Gau, TT Schattengerg, ER Giuliani, RG Tancredi: Atrial septal defect: Echocardiographic observations. Ann Intern Med 84:246, 1976.
6. Fraker TD, PJ Harris, VS Behar, JA Kisslo: Detection and exclusion of interatrial shunts by two-dimensional echocardiography and peripheral venous injections. Circulation 59:379, 1979.
7. Levin AR, MS Spach, JP Boineau, RV Canent, MP Capp, PH Jewet: Atrial pressure-flow dynamics in atrial septal defects (secundum type). Circulation 37:476, 1968.
8. Swan HJC, HB Burchell, EH Wood: Presence of venoatrial shunts in patients with interatrial communication. Circulation 10:705, 1954.
9. Alexander JA, JC Rembert, WC Sealy, JC Greenfield: Shunt dynamics in experimental atrial septal defects. J Appl Physiol 39:28, 1975.
10. Valdes-Cruz LM, DR Pieroni, JMA Roland, PH Varghese: Echocardiographic detection of intracardiac right-to-left shunts following peripheral vein injections. Circulation 54:558, 1976.
11. Seward JB, AJ Tajik, DJ Hagler, DG Ritter: Peripheral venous contrast echocardiography. Am J Cardiol 39:202, 1977.
12. Stewart JA, TD Fraker, DA Slosky et al.: Detection of persistent left superior vena cava by two-dimensional contrast echocardiography. J Clin Ultrasound 7:357, 1979.
13. Kronik G, J Slany, H Moesslacher: Contrast M-mode echocardiography in diagnosis of atrial septal defect in acyanotic patients. Circulation 59:372, 1979.
14. Cheng TO: Paradoxical embolism: a diagnostic challenge and its detection during life. Circulation 53:565, 1976.

15. Lieppe W, VS Behar, R Scallion, JA Kisslo: Detection of tricuspid regurgitation with two-dimensional echocardiography and peripheral vein injections. Circulation 57:128, 1978.
16. Weyman AE, LS Wann, RL Caldwell et al.: Negative contrast echocardiography: a new technique for detecting left-to-right shunts. Circulation 59:498, 1979.
17. Steinberg I, W Dubilier, D Lukas: Persistence of left superior vena cava. Dis Chest 24:479, 1953.
18. Campbell M, D Deuchar: The left sided superior vena cava. Br Heart J 16:423, 1954.
19. Sipila W, J Hakkila, P Keikel et al.: Ann Med Intern Fenn 44:241, 1955.
20. Winter FS: Persistent left superior vena cava. Angiology 5:90, 1954.

13. NEGATIVE CONTRAST ECHOCARDIOGRAPHY FOR THE DIAGNOSIS OF ATRIAL SEPTAL DEFECTS

ARTHUR E. WEYMAN

NEGATIVE CONTRAST ECHOCARDIOGRAPHY

In 1968, Gramiak et al., reported that rapid intracardiac injection of a variety of substances, including saline and indocyanine green dye, produced a cloud of echoes at the injection site which, one formed, would follow the path of blood flow downstream [1]. It was further noted that these intravascular echoes disappeared during passage through either the systemic or pulmonary capillary beds [2] and, thus, were normally confined to the side of the circulation in which they were generated. Based on these observations, it was suggested that the unexpected appearance of echocardiographic contrast crossing intracardiac septa might be used as evidence of an intracardia shunt. Subsequent reports confirmed the sensitivity of echocardiographic contrast as a means of detecting both intra and extracardiac shunts [3–7] and demonstrated that shunts as small as 5% of the systemic blood flow could be appreciated [5].

In patients with right-to-left shunts across atrial septal defects, peripherally injected contrast offered a direct method for detecting the abnormal blood flow and confirmed the presence of the defect [3–7]. When the shunt was from left to right, however, contrast appearance in the left atrium following peripheral injection was less consistent and in these cases, some other indicator of abnormal shunt flow appeared necessary.

Although not emphasized in early studies, interruption of the normal homogenous contrast pattern in areas where non-contrast-containing blood entered the contrast-containing blood pool was also noted. Gramiak and Shah, for example, observed that rapid saline injection into the proximal aorta filled the entire aortic root with a dense cloud of echoes during diastole [1]. During systole, a rectangular defect in this dense echo pattern appeared which was attributed to non-contrast-containing blood from the left ventricle entering the aorta and displacing the contrast near the valve orifice. Subsequently, it was emphasized that when contrast appeared in the left ventricle, following peripheral dye injection, examination of the area beneath the mitral leaflets was crucial in determining the location of the right-to-left shunt [5]. Specifically, when this area was echo-free, the blood flowing from the left atrium to the left ventricle did not contain contrast and by inference, the shunt must have been at the ventricular level. Conversely, if the area beneath the leaflets contained contrast, at least a portion of the shunt had to be at the atrial

level. The displacement of contrast or 'negative' contrast' effect therefore also provided information about the presence and direction of blood flow.

Role of the negative contrast effect in the diagnosis of atrial septal defect with predominant left-to-right shunting

The echocardiographic diagnosis of atrial septal defect with predominant left-to-right shunting is based on three primary features: 1) a right ventricular volume overload pattern, 2) direct visualization of a defect, or gap, in the echoes arising from the interatrial septum, and 3) the detection of abnormal flow patterns in the region of the suspected defect during echocardiographic contrast injection.

The right ventricular volume overload pattern, characterized by dilatation of the right ventricle and paradoxical motion of the interventricular septum, reflects the abnormal volume load imposed on the right heart by the atrial septal defect [8–13]. It is in no way specific, however, since a similar pattern may be seen in a variety of disorders, such as tricuspid regurgitation, pulmonary insufficiency, and anomalous pulmonary venous connection.

Direct visualization of a defect in the interatrial septum is far more specific and demonstration of an intact septum during cross-sectional recording can be considered to exclude an atrial septal defect [14]. Unfortunately, apparent defects in the interatrial septum are extremely common, particularly in the parasternal short-axis and apical four-chamber views in which the septum is aligned relatively parallel to the path of the scan plane. These false positives occur with sufficient frequency to limit the value of the cross-sectional echogram in the direct diagnosis of atrial septal defect [14].

Peripheral contrast injection offers a direct method for detecting shunt flow where there is a right-to-left component [15–17]. However, when right-to-left contrast flow is inapparent, additional supportive evidence may be necessary. This can be obtained by comparing the pattern of contrast flow along the right border of the intact atrial septum with that which occurs when a septal defect is present [16, 17].

Normal contrast flow in the area surrounding the interatrial septum

In normals following either direct injection of contrast into the right atrium or peripheral injection, the contrast material homogenously fills the right atrium, outlining its boundaries, particularly the right side of the interatrial septum [17]. Figure 1 is an example of an experimental study in which contrast was injected directly into the right atrium. In this figure, the continuous echoes from the interatrial septum before injection, as well as the homogenous opacification of the right atrium after the contrast injection can be visualized. Following contrast injection the septum is no longer visible, but the outline of the septal position can clearly be defined by the margin of the area of opacification. Figure 2 is a similar recording for a patient with a repaired atrial septal defect. In this example, the septal patch

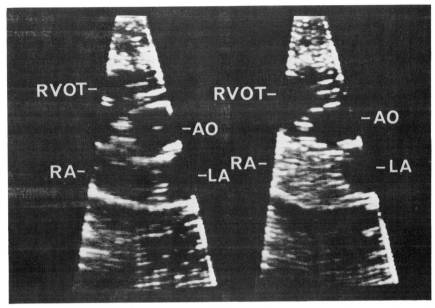

Figure 1. Short-axis cross-sectional recording of the interatrial septum and contiguous portions of the right and left atria. The left-hand panel is recorded prior to and the right-hand panel after direct contrast injection into the right atrium. Following the injection of contrast, there is homogenous opacification of the right atrial chamber, which delineates the position of the interatrial septum, despite the fact that the septum itself can no longer be visualized. RA = right atrium, LA = left atrium, AO = aorta, RVOT = right ventricular outflow tract. From ref. [17].

produces a dense vertical band of linear echoes between the right and left atria. After a peripheral injection of contrast material there is homogenous opacification of the right atrium, which again outlines the right septal border. The normal downstream path of contrast flow into the right ventricle and right ventricular outflow tract is also evident. In both Figures 1 and 2, the interatrial septum appears intact prior to the contrast injection and a defect would not have been suspected. In many normal subjects, however, it is possible either by improper transducer angulation or normal loss of echo production as the plane of the scanning transducer is aligned parallel to the interatrial septum to create an area of echo loss or drop-out in the mid-portion of the septum, simulating an atrial septal defect [14]. Figure 3A demonstrates such a false positive defect prior to contrast injection. In panel B, recorded after contrast injection, there is homogenous opacification of the right atrium without evidence of contrast flow into the left atrium. The contrast, therefore, serves to clearly delineate the separation between the two blood pools even though the actual membrane producing this separation cannot be recorded. The contrast confirms the presence and integrity of the interatrial septum despite the fact that the septum itself is not visualized.

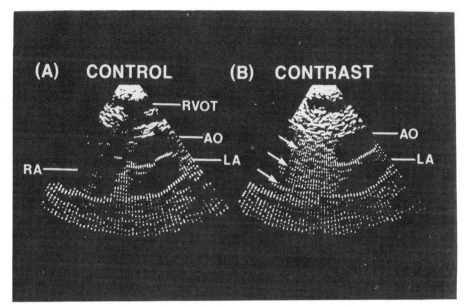

Figure 2. Short-axis cross-sectional study of the interatrial septum in a patient with a repaired atrial septal defect. The intensity of echo production from the septal patch is increased. Panel A is a control recording, while panel B is recorded after peripheral contrast injection. The injected contrast fills the right atrium and proximal portion of the right ventricular outflow tract, with a dense cloud of echoes. The left-sided aorta and the left atrium, however, remain echo-free. From ref. [17].

FLOW PATTERNS IN THE REGION OF AN ATRIAL SEPTAL DEFECT WITH LEFT-TO-RIGHT SHUNTING

To determine the flow patterns in the region of an atrial septal defect and hence, the expected path of contrast through the right atrium in patients with atrial septal defects and with left-to-right shunts, multiple injections of contrast material have been performed in the left and right atria [17]. Figures 4 and 5 illustrate the flow patterns observed during these injections. In panel A of Figure 4, a catheter has been passed from the right atrium through an atrial septal defect into the left atrium. In panel B, contrast has been injected through the catheter and flows back along the barrel of the cateter from the left atrium to the right, indicating that a defect is present and that shunt flow is from left to right. Panel C is taken several frames later and illustrates further displacement of the contrast toward the right atrium. If the interatrial septum had been intact, this contrast could have been expected to fill the left atrium and outline the position of the interatrial septum. Figure 5 compares the patterns of contrast flow which are recorded following left atrial and peripheral contrast injection. Panel A is a control recording obtained prior to contrast injection. In panel B, contrast has been injected directly into the left atrium and can be perceived to flow through the atrial septal defect from the left atrium to the right. In panel C, contrast has been injected peripherally. In this case, the contrast flows

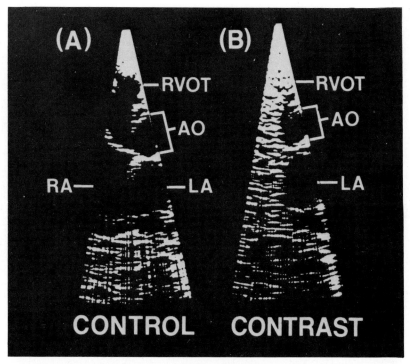

Figure 3. Panel A is a short-axis recording of the interatrial septum demonstrating an area of echo drop-out suggesting an atrial septal defect. In panel B, recorded after contrast injection, however, the right atrium is filled with a cloud of echoes which outlines the position and confirms the integrity of the interatrial septum, despite the fact that the septum itself cannot be visualized. From ref. [17].

through the right heart and can be perceived in the right atrium and right ventricular outflow tract superior to the aorta. At the right-hand margin of the atrial septal defect, however, there is a clear area in which no contrast is present, or an area of "negative contrast". This "negative contrast" is produced by the non-contrast-containing blood flowing from the left atrium to the right, displacing the contrast from the right margin of the atrial septal defect. This area of negative contrast brackets the atrial septal defect and confirms its presence.

CLINICAL STUDIES

To test the reproducibility of this pattern, peripheral contrast injection was carried out in 12 patients with atrial septal defects and with predominant left-to-right shunts [17]. Following peripheral injection, two different patterns of contrast flow were noted. In two of the 12, contrast was observed to pass from the right atrium to the left, due to mixing of blood at the atrial level. The appearance of contrast in the left atrium was considered specific for a defect in the atrial septum and no further study was felt to be necessary. In nine cases, peripheral injection of contrast did not

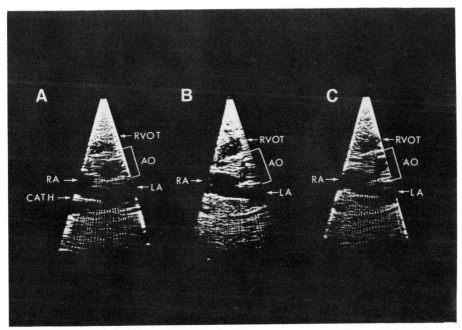

Figure 4. Short-axis cross-sectional studies of the interatrial septum during cardiac catheterization in a patient with an atrial septal defect. In panel A, the catheter (CATH) can be visualized traversing the atrial septal defect. In panel B, contrast has been injected slowly through the tip of the catheter and can be seen to flow back along the side of the catheter from the left atrium to the right atrium. From ref. [17].

produce any observable passage of dye from the right to the left atrium. In each of these cases, however, a negative contrast effect was produced in the right atrium due to the passage of non-dye-containing blood from the left atrium through the defect into the right atrium displacing the contrast-containing blood from the right side of the septum. Figure 6 shows this negative contrast pattern in a patient with an ostium secundum atrial septal defect. In panel A, the atrial septal defect is indicated prior to the injection of contrast material. Panel B is recorded following contrast injection. In this illustration, there is a large echo-free area within the right atrium which brackets the margins of the defect. Contrast can be visualized above and below this echo-free area. Figure 7 illustrates a similar phenomenon recorded in the subcostal long-axis view. In panel A of Figure 7, there is again a large defect in the interatrial septum indicated by the vertical arrow. In panel B, contrast has been injected directly into the left atrium and can be perceived to stream through the defect from left to right. In panel C, contrast has been injected peripherally and completely opacifies the right ventricle. The right atrium is echo-free and this large area of negative contrast results from the torrential shunt flow through the atrial septal defect. As a result, no contrast is seen in the right atrium even through it is obvious that it must have passed through the right atrium to get to the right ventricle. In the final case, no contrast could be detected despite repeated injections.

132

DISCUSSION

The initial observation of this negative contrast effect was an unexpected finding. In the original study, it was anticipated that when an atrial septal defect was present, mixing of blood at the atrial level would result in some contrast material crossing the septum from right to left, thereby confirming the presence of the defect [17]. Although passage of dye from right to left was routinely observed following both right atrial and high inferior vena cava injection, clearly defined right-to-left shunting was detected in only two cases after a peripheral injection. The unexpected observation that a nonopacified, or echo-free, area frequently appeared immediately to the right of the interatrial septum during at least a portion of the cardiac

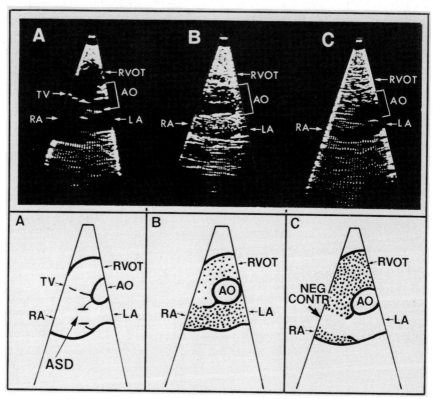

Figure 5. A series of recordings which contrast the pattern of echocardiographic contrast flow in the region of an atrial septal defect following left atrial and peripheral contrast injections. Panel A is a short-axis cross-sectional recording illustrating the defect. In panel B, contrast has been injected directly into the left atrium and flows back through the atrial septal defect from left to right. Panel C is recorded following peripheral injection. In this example, there is normal flow of contrast from the peripheral vein into the right atrium and right ventricular outflow tract. In the right atrium, bracketing the margin of the atrial septal defect, however, there is a clear, or echo-free, area which corresponds to the path of blood flowing from left to right through the atrial septal defect. This area of negative contrast is produced by the non-contrast-containing blood from the left atrium washing the contrast-containing blood in the right atrium away from the right septal margin. From ref. [17].

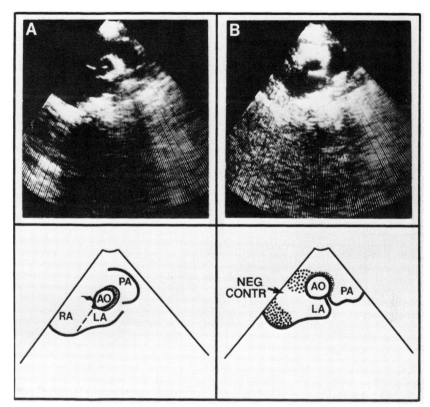

Figure 6. Panel A is a control recording of the interatrial septum from another patient with an ostium secundum atrial septal defect. Panel B, recorded after a peripheral injection, again illustrates an area of negative contrast (NEG CONTR) in the right atrium (RA) bracketing the region of the atrial septal defect From ref. [17].

cycle, suggested an alternative method for detecting these defects. Recognition of the area of negative contrast was further facilitated by the fact that this phenomenon occurred immediately to the right of a suspected defect and bracketed its margins. The relative incidence with which "positive contrast" (flow of peripherally injected contrast from right to left through a defect) and "negative contrast" occur in patients with atrial septal defect and with predominant left-to-right shunting has been questioned. Fraker et al., for example, suggested that some contrast may be seen crossing the interatrial septum in all patients with atrial septal defects, even those with predominant left-to-right shunts [15]. Gilbert et al., in a study of 22 patients with atrial septal defect, observed that either positive or negative contrast were present in all cases. In 12 of 22, both positive and negative contrasts were observed. Six patients, however, showed only positive contrast, while four showed only negative contrast [16].

The observation of "positive contrast" or contrast flow from right to left represents incontrovertible evidence that an atrial septal defect is present and can clearly be considered the primary method for detecting these anomalies. The role of negative contrast is that of a secondary or inferential finding. However, it does appear to be useful observation in patients in whom positive contrast is not evident; and it is particularly useful in excluding a false positive atrial septal defect. The negative contrast effect has also been observed in patients with ventricular septal defects. Farcot et al., for example, observed negative contrast within the right ventricular chamber in each of three patients with septal rupture and ventricular septal defect, following acute myocardial infarction [18]. In these cases, no right-to-left shunting was apparent and the only abnormal contrast pattern, therefore, was the negative phenomenon.

In patients with atrial septal defects, the area of negative contrast, when present, varies throughout the cardiac cycle, being greatest at the point of peak anterior motion of the aortic root, which corresponds to end systole or initial diastole. The timing of this peak negative contrast effect is consistent with the findings of Levin et al., who demonstrated that the maximum gradient across an atrial septal defect and peak shunt flow occurs during end systole and initial diastole [19].

Finally, it is important to remember that an atrial septal defect is not the only source of non-contrast-containing blood entering the right atrium. In normal patients, inflow from the inferior vena cava and coronary sinus will also be non-contrast containing, while various types of heart disease, such as tricuspid regurgi-

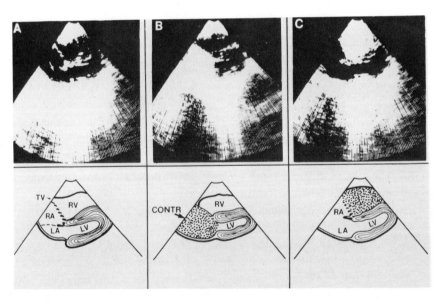

Figure 7. Cross-sectional recording of the interatrial septum and associated defect from the subcostal transducer location. Panel A is a control recording with the area of the defect indicated by the vertical arrow. In panel B, contrast has been injected into the left atrium. The cloud of echoes initially flows back across the defect from left to right following the path of the interatrial shunt. In panel C, contrast has been injected peripherally. The contrast-containing blood is now displaced from the right side of the interatrial septum by the non-contrast-containing blood flowing through the defect and produces a large area of negative contrast in the right atrium. From ref. [17].

tation, may also contribute non-contrast-containing blood to the right atrial blood pool.

The inferior vena cava represents a major source of non-contrast-containing blood in normal patients. This non-contrast-containing blood can be perceived in the lateral portion of the right atrium in the region of the confluence between contrast-containing blood from the superior vena cava and the non-contrast-containing blood from the inferior vena cava. Mixing of blood within the right atrial cavity, however, appears to occur very rapidly; and at the margin of the interatrial septum, the contrast pool appears homogenous. A second source of non-contrast-containing blood is the coronary sinus. In both normals and in patients with atrial septal defect, it is not uncommon to observe a discrete, non-contrast-containing area along the posterior margin of the right atrium. Though as yet unproven, we have always attributed this area of negative contrast to the inflow from the coronary sinus. This area is always bounded by the posterior wall of the atrium and, to date, has not caused confusion with the area of negative contrast which brackets an apparent atrial septal defect. Another possible source of non-contrast-containing blood is back flow through the tricuspid valve due to tricuspid insufficiency. The negative contrast effect does not become evident in the right atrium until the chamber is filled with contrast-containing blood which, as a rule, does not occur until several cycles after the initial appearance of the contrast material. By this time, the early flow of contrast has already passed through the tricuspid valve and regurgitant blood coming back through the tricuspid valve orifice will also contain contrast. Although we have not examined patients with associated atrial septal defect and tricuspid insufficiency, we have examined a number of patients with isolated tricuspid insufficiency and have not observed the negative contrast affect in the right atrium or above the tricuspid valve in any of these cases. Left-to-right shunting at the atrial level may also result from pathologic conditions other than ostium secundum or primum atrial septal defects (eg anomalous pulmonary venous connection or sinus venosus atrial septal defect). The potential for shunting at multiple levels within the right atrium mitigates against random injection of contrast in hopes of detecting left-to-right shunting. The negative contrast effect is helpful only when there is an apparent defect in the interatrial septum and the specific question can be asked:does this apparent defect represent a true or a false positive? In these cases, peripherally injected contrast should clearly outline the area of the apparent defect and when there is a false positive demonstrate the membrane separating the right and left atrial chambers. In the presence of a true atrial septal defect with right-to-left shunting, contrast will cross the septum providing a definitive diagnosis. When left-to-right shunting is present, the defect can still be detected by the effects of the non-contrast-containing blood passing from left to right, displacing the normal flow of contrast in the right atrium and creating an echo-free, or contrast free, space along the right side of the septum. This area of negative contrast indicates that blood is flowing through the area in question and confirms the presence of the defect.

136

REFERENCES

1. Gramiak R, PM Shah: Echocardiography of the aortic root. Invest Radiol 3:356, 1968.
2. Gramiak R, PM Shah, DH Kramer: Ultrasound cardiography: contrast studies in anatomy and function. Radiology 92:939, 1969.
3. Pieroni DR, PJ Varghese, RD Rowe: Echocardiography to detect shunt and valvular incompetence in infants and children. Circulation (Suppl IV) 48:IV–81, 1973.
4. Kerber RE, JM Kioschos, RM Lauer: The use of an ultrasonic contrast method in the diagnosis of valvular regurgitation and intracardiac shunts. Am J Cardiol 34:722, 1974.
5. Seward JB, AJ Tajik , JG Spangler, DG Ritter: Echocardiographic contrast studies: initial experience. Mayo Clin Proc 50:163, 1975.
6. Valdes-Cruz, LM, DR Pieroni, JM Roland, PJ Varghese: Echocardiographic detection of right to left shunts following peripheral vein injections. Circulation 54:588, 1976.
7. Valdes-Cruz LM, DR Pieroni, JM Roland, J-MA Shematek: Recognition of residual postoperative shunts by contrast echocardiographic techniques. Circulation 55:148, 1977.
8. Diamond MA, JC Dillon, CL Haine, S Chang, J Feigenbaum: Echocardiographic features of atrial septal defect. Circulation 43:129, 1971.
9. McCann WD, NB Harbold, BR Giuliani: The echocardiogram in right ventricular overload. J Am Med Assoc 221:1243, 1972.
10. Tajik AJ, GT Gau, DG Ritter, TT Schattenberg: Echocardiographic pattern of right ventricular diastolic volume overload in children. Circulation 46:36, 1972.
11. Popp RL, SB Wolfe, T Hirata, H Feigenbaum: Estimation of right and left ventricular size by ultrasound. A study of the echoes from the interventricular septum. Am J Cardiol 24:523, 1969.
12. Hagan AD, GS Francis, DJ Sahn, J Karliner, WF Friedman, R O'Rourke: Ultrasound evaluation of systolic anterior septal motion in patients with and without right ventricular volume overload. Circulation 50:248, 1974.
13. Weyman AE, S Wann, H Feigenbaum, JC Dillon: Mechanism of abnormal septal motion in patients with right ventricular volume overload: a cross-sectional echocardiographic study. Circulation 54:179, 1976.
14. Dillon JC, AE Weyman, H Feigenbaum, RC Eggleton, KW Johnston: Cross-sectional echocardiographic examination of the interatrial septum. Circulation 55:115, 1977
15. Fraker TD, S Myers, JA Kisslo: Detection and exclusion of interatrial shunts by contrast two-dimensional echo. Circulation (Suppl II) 58:II–187, 1978.
16. Gilbert BW, M Drobac: Contrast two-dimensional echocardiography in the interatrial shunts. Am J Cardiol 45:402, 1980.
17. Weyman AE, LS Wann, RL Caldwell, RA Hurwitz, JC Dillon, H Feigenbaum: Negative contrast echocardiography: a new method for detecting left to right shunts. Circulation 59:498, 1979.
18. Farcot JC, L Boiscento, M Rigoud, J Bardet, JP Bourdanas: Two-dimensional echocardiographic visualization of ventricular septal rupture after acute anterior myocardial infarction. Am J Cardiol 45:370, 1980.
19. Levin AR, MS Spach, JP Boineau, RV Canent, MP Capp, PH Jewett: Atrial pressure flow dynamics in atrial septal defects (secundum type). Circulation 37:476, 1968.

14. CONTRAST ECHOCARDIOGRAPHY IN PATENT FORAMEN OVALE

G. KRONIK

INTRODUCTION

Contrast echocardiography has been shown to be a very sensitive method for the diagnosis of hemodynamically significant interatrial communications (atrial septal defect). Shunting of contrast echoes from the right to the left heart can be detected by either M-mode [1, 2] or cross-sectional [3–5] contrast echocardiography in most patients with atrial septal defect even in the absence of Eisenmenger's reaction and cyanosis. The demonstration of atrial, left-to-right shunts requires the use of two-dimensional echocardiography. With this method the left-to-right shunt is seen during right atrial opacifications as a "negative contrast" effect at the site of the defect [6, 7]. The ability to detect right-to-left or left-to-right shunting is largely independent of the size of the atrial septal defect [1–3, 5–8]. We have therefore investigated if very small, hemodynamically insignificant interatrial communications could also lead to the same contrast echocardiographic phenomena. The occurrence of positive contrast studies in patients with only a patent foramen ovale would have important consequences for the diagnosis of atrial septal defect by contrast echocardiography; and furthermore the noninvasive detection of a patent foramen ovale may sometimes be clinically important, for example, in patients with unexplained cyanosis or in suspected paradoxical embolism.

PATIENTS

We performed peripheral contrast echocardiography on 21 patients with insignificant interatrial communications. In 20 cases the patent foramen ovale (PFO) was documented at cardiac catheterization, when a transvenous right atrial catheter was passed through the defect into the left atrium. The small size of the defect was documented at surgery in three of these cases, and was concluded from the clinical and catheterization data in 17. These patients had no oxymetric evidence of a significant interatrial left-to-right or right-to-left shunt exceeding two standard deviations of normal for our laboratory and no clinical sign of an atrial septal defect. The twenty-first patient had multiple pulmonary embolisms and well-documented paradoxical embolism in his left arm. He did not undergo cardiac catheterization, but the clinical findings, including auscultation, electrocardiogram, chest

X-ray, M-mode and cross-sectional echocardiography, did not reveal any evidence for a hemodynamically significant atrial septal defect or other shunt lesions.

Nine patients with PFO had right ventricular pressure overload (three with valvular pulmonic stenosis, one with cor pulmonale, one with idiopathic pulmonary hypertension, one with mitral insufficiency, one with ventricular septal defect, mitral insufficiency, and pulmonic stenosis, one with supravalvular aortic and peripheral pulmonic stenosis, and one with pulmonary embolism). Right-sided pressures were normal in the remaining 12 cases (one with small ventricular septal defect, one with anomalous drainage of a "scimitar" pulmonary vein into the inferior vena cava, one with congenital AV-block, four with coronary heart disease; five with no cardiac abnormality except PFO).

Interatrial communications may be of any size and thus there is a wide spectrum between PFO and a large atrial septal defect. In this chapter the terms patent foramen ovale (PFO) and hemodynamically insignificant interatrial communication, as defined above, will be used synonymously, while all atrial septal defects with oxymetrically detectable left-to-right shunts will be designated hemodynamically significant, even though the shunt was quite unimportant ($\leq 30\%$) from a clinical point of view in some patients.

The contrast echocardiographic findings in patients with PFO were compared to the results in 22 catheterized patients with atrial septal defect (ASD) and with left-to-right shunts ranging between 25% and 73% (mean = 54%) of total pulmonary blood flow. Eisenmenger's reaction with elevated pulmonary arteriolar resistance and with an oxymetrically demonstrable right-to-left shunt was present in five of them, but none had pure right-to-left shunting.

M-MODE STUDIES

M-mode contrast studies during normal quiet respiration were performed in all patients. Since it is known that transient right-to-left shunting may be provoked in patients with ASD or PFO by asking the patient to perform the Valsalva maneuver [1, 8, 9], contrast injections were repeated during the Valsalva maneuver in 16 cases including all with negative contrast studies at rest.

In order to produce a contrast effect, multiple 10 ml portions of normal saline solution stored at room temperature were rapidly injected by hand into an antecubital vein. During the contrast studies the sound beam was constantly directed towards the mitral valve. The gain controls of the echocardiograph were carefully adjusted to obtain a clear record, free of artifacts and background noise, but using as much gain and as little reject as possible. When analyzing the M-mode data, the following criteria and definitions were used.

"Contrast echoes" were defined as strong linear echoes that could be clearly differentiated from incomplete valve echoes and background noise. The appearance of contrast echoes in the left heart was termed "contrast shunting" and was semi-

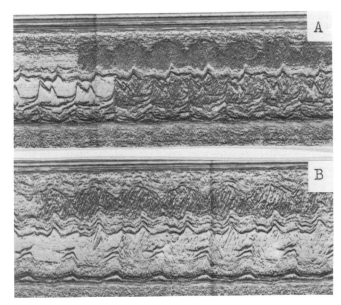

Figure 1. Massive (A) and strong (B) contrast shunting in a patient with PFO and severe valvular pulmonic stenosis. Both recordings were obtained during quiet respiration.

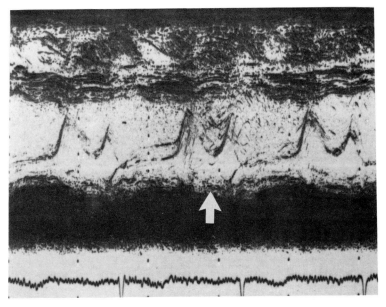

Figure 2. Strong contrast shunting at rest seen during one cardiac cycle (arrow) in the patient with paradoxical embolism.

quantitatively graded according to the following criteria: massive contrast shunting ($+++$), the mitral funnel is filled with contrast echoes (Figures 1A, 3C); strong contrast shunting ($++$), many contrast echoes are seen in the left heart (Figures 1B, 2); weak but definite contrast shunting ($+$), few (at least five) clearly identifiable contrast echoes are seen on the left side of the septum (Figures 3A, 3B, 10); questionable contrast shunting $\pm$), very few (≤ 4) contrast echoes in the left heart (Figure 4B) or recognition of contrast echoes is difficult because of artifacts and background noise; no contrast shunting (0), contrast echoes confined to the right heart (Figure 4A). Weak, strong and massive contrast shunting were considered "diagnostic" of an intracardiac defect (i.e. "positive contrast study"). Questionable and absent contrast shunting were both classified as "negative studies". When contrast shunting was variable during repeat injections in the same patient, which was a frequent occurrence, the maximal observed contrast shunting was counted.

One patient had to be excluded from the analysis of the M-mode data, because she had angiographic and cross-sectional contrast echocardiographic evidence of a right-to-left shunt through a large ventricular septal defect (VSD) and mitral insufficiency. Thus, the contrast echoes that were seen in her left atrium and mitral funnel could not be taken as proof for an atrial shunt.

Of the remaining 20 patients, eight (40%) had positive contrast studies at rest (five with elevated and three with normal right ventricular systolic pressure). Contrast shunting could be provoked by the Valsalva maneuver in another five patients. Positive contrast studies either at rest or during the Valsalva maneuver were thus obtained in 13 of 20 (65%) patients with PFO, including six out of eight (75%) with right ventricular systolic pressure overload (the ninth patient with PFO and right ventricular hypertension was the patient who had to be excluded) and seven out of 12 (58%) with normal resting right heart pressures. Seven patients had negative contrast studies at rest and during the Valsalva maneuver. Although questionable ($\pm$) contrast shunting was seen in two of these patients, this was considered insufficient for the diagnosis of a shunt. When studies at rest and during the Valsalva maneuver were compared, contrast shunting was usually more pronounced during the Valsalva maneuver (Figure 3), but there were exceptions.

The intensity of contrast shunting at rest and during the Valsalva maneuver was frequently variable when several injections were performed in the same patient (Figure 1). The variations in contrast shunting could often be explained by variable contrast generation in the right heart or by differences in the quality of the Valsalva maneuver, but sometimes there was no obvious reason discernible. Maximal contrast shunting in different patients was even more variable, ranging from 0 to $+++$ (Figures 1–4).

Since the size of the defect was similar and very small by definition in all cases, one might have expected that the presence or absence of right-to-left shunting should be primarily dependent upon intracardiac pressures.

A comparison between the contrast echocardiographic results and the hemodynamic findings revealed that all eight patients with contrast shunting at rest had

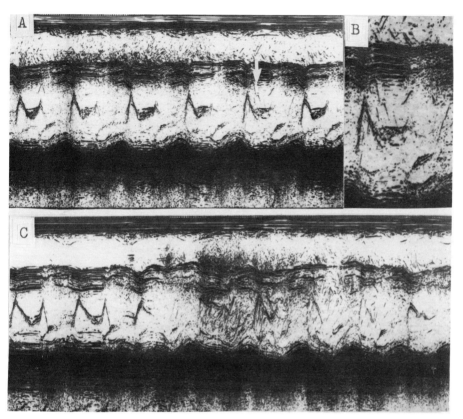

Figure 3. Weak contrast shunting at rest (A, B) and massive contrast shunting during the Valsalva maneuver (C) in a patient with coronary heart disease and normal right heart pressures. The diastole showing most contrast echoes in the left heart at rest is marked with a white arrow in panel A and shown in a close-up presentation in panel B.

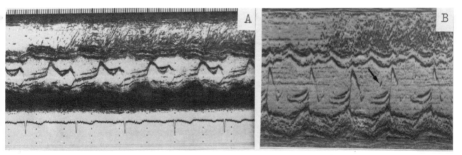

Figure 4. Negative contrast studies in PFO. No contrast shunting at all is seen in the left panel (A), although this patient had moderate idiopathic pulmonary hypertension. One single probably contrast echo marked by an arrow (questionable contrast shunting ($\pm$)) is visible in the left heart, in the right panel from a patient with normal right heart pressures (B). Valsalva studies were also negative in both patients.

142

either right ventricular systolic pressure overload or very similar mean pressures in the right and left atrium or both. All four patients with intense contrast shunting (+ + or + + +) had right ventricular pressure overload. However the relationship between contrast shunting and intracardiac pressures was quite imperfect. Pressures in patients with and without contrast shunting showed considerable overlap and there were patients with elevated right ventricular systolic pressure, low interatrial pressure difference or both, in whom contrast shunting could not be detected during quiet, normal respiration (Figure 5).

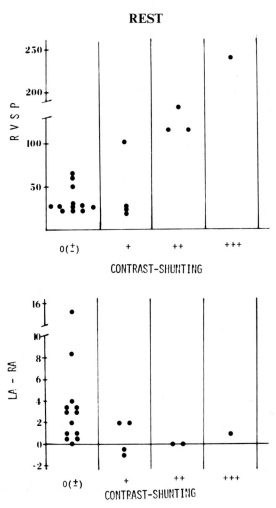

Figure 5. Correlation between resting intracardiac pressures and contrast shunting during normal respiration in patients with PFO. RVSP = right ventricular systolic pressure in mm Hg; LA–RA = difference between left atrial and right atrial mean pressure in mm Hg; 0 (±) = negative contrast study; + = weak; + + = strong; + + + = massive contrast shunting, as defined in the text. The patient with pulmonary and paradoxical embolism, in whom no catheterization data were available, has been plotted in the blank RVSP zone in the upper panel and has been left out in the lower panel.

During the Valsalva maneuver the presence or absence and the intensity of contrast shunting were entirely independent of the resting intracardiac pressures. In particular, strong and massive contrast shunting during the Valsalva maneuver was compatible with completely normal right heart hemodynamics and did not necessarily indicate right ventricular hypertension (Figure 6).

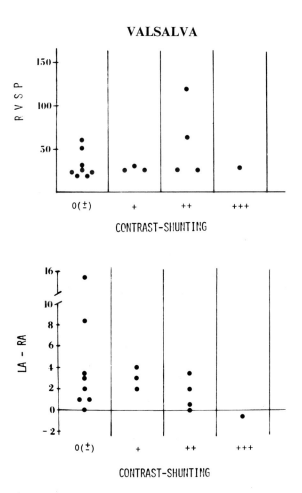

Figure 6. Correlation between resting intracardiac pressures and contrast shunting during the Valsalva maneuver in 16 patients with PFO, in whom Valsalva studies were performed. Abbreviations as in Figure 5.

CROSS-SECTIONAL STUDIES

Cross-sectional contrast echocardiograms were performed on 20 patients with PFO using two different mechanical sector scanners (ATL and Picker). Contrast was injected while the interatrial septum was visualized either from the parasternal [10] or from the apical approach (four-chamber view) [11, 12] and occasionally from the subxiphoid transducer position [13, 14]. The two-dimensional contrast studies were analyzed for any right-to-left or left-to-right shunt.

An interatrial right-to-left shunt, that is to say, the unequivocal appearance of contrast echoes in the left atrium was seen during normal respiration in only three patients (Figure 7), two with pulmonary stenosis and one with normal right-sided pressures. Cross-sectional echocardiography was negative in five patients with positive M-mode studies at rest. The lower sensitivity of cross-sectional as compared to M-mode echocardiography in detecting small right-to-left shunts in patients with PFO and ASD, which has been repeatedly noted in our laboratory [7], may be due to the superior resolution capabilities of the M-mode technique, which permits the reliable recognition of even very few scattered contrast echoes in the left heart. However, the ability to detect single contrast echoes by two-dimensional echocardiography may depend upon the instrument used, for others have reported considerably better results with the cross-sectional method [2, 4, 5] and we have noted that one of our two sector scanners seems to be better suited for this purpose than the other.

Interatrial left-to-right shunting can be seen in patients with ASD as a stream of contrast-free blood flowing from the left atrium through the defect into the right atrium and washing away the contrast echoes near the defect [6, 7]. This "wash out" or "negative contrast" effect (Figure 8) is accompanied by turbulence within the right atrium. In the majority of our patients with PFO the cross-sectional studies

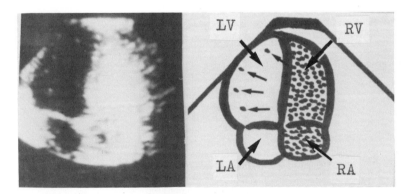

Figure 7. Contrast shunting as viewed by two-dimensional echocardiography in a patient with PFO and moderate pulmonic stenosis. The heart is visualized in the apical four-chamber view. A few scattered contrast echoes (small arrows) are seen in the left ventricle (LV). There is no "negative contrast" effect in the right atrium (RA). RV = right ventricle; LA = left atrium.

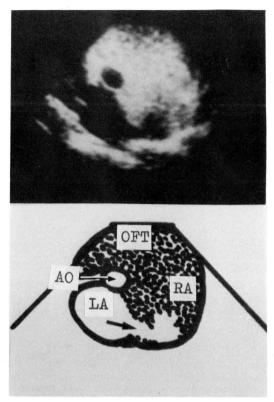

Figure 8. "Negative contrast" effect due to left-to-right interatrial shunting in a patient with hemo-dynamically significant ASD. The arrow points to the defect through which contrast-free left atrial blood flows into the contrast-filled right atrium. LA = left atrium; RA = right atrium; OFT = right ventricular outflow tract, AO = aortic root.

were clearly negative for left-to-right shunting (Figures 7, 9A). Some had inhomo-genous contrast filling of the right atrium, but in the absence of other evidence for a left-to-right shunt this is a nonspecific finding in our experience, which may also be seen in patients with an intact interatrial septum [7]. In two patients the two-dimensional contrast study showed very prominent turbulence in the right atrium, which was quite suspicious for possible left-to-right shunting (Figure 9B). One of these patients had actually been diagnosed as having a left-to-right shunt during a blind analysis of his video tape [7]. The possibility cannot be excluded that these two patients actually had very small left-to-right shunts, which were not detected by oxymetry, because oxymetry is relatively insensitive for the diagnosis of small shunts [15]. It is also possible, however, that the prominent turbulence, inhomog-enous contrast filling and questionable wash out effect was due to contrast-free blood from the inferior vena cava. Thus, none of our patients with PFO had the full blown, unequivocal findings of an interatrial left-to-right shunt, but in individual cases the decision whether or not a left-to-right shunt is present may be difficult.

DIFFERENTIAL DIAGNOSIS

Artifacts

The diagnosis of a PFO by contrast echocardiography frequently rests upon the recognition of just a few contrast echoes in the left heart, which sometimes appear only briefly and only after multiple injections. Thus, even a few contrast echoes must be reliably differentiated from artifacts and other intracardiac structures. Use of excessive gain may lead to multiple fuzzy "noise echoes" on the tracing and to the "overload" effect, which is a homogenous opacification of the whole tracing due to reverberations of the contrast echoes (Figure 10). Both of these phenomena are usually easily differentiated from the typical short linear contrast echoes. Incom-

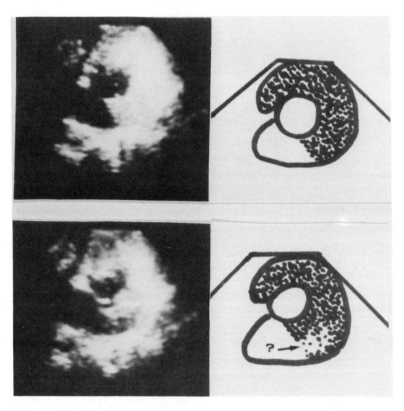

Figure 9. Questionable "negative contrast" effect in a patient with PFO and only an insignificant atrial left-to-right shunt by oxymetry (anatomic situation as in Figure 8). A clear demarcation between the contrast-free left atrium and the contrast-filled right atrium is seen in the upper panel. Intermittently there is very inhomogenous right atrial opacification (lower panel) which resembles the "negative contrast" effect in Figure 7. It should be noted, however, that the differentiation between true and false "negative contrast" effects is much easier when watching the moving pictures on the screen. When seen in real time the "negative contrast" effect in the patient with PFO was much less impressive than in the patient with ASD (Figure 7).

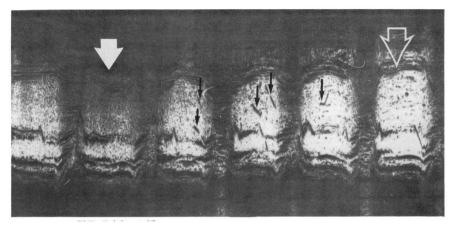

Figure 10. Weak contrast shunting during the Valsalva maneuver in a patient with PFO and normal right-sided pressures. The tracing quality is definitely suboptimal due to excessive gain. There is an intense overload effect (solid white arrow) and fuzzy noise echoes are seen everywhere (for example in the area denoted with an open white arrow). Nevertheless several linear contrast echoes (some marked with small black arrows) are recognizable in the left heart.

plete mitral echoes may sometimes resemble contrast echoes; but when these "contrast echoes" repeatedly appear in the same position on successive beats, the diagnosis should be seriously doubted, for true contrast echoes always show a random motion pattern. Although these criteria have been found to be very reliable [1], the possibility cannot be excluded that once in a while an artifact will erroneously be considered a contrast echo. However, it is extremely unlikely that several contrast echoes would be confused with artifacts and incomplete mitral echoes. Thus, the detection of at least five typical contrast echoes in the left heart following one contrast injection proves the presence of a shunt, for peripherally injected contrast can never pass through the pulmonary circulation and reach the left heart under normal conditions [17].

Other shunt lesions

Contrast shunting through a PFO must be differentiated from other shunt lesions. Contrast shunting through a ventricular septal defect (VSD) typically opacifies the aortic root and most of the left ventricle, but spares the left atrium and the mitral funnel (VSD-type of contrast shunting). When contrast shunting occurs through an interatrial communication, contrast echoes are also seen in the left atrium and between the mitral leaflets (ASD-type of contrast shunting) (Figures 1–3). When just a few contrast echoes appear in the left heart with just an occasional echo behind the mitral valve, these two types of contrast shunting cannot be recognized. We call this an indeterminate type of contrast shunting. Such weak, indeterminate contrast shunting is quite frequent in patients with ASD and PFO (Figure 10), but sometimes also occurs in small ventricular septal defects. Directing the sound beam towards the aortic root and left atrium would facilitate the localization of the shunt in cases with weak contrast shunting. However, interatrial contrast shunting may be missed altogether in the aortic position [18], when the sound beam traverses a high portion of the left atrium, and furthermore it is usually easier to obtain a good artifact-free record in the mitral position.

The differentiation between PFO and ASD is difficult by M-mode contrast echocardiographic criteria. Many patients with ASD, including cases with a large left-to-right shunt and an obviously large defect, have only weak contrast shunting at rest and during the Valsalva maneuver (Figure 11). On the other hand, patients with PFO may have strong or even massive contrast shunting, particularly during the Valsalva maneuver or with severe right ventricular hypertension. Intense contrast shunting (+ + and + + +) through a PFO at rest seems to be unusual in the absence of additional right-sided heart disease. When other right-sided problems (e.g. pulmonary valve stenosis, Ebstein's disease, pulmonary hypertension) can be excluded, strong contrast shunting during normal respiration favors the diagnosis of an ASD rather than a PFO. The value of this sign is limited, however, because contrast shunting may be variable in the same patient, depending upon the amount of contrast generated in the right heart and other factors (Figures 1A, B).

The detection of an interatrial left-to-right shunt by cross-sectional contrast echocardiography may also aid in the differential diagnosis. Unequivocal left-to-right shunting was detected by two-dimensional contrast echocardiography in over 80% of our ASD patients [7], but was not found in any of the PFO patients. However, two cases with PFO had questionable evidence for a left-to-right shunt. Therefore, a definite wash out effect indicates a hemodynamically significant leak, but there are patients in whom cross sectional contrast echocardiography is not very helpful, because the findings are neither clearly positive nor clearly negative for a left-to-right shunt (Figure 9).

Despite these moderately different contrast echocardiographic findings in patients with PFO and ASD, contrast echocardiography should be primarily used to diagnose the existence, but not the size, of an interatrial communication. The differential diagnosis between PFO and ASD and the recognition of additional heart disease is much better accomplished by looking at the clinical findings and other echocardiographic criteria. For example, the simple measurement of right ventricular dimension allows excellent separation of insignificant and hemodynamically important leaks. Right ventricular dilatation is found in virtually all patients with ASD [1, 5, 19, 20], but not in uncomplicated PFO.

Pulmonary arteriovenous fistula is another rare cause for contrast shunting of the ASD type [18, 21–23]. In this disease the contrast echoes, which flow through the fistula bypassing the pulmonary capillary bed, escape the usual entrapment and destruction in the pulmonary circulation and finally appear in the left atrium. An important criterion for the differential diagnosis between an interatrial and an intrapulmonary shunt is the delay between the arrival of contrast in the right and

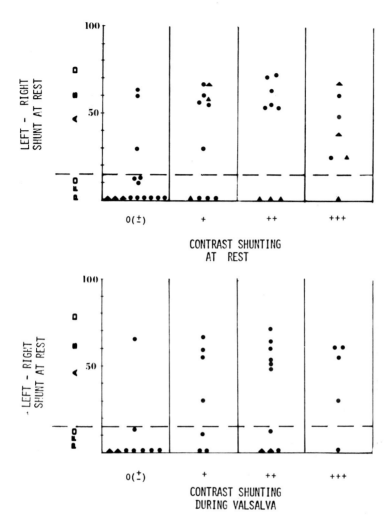

Figure 11. Contrast shunting in patients with ASD and PFO at rest (upper panel) and during the Valsalva maneuver (lower panel). Patients with PFO and right ventricular hypertension and patients with ASD and Eisenmenger's reaction are marked with ▲; uncomplicated cases with ●. The lower panel contains fewer data points, because Valsalva studies were not performed in all patients. Note the complete absence of any correlation between the left-to-right shunt at rest and contrast shunting either at rest or during the Valsalva maneuver.

left heart. This delay should be longer when the contrast echoes have to travel through the pulmonary circulation than when they cross through an interatrial leak. Furthermore, contrast shunting should be a constant consequence of every success-ful contrast injection in patients with pulmonary arteriovenous fistula, while it is a chance occurrence and should therefore be more variable in acyanotic patients with ASD and PFO.

In the few reported cases with pulmonary arteriovenous fistula [18, 21–23] and in two patients from our laboratory, the "arrival time" between the appearance of the first contrast echo in the right heart and the first contrast echo in the left heart has ranged between 2.5 and 10 cardiac cycles and has shown moderate variations of up to two heart beats in some cases [18].

In patients with interatrial communications the arrival time after injections leading to diagnostic contrast shunting (+, + +, + + +) at rest has been from 0 to 2.5 (mean 1.3) heart beats for PFO and from 0 to 5 (mean 1.5) beats for ASD in our laboratory. Thus, contrast shunting in interatrial communications may occur as late as in pulmonary arteriovenous fistula and may be somewhat variable. Though early (≤ 2 cardiac cycles) arrival seems to indicate an interatrial leak, late arrival is no proof for a pulmonary arteriovenous fistula. Many more patients will have to be studied before reliable criteria for the differentiation between intrapulmonary and interatrial contrast shunting will be available.

CLINICAL SIGNIFICANCE OF PFO

A patent foramen ovale is not a disease, but rather a variation of normal, which is fully compatible with normal longevity. Nevertheless the ability to detect PFO noninvasively by contrast echocardiography may be of clinical significance in individual cases. In patients with severely abnormal right heart hemodynamics, significant right-to-left shunting through even a small interatrial leak may be a cause of central cyanosis. These patients will always have strongly positive contrast studies. Secondly, a PFO in a patient with venous thromboembolism may allow the passage of thrombi into the left heart with consequent paradoxical embolism in the major circulation (Figure 2). Of course, the demonstration of a PFO in a patient with systemic embolism does not prove that the embolism is indeed paradoxical in origin; but if paradoxical embolism is suspected clinically, a positive contrast study strongly supports this suspicion. Thirdly, when contrast echocardiography is used for the diagnosis of atrial septal defect, it is important to know that a positive study does not prove an ASD, but may also be due to a PFO. Therefore, when patients are sent to the echocardiographic laboratory to exclude ASD, it is more important to look for signs of right ventricular volume overload in the baseline echocardiogram than to perform a contrast study. When the right ventricular diameter and septal motion are normal, contrast injections are unnecessary, for even a positive study would only indicate a PFO, but not a hemodynamically significant ASD. When echocardiographic evidence of right ventricular volume overload is demonstrable, the contrast study may aid in the differentiation between the various causes of right ventricular dilitation.

CONCLUSION

Peripheral M-mode contrast echocardiography, when properly performed with multiple injections during normal respiration and during the Valsalva manuever, can demonstrate the existence of an intracardiac shunt in about two-thirds of patients with patent foramen ovale, even when there is no coexisting right heart disease. Positive contrast studies, though proving the presence of a defect, do not allow any conclusions with respect to its size. The noninvasive diagnosis of PFO may have clinical significance in selected patients.

REFERENCES

1. Kronik G, J Slany, H Mösslacher: Contrast M-mode echocardiography in diagnosis of atrial septal defect in acyanotic patients. Circulation 59:372, 1979.
2. Kronik G, H Mösslacher, J Slany: Ein- und zweidimensionale Kontrastechokardiographie bei acyanotischen Patienten mit ASD. Z Kardiol 68:268, 1979 (abstract).
3. Fraker JD, PJ Harris, VS Behar, JA Kisslo: Detection and exclusion of interatrial shunts by two-dimensional echocardiography and peripheral venous injections. Circulation 59:379, 1979.
4. Bourdillon PDV, RA Foale, AF Rickards: Assessment of atrial septal defects by cross-sectional echocardiography. In: Lancée CT (ed), Echocardiology p 61. Martinus Nijhoff, The Hague 1979.
5. Serruys PWM, M van den Brand, PG Hugenholtz, J Roelandt: Intracardiac right to left shunts demonstrated by two-dimensional-echocardiography after peripheral vein injection. Br Heart J 42:429, 1979.
6. Weyman AE, LS Wann, RL Caldwell, RA Hurwitz, JC Dillon, H Feigenbaum: Negative contrast echocardiography: a new method for detecting left to right shunts. Circulation 59:498, 1979.
7. Kronik G, B Hutterer, H Mösslacher: Diagnose atrialer Links-rechts-Shunts mit Hilfe der zweidimensionalen Kontrastechokardiographie. Z Kardiol 70:138, 1981.
8. Kronik G, H Mösslacher, R Schmoliner, B Hutterer: Kontrastechokardiographie bei Patienten mit kleinen interatrialen Kurzschlußverbindungen (offenes Foramen ovale). Wien Klin Wochenschr 92:290, 1979.
9. Cheng TO: Paradoxical embolism: a diagnostic challenge and its detection during life. Circulation 53:565, 1976.
10. Dillon JC, AE Weyman, H Feigenbaum, RC Eggleton, K Johnston: Cross-sectional echocardiographic examination of the interatrial septum. Circulation 55:115, 1977.
11. Grube E, V Sarrasch, W Fehske, H Simon: Apex-echokardiographie: Darstellung kardialer Strukturen von der Herzspitze mit Hilfe zweidimensionaler Sektor-Echokardiographie. Z Kardiol Suppl 5:137, 1978.
12. Schiller N, NH Silverman: Apex echocardiography: a new method of imaging the adult heart using a phased array real time two-dimensional 80° sector scanner. Am J Cardiol 38:279, 1977.
13. Lange LW, DJ Sahn, HD Allen, SJ Goldberg: Subxiphoid cross-sectional echocardiography in infants and children with congenital heart disease. Circulation 59:513, 1979.
14. Biermann FZ, RG Williams: Subxiphoid two-dimensional imaging of the interatrial septum in infants and neonates with congenital heart disease. Circulation 60:80, 1979.
15. Just H: Herzkatheterdiagnostik: Methodik, Messungen, Formeln, Nomogramme, p 140. Mannheimer Morgen, Darmstadt, 1976.
16. Valdes-Cruz LM, DR Pieroni, JA Roland, PJ Varghese: Echocardiographic detection of intracardiac right to left shunts following peripheral vein injections. Circulation 54:558, 1976.

17. Gramiak R, PM Shah, DH Kramer: Ultrasound cardiography: Contrast studies in anatomy and function. Radiology 92:939, 1969.
18. Seward JB, AJ Tajik, DJ Hagler, DG Ritter: Peripheral venous contrast echocardiography. Am J Cardiol 39:202, 1977.
19. Diamond MA, JC Dillon, CL Haine, S Chang, H Feigenbaum: Echocardiographic features of atrial septal defect. Circulation 43:129, 1971.
20. Meyer RA, DG Schwartz, G Benzing, S Kaplan: Ventricular septum in right ventricular volume overload: an echocardiographic study. Am J Cardiol 30:349, 1972.
21. Lewis AB, GF Gates, P Stanley: Echocardiography and perfusion scintigraphy in the diagnosis of pulmonary arterio-venous fistula. Chest 73:675, 1978.
22. Shub C, A Tajik, JB Seward: Detecting intrapulmonary right to left shunt with contrast echocardiography. Observations in a patient with diffuse pulmonary arteriovenous fistula. Mayo Clin Proc 51:81, 1976.
23. Most E: personal communication.
24. Duff DF, HP Gutgesell: The use of saline or blood for ultrasonic detection of a right to left intra cardiac shunt in the early postoperative patient. Am Heart J 94:402, 1977.

15. ECHO CONTRAST STUDIES IN THE EARLY POSTOPERATIVE PERIOD AFTER ATRIAL SEPTAL DEFECT CLOSURE

LILLIAM M. VALDES-CRUZ, DANIEL R. PIERONI, MICHAEL JONES, J.-MICHEL A. ROLAND, and JON P. SHEMATEK

INTRODUCTION

Contrast echocardiographic injections, performed through surgically positioned central venous and left atrial lines, have been shown to be valuable in detecting and localizing right-to-left and left-to-right intracardiac shunting respectively, during the early postoperative period. When applied serially over the first few days after surgery, this technique differentiates flow through surgical patches from shunting across true residual defects [1].

The purpose of this chapter is to review and summarize our experience with contrast echocardiography, validated with indocyanine green indicator dilution curves, during the early postoperative period following closure of simple and complex atrial septal defects. The data are based on a study of 44 patients operated on at the Johns Hopkins Hospital or the Clinic of Surgery, National Heart, Lung and Blood Institute.

The first section summarizes technical aspects of surgery, dye curves, and contrast studies. The second section reviews the different qualitative patterns observed on the echo after contrast injections from the right and left sides of the heart. The third section compares results of indicator dilution curves to those of echo contrast and discusses sensitivity of the techniques. Finally, the last section discusses the surgical implications of our observations.

TECHNICAL ASPECTS

Three surgical methods were used to close the atrial defects: (a) primary suture closure (n = 7); (b) patching with thin, knit Teflon^R fabric, 0.3 mm thick* (n = 13); and (c) patching with thicker, knit Teflon 0.5 mm thick, specially treated to have very low porosity* (n = 24). Standard in vitro tests of patch leakage under 120 mm Hg pressure showed the thinner Teflon to have a flow of 2800 $cm^3/cm^2/min$ while the thicker Teflon had flows of 500 $cm^3/cm^2/min$ (personal communication, United States Catheter and Instruments Co., Billerica, Mass., January, 1981).

Central venous and left atrial lines were routinely placed at the time of surgery for

---

* United States Catheter and Instruments Co., Billerica, Mass.

postoperative monitoring purposes. These catheters usually have smooth flow on withdrawal of blood for several days after insertion and, with precautions to avoid air or clots, should not offer complications.

Indocyanine green dye curves were performed either in the operating room following chest closure, or upon arrival in the intensive care unit. Indicator was injected into the central venous line and sampled from a peripheral artery. The magnitude and direction of shunts were calculated by established methods [2–4].

Following the dye curves, contrast echocardiographic studies were done by injecting $1-2 \, cm^3$ of the patient's blood through the central venous and/or left atrial catheters while recording a strip chart echocardiogram. Timing was accomplished with a lead II electrocardiogram and an injection marker.

Four areas are examined when looking for bidirectional shunting: (a) aortic; (b) mitral; (c) ventricular; and (d) tricuspid positions. A technically acceptable study is one where the contrast effect completely opacifies cardiac structures located on the side into which the injection is made. To accomplish this, the echocardiograph is usually set at the highest gain settings which still allow definition of structures. Damping out of microbubbles is a problem often encountered with M-mode and two-dimensional echocardiographic contrast studies. As a result of this technical difficulty, several trial injections may be necessary before appropriate settings are obtained.

Blood has been tested both in vivo and in vitro and has been found adequate for causing microbubbles. In postoperative conditions, blood is preferred to other substances like 5% dextrose water or saline because of fluid restrictions commonly necessary, especially in infants [5, 6].

QUALITATIVE PATTERNS

A contrast study is considered negative when microbubbles are confined to the side into which the injection is made (Figures 1–4). In the presence of a right-to-left atrial shunt, the central venous injection produces contrast echoes appearing in the left atrium and within the mitral orifice followed by filling of the left ventricular cavity and aortic root (Figures 5, 6). With left-to-right shunts, left atrial injections produce microbubbles which fill the tricuspid valve orifice, right ventricular cavity, and then the right ventricular outflow area (Figures 7, 8, 9). With bidirectional shunting, both patterns are observed.

Filling of the area defined by the atrioventricular valve leaflets is the hallmark of atrial level shunting. Opacification of a ventricular cavity while sparing its atrioventricular valve orifice indicates the presence of a shunt at ventricular level [7].

Technical false positives occur when the field is "overloaded" with contrast echoes. Normally, the microbubbles are confined to cavities by delineating intracardiac structures such as the right ventricular wall and interventricular septum. With overload, contrast is seen within as well as through delineating walls and then

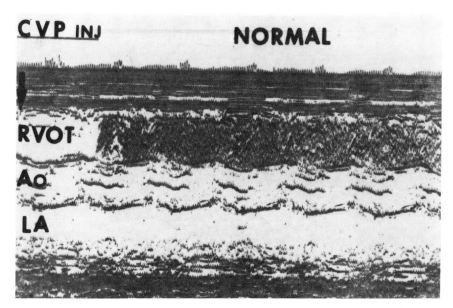

Figure 1. Central venous injection in a patient with no residual intracardiac communication. The contrast echo effect is confined to the right ventricular outflow tract (RVOT). The left atrium (LA) and aortic root (ao) are echo-free. Reproduced by permission of the American Heart Association from Valdes-Cruz et al. [1].

tapers rapidly (Figure 10). These studies can be falsely interpreted as indicative of intracardiac shunting as "microbubbles" do appear on the side opposite that of injection. This overloading effect is corrected by reducing the pressure of injection and/or modifying the gain settings of the echocardiograph [7].

SENSITIVITY OF CONTRAST

During the first postoperative day, residual atrial defects were documented by indicator dilution in ten out of the 44 patients: six had isolated right-to-left, one had isolated left-to-right, and three had bidirectional shunting. The remaining 34 patients had normal dye dilution curves. In all patients with positive shunts, thin knit Teflon had been used to close the atrial septal defects. The results of the contrast studies agreed with those of the dye curves.

Forward green dye curves detect right-to-left intracardiac shunting as small as 3–5% of systemic blood flow, while reverse curves demonstrate left-to-right shunts in the order of 5% of pulmonary blood flow [2–4].

In 1973, Pieroni et al. reported 12 cases of simultaneous forward and reverse indicator dilution curves and contrast studies conducted in the cardiac catheterization laboratory; the results showed equal sensitivity of both techniques in detecting right-to-left and left-to-right intracardiac shunts [8]. Later, in 1976 and 1977, we

156

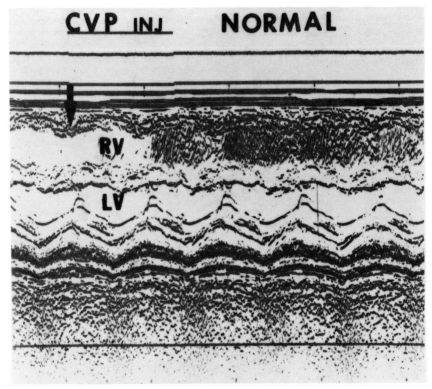

Figure 2 (Legend: see p. 157).

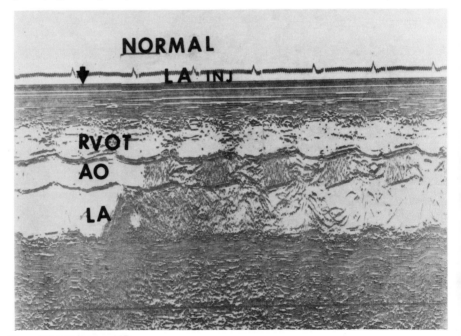

Figure 3 (Legend: see p. 157).

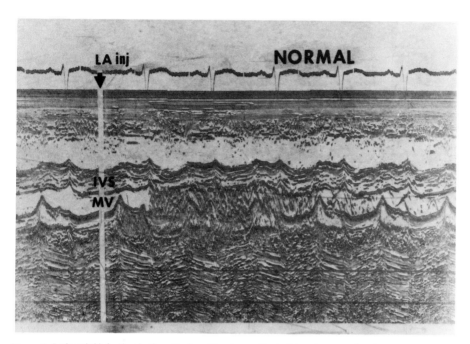

Figure 4. Left atrial injection in the mitral position in a patient with no intracardiac shunting. Following a left atrial injection, the left ventricular cavity fills through the mitral valve with no evidence of microbubbles appearing in the right ventricle. IVS = interventricular septum; MV = mitral valve. Reproduced by permission of the American Heart Association from Valdes-Cruz et al. [1].

reported contrast techniques from peripheral vein, central venous, and left atrial injections which proved at least as sensitive as dye curves for shunt detection [1,7]. The expanded series, which forms the basis of this chapter, supports these previous reports and confirms the sensitivity of contrast to detect shunts as small as 3–5%.

SURGICAL IMPLICATIONS

Table 1 summarizes our experience. No patient whose ASD was closed by either direct suturing or thick Teflon had shunting in the first postoperative day. Of the 13

Figure 2 (see facing page, top). Central venous injection in a patient with no residual atrial defect. The right ventricular cavity (RV) fills with contrast echoes, but the left ventricle (LV) remains clear. Reproduced by permission of the American Heart Association from Valdes-Cruz et al. [1].

Figure 3 (see facing page, bottom). Left atrial injection in a patient with no residual atrial defect. The microbubbles are observed within the left atrium and aortic root. The right ventricular outflow tract is free of contrast echoes. Reproduced by permission of the American Heart Association from Valdes-Cruz et al. [1].

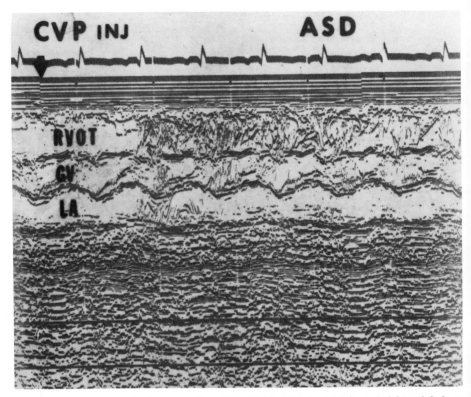

Figure 5. Central venous injection in a patient with a right-to-left interatrial shunt. A right-to-left shunt at the atrial level is confirmed by the appearance of contrast echoes in the left atrium. This patient had a Mustard operation for transposition of the great arteries. GV = great vessel. Reproduced by permission of the American Heart Association from Valdes-Cruz et al. [1].

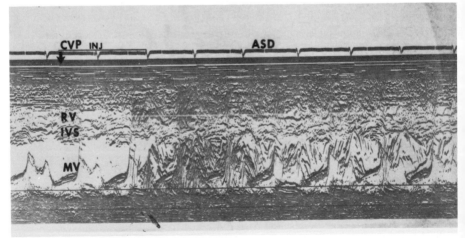

Figure 6. Central venous injection in the mitral position in a patient with a right-to-left interatrial shunt. Following opacification of the right ventricle, the left ventricle fills with microbubbles which opacify the mitral valve orifice in diastole. This is the hallmark of an atrial level shunt. Reproduced by permission of the American Heart Association from Valdes-Cruz et al., [1].

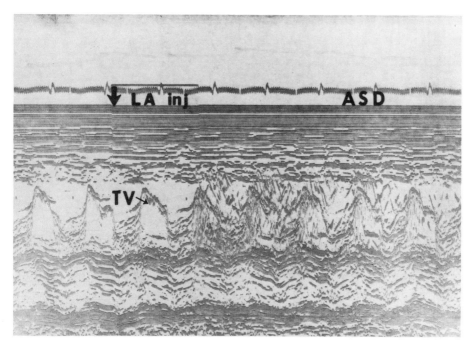

Figure 7. Left atrial injection in the tricuspid position on a patient with left-to-right shunt across an atrial septal defect. Complete filling of the right ventricular inflow area through the orifice of the tricuspid valve (TV) establishes the presence of a left-to-right shunt at atrial level. Reproduced by permission of the American Heart Association from Valdes-Cruz et al. [1].

Table 1. Summary of results in the first postoperative day.

	Suture closure (n = 7)	Thin teflon (n = 13)	Thick teflon (n = 24)
Negative shunt	7	3	24
Positive shunt	0	10	0

patients in whom thin Teflon was used, ten had shunting during the day of surgery. Of these, five demonstrated progressive diminution in shunting by repeated contrast studies over 3–5 consecutive days; these patients had benign recovery. The remaining five patients had evidence of persistent shunting by contrast echo and their clinical courses were more complex, some requiring additional surgery.

These data confirm the commonly accepted phenomenon of temporary leakage across new patches and stress the need for followup contrast studies when evidence of shunting is found immediately after surgery. Further, direct suturing of small defects or patching larger or complex defects with thicker Teflon seems to prevent early leakage and indicates that in patients with complex lesions in whom continued shunting during the early postoperative period may cause serious hemodynamic embarrassment, use of heavier patch material or primary closure is advisable.

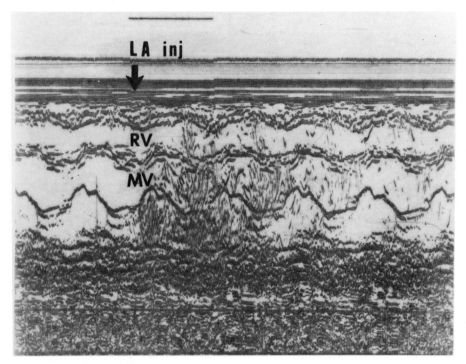

Figure 8 (Legend: see p. 161).

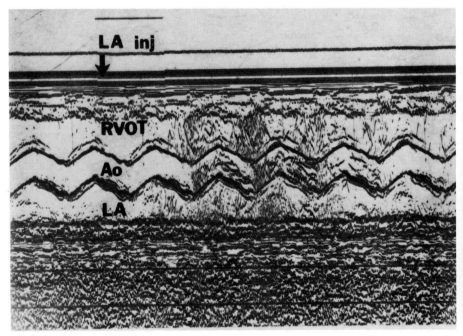

Figure 9 (Legend: see p. 161).

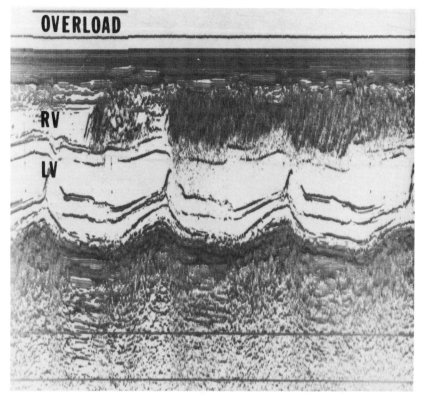

Figure 10. Example of overload. The contrast echoes are seen within as well as through the walls of the interventricular septum and then taper rapidly. This is a technical false positive. Reproduced by permission of the American Heart Association from Valdes-Cruz et al. [1].

CONCLUSIONS

Contrast echocardiography is a sensitive and minimally invasive technique which, when used in the early postoperative period, provides valuable information on the integrity of septal defect repairs. It can prove to be a useful adjunct in early postoperative monitoring, particularly to evaluate the need for early catheterization and further surgery in patients with postoperative complications.

Figure 8 (see facing page, top). Left atrial injection in a patient with a left-to-right intracardiac communication. The left ventricle fills with microbubbles which then appear in the right ventricular cavity. Reproduced by permission of the American Heart Association from Valdes-Cruz et al. [1].

Figure 9 (see facing page, bottom). Left atrial injection in the presence of a left-to-right intracardiac shunt. Following the injection, microbubbles not only opacify the left atrium root, but also fill the right ventricular outflow tract area, confirming the presence of a left-to-right shunt. Reproduced permission of the American Heart Association from Valdes-Cruz et al. [1].

162

ACKNOWLEDGMENTS

The authors acknowledge with thanks the technical assistance of Virginia A. Kuentz, B.S.

REFERENCES

1. Valdes-Cruz LM, DR Pieroni, J-M Roland, JP Shematek: Recognition of residual post-operative shunts by contrast echocardiographic techniques. Circulation 55:148, 1977.
2. Swan HJC: Indicator dilution methods in the diagnosis of congenital heart disease. Prog Cardiovasc Dis 2:143, 1959.
3. Carter SA, DF Bajec, E Yannicelli, EH Wood: Estimation of left-to-right shunt from arterial dilution curves. J Lab Clin Med 55:77, 1960.
4. Krovetz LJ, IH Gessner: A new method utilizing indicator dilution techniques for estimation of left-to-right shunts in infants. Circulation 32:772, 1965.
5. Ziskin MC, A Bonakdarpour, DP Weinstein, PR Lynch: Contrast agents for diagnostic ultrasound. Invest Radiol 7:500, 1972.
6. Valdes-Cruz LM, DR Pieroni, J-M Roland, PJ Varghese: Peripheral vein injections as a means of producing microcavitations detectable by echocardiography. Pediatr Res 9:273, 1975 (abstract).
7. Valdes-Cruz LM, DR Pieroni, J-M Roland, PJ Varghese: Echocardiographic detection of intracardiac left-to-right shunts following peripheral vein injections. Circulation 54:558, 1976.
8. Pieroni DR, PJ Varghese, RD Rowe: Echocardiography to detect shunt and valvular incompetence in infants and children. Circulation 48:81, 1973 (abstract).

16. TWO-DIMENSIONAL CONTRAST ECHOCARDIOGRAPHY IN THE STUDY OF VENTRICULAR SEPTAL DEFECTS

G.J. van Mill, A.J. Moulaert, and E. Harinck

INTRODUCTION

Isolated ventricular septal defects (VSDs) can usually be diagnosed under normal circumstances by physical examination, electrocardiogram, phonocardiogram, and chest X-ray. If necessary, confirmation is obtained by cardiac catheterization and angiocardiography. The exact location of the defect may be obtained by angled left ventricular angiocardiography [1]. To achieve angiocardiographic localization several X-ray films are often necessary.

Recent developments in echocardiology have enabled us to visualize haemo-dynamically important VSDs and to determine their exact localization in the interventricular septum (IVS). M-mode echocardiography (M-mode echo) provides some information about the degree of volume overload of the left heart and the pulmonary vascular resistance [2–7], but is not really suitable for visualizing isolated VSDs. Initially it was thought that these defects could not be visualized by the two-dimensional echocardiogram (2D echo) either [8]; but with the improvement of electronic devices and the introduction of the 5 mHz transducer, VSDs can now be visualized by 2D echo in most cases, particularly in small children. It has been our experience that besides visualizing the VSD the exact site of the IVS can also be accurately recognized [15]. Two-dimensional contrast echocardiography (2D contrast echo) complements the results obtained by direct 2D echo visualization. It distinguishes between real defects and septal dropouts which falsely simulate a VSD. If a VSD constitutes a part of the complex structural cardiac defect, then the common clinical features of an isolated VSD are usually missing. In these cases the M-mode echo may reliably reveal the localization of the VSD, in for example, Fallot's tetralogy with the typical overriding of the aorta [16]. Another example is the complete atrioventricular canal defect with its peculiar discontinuity between the aorta and the IVS caused by the single atrioventricular valve. This discontinuity is particularly striking on the subcostal M-mode scans and confirms the presence of a large VSD [17]. 2D echo is generally also more suitable for imaging complex VSDs than M-mode echo.

This chapter deals with the present role of 2D contrast echo in the localization of the VSD as an isolated entity and as part of a complex cardiac defect.

164

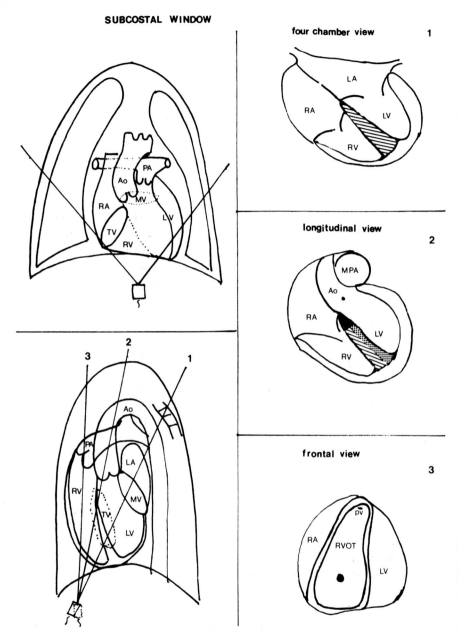

SUBCOSTAL WINDOW

four chamber view   1

longitudinal view   2

frontal view   3

Figure 1. Diagrammatic representation of the use of the subcostal window. The posterior four-chamber view is indicated by (1). In this cross-section the posterior inlet septum is visualized with its atrio-ventricular part between the insertion of septal tricuspid and mitral leaflets. Angulation of the transducer to plane in (2) provides a longitudinal view of the left ventricle showing the origin of the posterior great artery. In this plane the proximal part of the interventricular septum (IVS) represents the membranous septum and the large distal part, the transition region between inlet and trabecular septum. In the frontal view (3) the IVS is not visible. RA = right atrium; RV = right ventricle; PA = pulmonary artery; LA = left atrium; LV = left ventricle; Ao = aorta; MV = mitral valve; TV = tricuspid valve; PV = pulmonary valve; MPA = main pulmonary artery; RVOT = right ventricular outflow tract.

THE ISOLATED VSD

For an accurate description of the localization of VSDs, it is advisable to classify the IVS into four components: membranous, inlet, trabecular, and outlet [18,19]. A number of standard two-dimensional cross-sections should be routinely used (Figures 1, 2). A VSD is considered to be present when there is discontinuity in the IVS during the whole or a particular period of the cardiac cycle. Such discontinuity should preferably be observed in corresponding parts of the IVS in different cross-sections and the outline of the IVS should be clearly demarcated. The size of the VSD may change during the cardiac cycle [13]. Usually the defect is largest during diastole. If a defect appears to vary in size or disappears entirely during the cardiac cycle the examiner should be aware of a possible artifact. Because of movements of the heart within the chest the defect may move in and out of the selected cross-section. Such movements may remove the discontinuity from a certain cross-section on which its presence had previously been obvious. If cardiac catheterization is indicated, the 2D echo findings should be confirmed in the catheterization laboratory. For instance, if the cardiac catheter is manipulated through the VSD, it will show on the echocardiogram; thus the location of the VSD can be verified.

Usually a left ventricular contrast echocardiogram (LV contrast echo) is required to confirm the exact site of the shunting. In the presence of a concomitant right-to-left shunt, venous contrast injections may suffice. To provide echocontrast, or microbubbles which reflect ultrasound, we normally use saline or cardiogreen. As the microbubbles pass with the blood flow through the VSD, the site of the septal interruption can be precisely identified on the appropriate cross-section. If echo contrast enters the right ventricle from the left without obvious passage through the suspected septal deficiency, a VSD cannot be diagnosed with confidence. False positive 2D echo findings rarely occur providing a number of conditions are strictly adhered to. The quality of the echocardiogram must of course be adequate. The IVS must be identified on several standard cross-sections. Cross-sections that do not clearly show the right ventricular cavity should be avoided, as they easily lead to erroneous conclusions. In our experience the subcostal longitudinal cross-section (Figures 1, 2) can be used to recognize the relatively small membranous VSDs. In this view the medial wall of the left ventricular outflow region and the septal insertion of the tricuspid leaflet are clearly demarcated. It should be realized that VSDs smaller than approximately 3–4 mm in diameter cannot be reliably visualized.

Figure 3 shows the 2D echo of a membranous VSD. The defect is covered on the right side by the septal tricuspid leaflet. LV contrast echo confirms the defect at the suspected site. Large membranous defects often extend into the surrounding muscular septum. When the defect spreads anteriorly to the outlet septum, the VSD is also visible in the parasternal short-axis view through the outflow region of the left ventricle. In this view the defect is not always visible throughout the whole cardiac cycle, probably due to cyclic cardiac movement. Figure 4 shows a parasternal short-axis view through the left ventricular outflow tract of a large membranous VSD

166

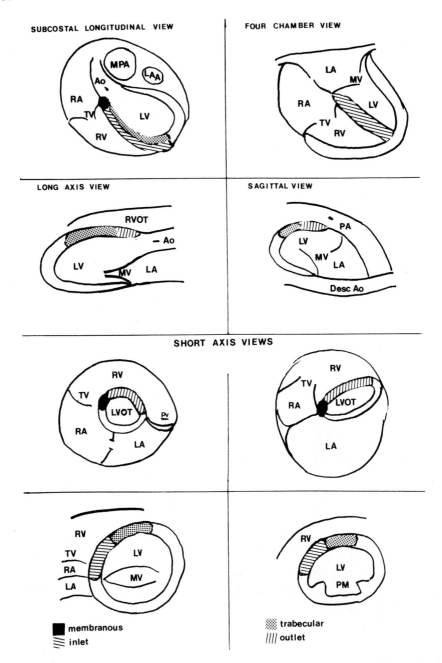

Figure 2. Diagrammatic representation of all the matching cross-sectional planes showing the different parts of the IVS. Short-axis views are shown at the level of the left ventricular outflow tract, the mitral valve, and the papillary muscles in the left ventricle. LAA = left atrial appendage; Desc Ao = descending aorta; LVOT = left ventricular outflow tract; PM = papillary muscles; for other abbreviations see Figure 1.

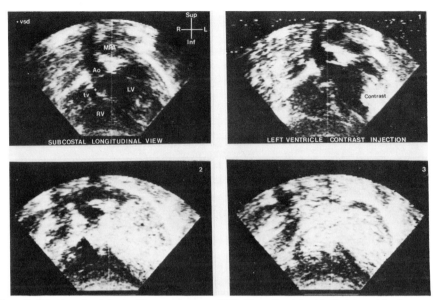

Figure 3. 2D echo of an infant with a membranous VSD. From the right side the tricuspid valve covers the defect. LV contrast echo was carried out with 2–3 ml saline injections into the left ventricle. The echo contrast appeared at first in the apex of the left ventricle (1). Next (2) the whole left ventricle was filled and through the VSD echo contrast reached the septal tricuspid leaflet. Finally the entire right ventricle was filled with echo contrast as a result of the large left-to-right shunt (3) VSD = ventricular septal defect; for other abbreviations see previous figures.

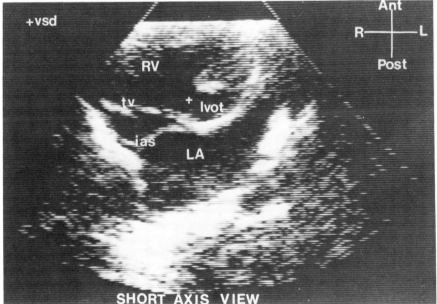

Figure 4. 2D echo of an infant with a membranous VSD extending into the outlet septum. The left ventricular outflow tract has on the right side a large communication with the right ventricle. The defect extends dorsally to the tricuspid valve. lvot = left ventricular outflow tract; ias = interatrial septum; for other abbreviations see previous figures.

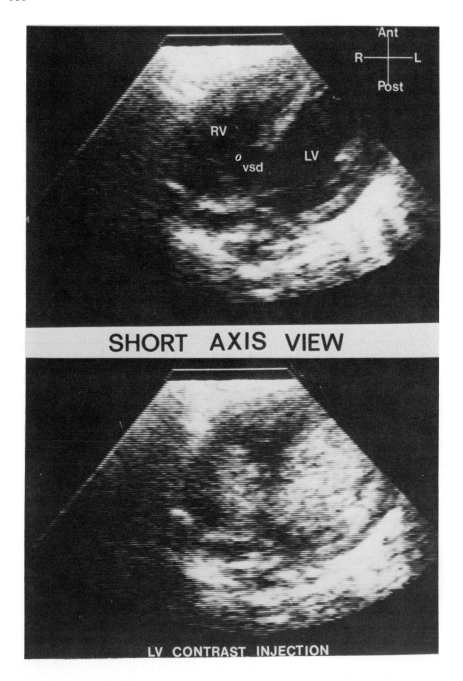

Figure 5. 2D echo of an infant with a large muscular defect of the posterior or inlet septum. A left ventricular contrast injection shows filling of the right ventricle through the defect. For abbreviations see previous figures.

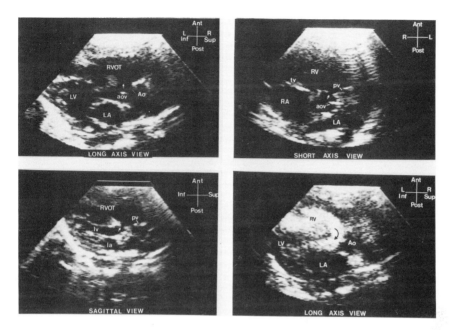

Figure 6. 2D echo of an infant with a subarterial infundibular, supracristal or subpulmonary VSD. Upper left panel: in the long-axis view the defect is located at the level of the aortic valve (arrow). Upper right panel: in the short-axis view the defect (arrow) is on the left side of the aortic ring and shows a close relation to the pulmonary valve. Lower left panel: the sagittal view also exhibits the close relation of the defect with the subpulmonary area (arrow). Lower right panel: the long-axis view on the right side shows a right-to-left shunt through the VSD, visualized by a venous contrast injection. AOV = aortic valve; for other abbreviations see previous figures.

which was confirmed by LV contrast echo. The side of these large VSDs hardly alter during the cardiac cycle. Figure 5 shows, in short-axis view, a large posterior defect of the inlet septum. The same large defect was also visualized at a corresponding site on the subcostal and apical four-chamber views. LV contrast echo confirmed this defect. In Figure 6 a supracristal, also called subpulmonary or subarterial infundibular, VSD is shown in different cross-sections. Because of equal pressures in the ventricles the diagnosis could be confirmed by a venous contrast injection. Echo contrast passes through the VSD from the right ventricle to the left during diastole, as shown in the long-axis view (Figure 6, lower right panel). A trabecular VSD visualized in the subcostal transverse view is demonstrated in Figure 7. This cross-section is situated in a sagittal plane and simulates a lateral angiocardiogram. It shows the anterior part of the IVS and should also be regarded as one of the standard views. The echo contrast enters the right ventricle through the VSD.

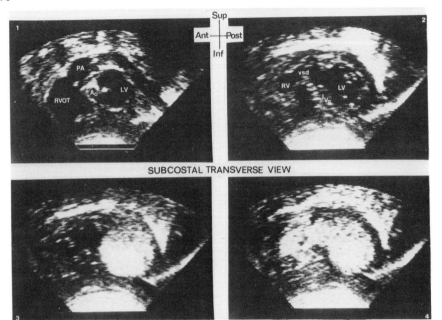

SUBCOSTAL TRANSVERSE VIEW

Figure 7. 2D echo of an infant with a large muscular defect of the trabecular septum. The heart is visualized in a sagittal plane through the right ventricular outflow tract and the pulmonary artery (1). Slight angulation of the transducer to the left shows the trabecular septum and an arteriorly located VSD (2). A left ventricular echo contrast injection shows filling of the right ventricle through the defect (3), (4). For abbreviations see previous figures.

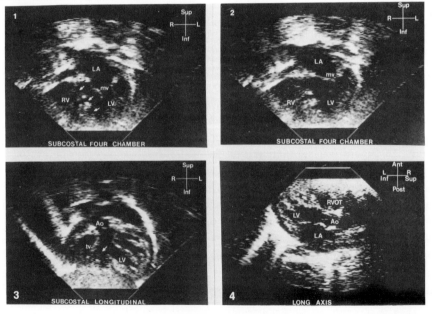

Figure 8. 2D echo of an infant with multiple VSDs of the posterior or inlet septum. (1) The subcostal four-chamber view shows three defects (arrows) when the mitral valve is open. (2) In the subcostal four-chamber view with the mitral valve closed, the VSDs are of equal size. (3) In the subcostal longitudinal view one large VSD is visible. (4) The anterior septum in the long-axis view is intact. For abbreviations see previous figures.

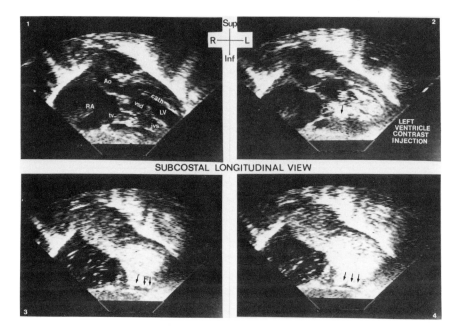

Figure 9. 2D echo of an infant with a large muscular defect in the transition region between inlet and trabecular part of the IVS. (1) Pre-injection: (2) a left ventricular echo contrast injection opacifies the VSD. (3), (4) In the subsequent systole several small "echo flows," parallel to each other, are visible in the more distal and thickened part of the IVS indicating several small VSDs (arrows). cath = catheter; for other abbreviations see previous figures.

MULTIPLE VSDs

When a VSD is seen in different cross-sections, but at non-corresponding sites, more than one VSD should be suspected. Careful analysis may reveal whether or not these defects communicate with each other. Multiple VSDs of the inlet septum may often be seen in one single cross-section (Figure 8). In the "Swiss cheese" VSD there usually are a few large defects and several smaller ones between the trabeculae. These small ones may be identified only by LV contrast echo (Figure 9).

VSD IN COMPLEX STRUCTURAL HEART DISEASE

When a VSD is part of a complex structural heart disease, particularly in the presence of malalignment defects, confirmation by 2D contrast echo is not always needed. For instance, if 2D echo shows overriding of a great artery across the IVS, the subarterial VSD is obvious. Figure 10 demonstrates the 2D echo of a small child with transposition of the great arteries (TGA) and VSD with overriding of the main pulmonary artery. This overriding inevitably indicates a large subpulmonary VSD. There is a striking malalignment between outlet and trabecular septum, as demonstrated in the subcostal frontal and transverse views. When the aorta overrides the

172

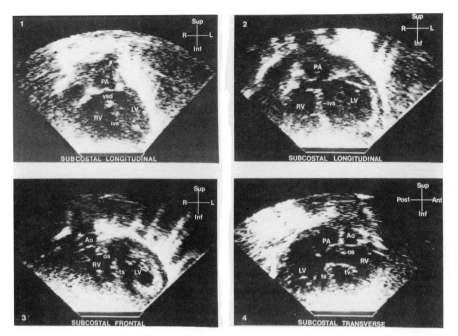

Figure 10. 2D echo of an infant with transposition of the great arteries and ventricular septal defect. (1) In the subcostal longitudinal view the posterior great artery is visualized through its branching pattern identified as the pulmonary artery (arrows). (2) The main pulmonary artery overrides the interventricular septum indicating a subpulmonary VSD. (3) The subcostal frontal view shows the anteriorly located aorta and the outlet septum. (4) In the subcostal transverse view the outlet septum is also visualized as an extension of the aortopulmonary septum. The displacement of the outlet septum in relation to the trabecular septum is most marked in the transverse view. ts = trabecular septum; os = outlet setptum; for other abbreviations see previous figures.

IVS as for instance in Fallot's tetralogy, pulmonary atresia with VSD, and truncus arteriosus, the presence of the subaortic VSD is also clear and analysis with contrast echo does not provide useful additional information. VSDs other than the malalignment type also occur with TGA. In Figure 11 a tunnel-like subpulmonary VSD is shown in association with TGA without overriding of the posterior great artery. This type of VSD is referred to as a paratricuspid VSD [20]. This VSD may require confirmation by 2D contrast echo.

An inlet VSD is indicated when an atrioventricular valve overrides the IVS (Figure 12). The VSD component of complete atrioventricular defect Rastelli type C [21] cannot be overlooked on a good quality four-chamber echo. The anterior bridging leaflet of the common atrioventricular valve touches the proximal part of the septum during diastole, whereas during systole it is seen to be distinct from the septum revealing a large VSD. Occasionally some echocardiographic problems may be encountered when trying to differentiate between partial and Rastelli type A complete atrioventricular canal because in the latter short and thick chordae reach the most proximal part of the IVS. In this situation LV contrast echo may establish or refute the presence of a VSD. If a VSD is present, the echocontrast will flow from

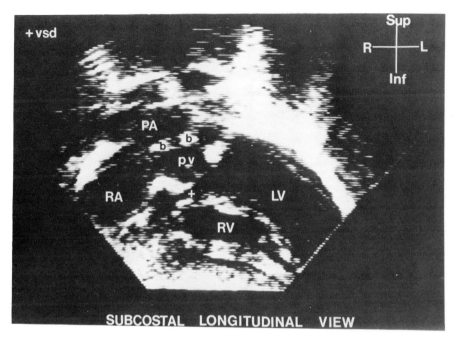

Figure 11. 2D echo of an infant with transposition of the great arteries and VSD. To diminish the pulmonary bloodflow and to reduce the pulmonary artery pressure, a pulmonary artery banding was done. In the subcostal longitudinal view the banding of the pulmonary artery is visualized. Just beneath the pulmonary valve a channel-like VSD is seen. There is no overriding of the pulmonary artery over the IVS. b = region of banding; for other abbreviations see previous figures.

the left ventricle through the chordae to the right. Hagler et al. [22] were able to diagnose atrioventricular canal correctly in 96% of their cases with the 2D echo and in all cases in combination with 2D contrast echo. Left ventricular-right atrial incompetence, commonly observed in atrioventricular canal defect, is remarkably well demonstrated by LV contrast echo in the four-chamber view.

UNIVENTRICULAR HEART

In univentricular heart the IVS is entirely absent or consists of small fragments of the outlet and/or trabecular septum which separate the main double inlet chamber from the outlet chamber. The correct diagnosis can usually be derived by 2D echo alone [23]. However, occasionally 2D echo contrast studies may add useful information. The 2D echo of the patient shown in Figure 13 was at first erroneously diagnosed as a univentricular heart. Venous contrast injections during visualization of the possible outlet foramen, forced this diagnosis to be discarded, since echo contrast reached the anterior right ventricular outflow tract before the posterior ventricle (Figure 14).

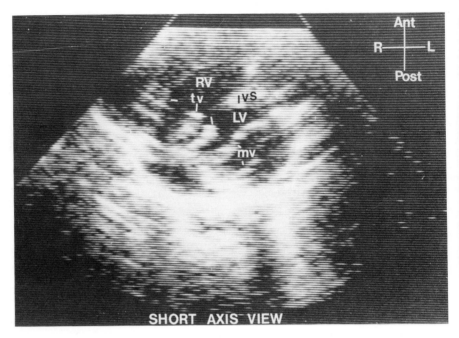

Figure 12. 2D echo of a child showing overriding of the tricuspid valve indicating a large inlet septal defect. The anterior portions of the IVS only are visible. For abbreviations see previous figures.

CONCLUSIONS

Nowadays serious complaints due to isolated VSDs are almost entirely confined to infants. Therefore, our experience with these large defects is for the greater part limited to this age group. We believe that it is possible to gain sufficient expertise with 2D echo to accurately visualize hemodynamically important VSDs and to locate their exact positions in these infants. 2D contrast echo often provides additional confirmative information. Presently, 2D contrast echo is a routine procedure in our catheterization laboratory in cases with isolated VSD. In the future 2D contrast echo may be preferred to angiocardiography in these cases. The presence and location of these VSD can be accurately established by 2D echo before angiocardiography; and as such we believe that it has already reduced the number and length of angiocardiograms, and consequently the amount of X-ray exposure in our laboratory. With advancing experience the necessity to confirm the 2D echo diagnosis by 2D contrast echo probably will decline to some extent. Some authors describe the value of pulsed Doppler in combination with the M-mode echo in the diagnosis of VSDs, particularly when a left-to-right shunt is involved [24, 25]. Muscular inlet VSDs and subpulmonary defects may be difficult to locate by this method. It is to be expected that if pulsed Doppler is used together with 2D echo, better results will be obtained. If this technique can be reliably applied for confirmation of the localization if isolated VSDs, it may diminish the need for contrast

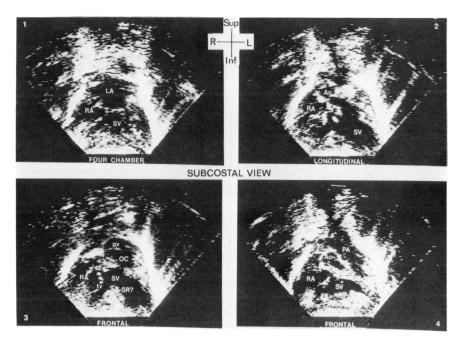

Figure 13. 2D echo of an infant diagnosed as univentricular heart with an anteriorly located outflow chamber and a normal relation of the great arteries. (1) In the subcostal four-chamber view the inlet septum is entirely absent. (2) The region of the ventricular outflow tract and aorta has a goose neck appearance in the longitudinal view (3), (4). The more anteriorly located frontal views visualize the pulmonary artery which traverses abnormally from a left inferior to a right superior direction (4). A septal remnant (SR) is suggested in the frontal view (3), but it may also be the posterior medial muscle bundle. SV = single ventricle; SR = septal remnant; OC = outlet chamber; for further abbreviations see previous figures.

echo because the latter, in contrast to pulsed Doppler echo, often involves an invasive catheter technique.

In our experience, 2D contrast echo is needed in the multiple "Swiss cheese" VSD to localize the small defects in addition to the larger ones. In VSDs associated with complex structural heart disease, direct visualization by 2D echo alone is often enough to establish the defect. In the diagnosis of univentricular heart contrast echo is also helpful in a minority of the cases.

REFERENCES

1. Soto B, CH Coghlan, LM Bargeron Jr: Angiography of ventricular septal defect. In: Anderson RH, EA Shinebourne (eds) Paediatric Cardiology 1977, pp 125–137, Churchill Livingstone, Edinburgh, 1978.
2. Lewis AB, M Takahashi: Echocardiographic assessment of left-to-right shunt volume in children with ventricular septal defect. Circulation 54:78–82, 1976.
3. Ahmad M, KA Hallidie-Smith: Assessment of left to right shunt and left ventricular function in isolated ventricular septal defect. Echocardiographic study. Br Heart J

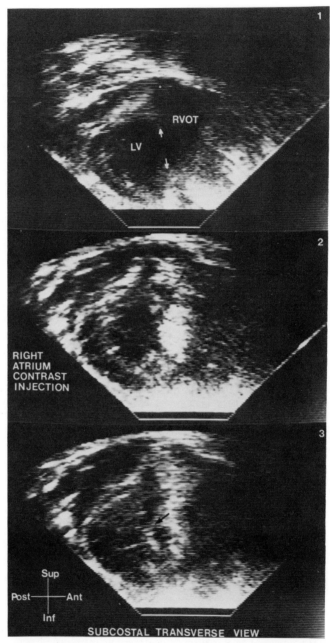

Figure 14. Subcostal transverse views from the same patient as in Figure 13. A large communication is visualized between the left ventricle (LV) and right ventricular outflow tract (RVOT). (1) The edges of the communication are marked with arrows. (2) After a right atrial contrast injection, the contrast appeared first in the RVOT, and subsequently (3) through the large communication in the LV. Therefore, there must be an inlet into the anterior chamber. The diagnosis of univentricular heart was thus discarded and changed to a very large VSD or multiple VSDs (inlet and trabecular). For abbreviations see previous figures.

41:147–158, 1979.

4. Lester LA, D Vitullo, P Sodt, N Hutcheon, R Arcilla: An evaluation of the left atrial/ aortic root ratio in children with ventricular septal defect. Circulation 60:364–372, 1979.

5. Hirschfeld S, R Meyer, D Schwartz, J Korfhagen, S Kaplan: The echocardiographic assessment of pulmonary artery pressure and pulmonary vascular resistance. Circulation 52:642–650, 1975.

6. Riggs Th, S Hirschfeld, J Borkat, J Knoke, J Liebman: Assessment of the pulmonary artery vascular bed by echocardiographic right ventricular systolic time intervals. Circulation 57:939–947, 1978.

7. Silverman NH, AR Snider, AM Rudolph: Evaluation of pulmonary hypertension. By M-mode echocardiography in children with ventricular septal defect. Circulation 61: 1125–1132, 1980.

8. Goldberg SJ, HD Allen, DJ Sahn: Pediatric and Adolescent Echocardiography. Year Book Medical Chicago, 1975.

9. King DL, CN Steeg, K Ellis: Visualization of ventricular septal defects by cardiac ultrasonography. Circulation 48:1215–1220, 1973.

10. Seward JB, AJ Tajik, DJ Hagler, DD Mair: Visualization of isolated ventricular septal defect with wide-angle two-dimensional sector echocardiography. Circulation (Suppl II) 58:II–202, 1978 (abstract).

11. Silverman NH, NB Schiller: Apex echocardiography: a two-dimensional technique for evaluating congenital heart disease. Circulation 57:503–511, 1978.

12. Cheatham JP, LA Latson, HP Gutgesell: Ventricular septal defect in infancy: detection by two-dimensional echocardiography. Am J Cardiol 47:85–89, 1981.

13. Canale JM, DJ Sahn, HD Allen, SJ Goldberg: Factors affecting real-time cross-sectional echocardiographic imaging of ventricular septal defects. Am J Cardiol 45:467, 1980 (abstract).

14. Bierman FZ, K Fellows, RG Williams: Prospective identification of ventricular septal defects in infancy using subxiphoid two-dimensional echocardiography. Circulation 62:807–817, 1980.

15. Van Mill GJ, AJ Moulaert, E Harinck: Two-dimensional echocardiographic localisation of isolated ventricular septal defects. In: Hunter S (ed) Echocardiography 1980. Churchill Livingstone, Edinburgh (in press).

16. Caldwell RL, AE Weyman, RA Hurwitz, DA Girod, H Feigenbaum: Right ventricular outflow tract assessment by cross-sectional echocardiography in tetralogy of Fallot. Circulation 59: 395–402, 1979.

17. Sutherland GR, Van Mill GJ, RH Anderson, S Hunter: Sub-xiphoid echocardiography – a new approach to the diagnosis and differentiation of atrioventricular defects. Eur Heart J 1:45–54, 1980.

18. Anderson RH: Embryology of the ventricular septum. In: Anderson RH, EA Shinebourne (eds) Paediatric Cardiology 1977, pp 103–112. Churchill Livingstone, Edinburgh, 1978.

19. Soto B, AF Becker, AJ Moulaert, JT Lie, RH Anderson: Classification of isolated ventricular septal defects. Br Heart J 43:332–343, 1980.

20. Oppenheimer-Dekker A: Interventricular communications in transposition of the great arteries. In: van Mierop LHS, A Oppenheimer-Dekker, CLDC Bruins (eds) Embryology and Teratology of the Heart and the Great Arteries, pp. 139–159 Leiden University Press, The Hague, 1978.

21. Rastelli GC, JW Kirklin, JL Titus: Anatomic observations on complete form of persistent common atrioventricular canal with special reference to atrioventricular valves. Mayo Clin Proc 41:296–308, 1966.

22. Hagler DJ, AJ Tajik, JB Seward, DD Mair, DG Ritter: Real-time wide-angle sector

echocardiography: atrioventricular canal defects. Circulation 59:140–150, 1979.

23. Sahn DJ, J Harder, R Freedom, W Duncan, R Rowe: Cross-sectional echocardiographic recognition of septal structures in univentricular hearts. In: Moulaert AJ, A Oppenheimer-Dekker, A Wenink (eds), The Ventricular Septum. Leiden University Press, The Hague (in press).
24. Stevenson JG, I Kawabori, T Dooley, WG Guntheroth: Diagnosis of ventricular septal defect by pulsed Doppler echocardiography. Circulation 58:322–326, 1978.
25. Magherini A, G Azzolina, V Wiechmann, F Fantini: Pulsed Doppler echocardiography for diagnosis of ventricular septal defects. Br Heart J 43:143–147, 1980.

17. CONTRAST ECHOCARDIOGRAPHY FOR EVALUATION OF RIGHT VENTRICULAR HEMODYNAMICS IN THE PRESENCE OF VENTRICULAR SEPTAL DEFECTS*

GERALD A. SERWER and BRENDA E. ARMSTRONG

INTRODUCTION

The use of a contrast agent is uniquely suited for describing intracardiac flow hemodynamics as it allows description of blood flow patterns within cardiac structures. While contrast echocardiography has been used to detect the presence of phenomena such as valvular insufficiency and right-to-left shunting across atrial or ventricular septal defects [1–3], it can further be used to evaluate abnormal pressure and flow states which may vary even in the presence of similar structural defects. As intracardiac pressure–flow relationships are altered by factors in addition to the size of the ventricular septal defect (VSD) itself, knowledge of the specific intracardiac flow pattern present can provide information permitting evaluation of the pulmonary vascular resistance and the presence or absence of pulmonic stenosis. In this chapter, contrast echocardiographic flow patterns present in varying hemodynamic states associated with a ventricular septal defect will be described to enable one to semiquantitatively assess right ventricular and pulmonary artery pressures. Such information coupled with estimation of total shunt size by techniques such as radionuclide angiography provides a very thorough evaluation of such a patient which in many instances would obviate the need for serial catheterizations.

The intracardiac pressure–flow relationships encountered in the presence of a ventricular septal defect and alterations produced by the changing size of the defect or superimposed conditions such as pulmonic stenosis will first be discussed. These hemodynamic states will then be compared to contrast echocardiographic patterns seen. Finally, a discussion of complicating factors will be presented which may prevent, in some cases, utilization of this technique. This is extremely important as awareness of such potential problems can markedly reduce the number of false positive or false negative studies obtained.

PRESSURE–FLOW HEMODYNAMICS

The degree of pressure elevation of the right ventricle and the degree of pulmonary

* This work is supported in part by grants: HL11307, HL20677, HL00718.

overperfusion which exists in the presence of a ventricular septal defect are influenced by not only resistance to blood flow through the lungs themselves, as a consequence of pulmonary vascular resistance, but also by the obstruction of blood flow proximal to the lungs, that is to say, in pulmonic stenosis or resistance across the VSD itself. Defects of less than $1 \text{ cm}^2/\text{m}^2$ in body surface area have been felt to offer significant resistance to flow across them; whereas, defects greater than this in size essentially offer no resistance to flow [4]. Patterns of flow across the defect in varying hemodynamic situations were evaluated by Levin and co-workers [5]. They showed that patients who had right ventricular peak pressures less than 70% of left ventricular pressure demonstrated persistant left-to-right shunting across the defect throughout the cardiac cycle. Even though total shunt size varied between 40 and 60% of total pulmonary blood flow, the interventricular pressure–flow relationships were unaltered. At the end of isovolumic relaxation left ventricular pressure transiently fell below that of the right ventricle but no right-to-left flow of contrast material was demonstrated. Thus, while left-to-right flow may stop at this time in the cardiac cycle, no right-to-left flow occurred.

With further elevation of the right ventricular peak pressure so that it was approximately 80% that of the left ventricular pressure, the transient pressure gradient favoring the right ventricle during isovolumic relaxation was increased in magnitude and now flow from the right to the left ventricle occurred (Figure 1C). This was due to a more rapid pressure fall in the left ventricle than in the right producing a right-to-left gradient when all cardiac valves were closed. This resulted in a right-to-left shunt of blood into the outflow tract of the left ventricle. During diastole the left-to-right gradient was reestablished and the small volume of blood which was shunted into the left ventricle rapidly returned to the right ventricle so that no patient exhibited evidence of systemic right-to-left shunting (Figure 1D). With the onset of isovolumic contraction the left-to-right shunt increased (Figure 1A) and reached its maximum during ventricular ejection (Figure 1B). The phonocardiogram also showed a similar pattern with a holosystolic murmur which began during isovolumic contraction, peaked during ejection, and tapered off during late isovolumic relaxation as the pressure gradient reversed.

With large defects the right and left ventricular peak systolic pressures become equal. Pressure–flow relationships were altered from the previous state. Left-to-right shunting still occurred during isovolumic contraction. During ventricular ejection it was maintained again reaching maximal magnitude (Figure 2A and B). With the onset of isovolumic relaxation a right-to-left pressure gradient was established again as a consequence of the more rapid fall in the left ventricular pressure creating right-to-left shunting into the left ventricle (Figure 2C). This blood was shown to mix in the upper portion of the left ventricle and remained there during diastole despite a small left-to-right gradient (Figure 2D). On the subsequent systole it was ejected into the aorta. Thus, in contrast to the prior group, this situation resulted in right-to-left systemic shunting even though pulmonary vascular resistance might be low and the net left-to-right shunt large.

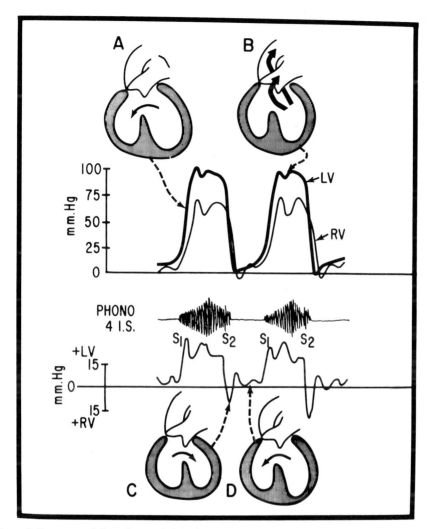

Figure 1. Pressure and flow characteristics of a patient with a ventricular septal defect and LV/RV pressure ratio of 0.75. With the onset of isovolumic contraction (A) a left-to-right shunt is established which reaches its maximal flow during ventricular ejection (B). Phonocardiography shows accentuation of the murmur which reaches its maximum intensity during maximal left-to-right shunting. During isovolumic relaxation a right-to-left pressure gradient is established (C) with right-to-left shunting. Left-to-right pressure gradient is reestablished during late diastole (D). Courtesy of Dr. M.S. Spach.

Finally, children with tetralogy of Fallot with significant pulmonic stenosis exhibited a related, but distinctly different pattern [6]. Again, during isovolumic contraction, the more rapid rise of left ventricular pressure resulted in a left-to-right pressure gradient which rapidly reversed during early ventricular ejection (Figure 3). However, even though a small right-to-left gradient was established, right-to-left flow from the right-to-left ventricle could not be demonstrated. Shunting did occur from the right ventricle directly into the aorta during early ventricular ejection

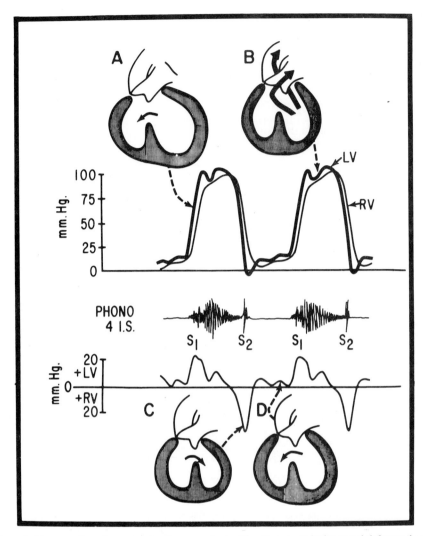

Figure 2. Pressure–flow characteristics from a patient with a large ventricular septal defect and equal right and left ventricular pressures. In (A) a left-to-right gradient is established initially during iso-volumic contraction which again is maximal during ventricular ejection. Again, phonocardiography shows the murmur to be maximal at the time of maximal shunt, but with a more rapid diminution compared to the patient with less than systemic right ventricular pressure. Again, during isovolumic relaxation (C), a right-to-left pressure gradient is established with right-to-left shunting. In late diastole (D), left-to-right shunting is again reestablished. Courtesy of Dr. M.S. Spach.

rather than into the body of the left ventricle. With the commencement of iso-volumic relaxation, the right-to-left pressure gradient was again established which now did result in significant right-to-left shunting from the right to the left ventricle. The establishment of the right-to-left gradient appeared somewhat earlier in the cardiac cycle than it did in the situation of an isolated ventricular septal defect with equal right and left pressures, and initial flow of contrast from the right-to-left

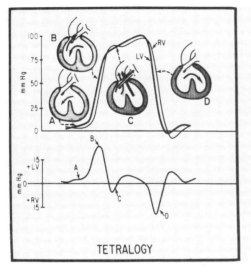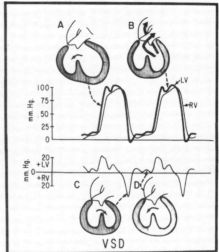

Figure 3. Comparison of pressure–flow characteristics present in tetralogy of Fallot versus a large isolated VSD. Note the transient right-to-left pressure gradient established during early ventricular ejection (C). However, this is associated with direct shunting from the right ventricle into the aorta rather than into the body of the left ventricle. During isovolumic relaxation (D), a right-to-left pressure gradient is established with now right-to-left flow into the body of the left ventricle. Courtesy of Dr. M.S. Spach.

ventricle occurred earlier than had been found for isolated ventricular septal defects. Thus, in children with tetralogy of Fallot, right-to-left shunting occurred during two phases of the cardiac cycle and in two different sites. During ventricular ejection the shunt occurred directly into the aorta while during isovolumic relaxation it occurred across the ventricular septal defect into the left ventricle. There was no shunt from the right to the left ventricle during ejection.

In summary, right-to-left ventricular shunting occurred predominantly during isovolumic relaxation as a consequence of the asynchronous nature of right and left ventricular contraction and relaxation. Right-to-left shunting was a consequence of an earlier fall in left ventricular pressure. This was accentuated in severe obstruction due to tetralogy of Fallot. The reasons for this are not fully understood, but it is logical to assume that conditions in which right ventricular ejection is prolonged, such as with right ventricular outflow, obstruction would produce a right-to-left ventricular shunt earlier within the cardiac cycle. It must also be realized that if right ventricular ejection is significantly delayed, such as with right bundle branch block, then a right-to-left shunt could occur even in situations in which the peak right ventricular pressure is less than peak left ventricular pressure.

CONTRAST ECHOCARDIOGRAPHIC PATTERNS

Based upon the pressure–flow hemodynamics discussed above one might anticipate the ability of contrast echocardiography to distinguish between the various hemodynamic states associated with a VSD. Contrast echocardiographic patterns obtained utilizing peripheral injections do not directly demonstrate left-to-right shunting. Therefore, the important distinguishing considerations revolve around the period of right-to-left ventricular shunting. Echocardiographic contrast patterns to be presented were obtained utilizing standard contrast echocardiographic techniques [7]. All injections were performed into a peripheral vein in either the arm or leg. Saline or the patient's own blood was utilized in all cases with injections not exceeding 2 cm^3 of injectate. Agents such as indocyanine green were not used. Initially, injections were performed while visualizing the right ventricle, interventricular septum, left ventricle, and mitral valve apparatus. Recordings were obtained at a paper speed of 50 mm/s. If contrast material was found to be present in the left ventricle, a second injection was performed while recording at a paper speed of 100 mm/s. A third injection was also performed while visualizing the right ventricular outflow tract, aorta, and left atrium to be certain that the right-to-left shunting visualized previously was not due to right-to-left atrial shunting. A limb lead II electrocardiogram was simultaneously obtained in order to calculate the appearance time.

Appearance time was calculated for all instances of contrast appearing in the left ventricle (Figure 4). The time from the onset of QRS to the first appearance of echo dense material within the left ventricle (AT) was measured. It is emphasized that only the first appearance can be utilized as the presence of contrast material in the left ventricle from prior cardiac cycles interferes with accurate measurement of the true appearance time. All measurements were made at the level of the interventricular septum, since the appearance time measures the earliest time at which any echogenic material is seen in the left ventricle. As this time in seconds varies depending upon heart rate, it is expressed as percentage of the RR interval. Thus, the appearance time/RR interval ratio (AT/RR) becomes independent of heart rate [7].

Five distinct patterns were described. Patients in whom the ratio of right-to-left ventricular pressure was less than 60% did not show any flow of contrast material from the right to the left ventricle. Thus, by this technique, they were indistinguishable from a patient with no ventricular septal defect. Based upon the hemodynamic pressure–flow relationships described previously, this is anticipated as there was no angiographic flow from the right to left ventricle seen in such patients.

The second pattern seen consisted of a transient flow of contrast material from the right to left ventricle commencing during early ventricular filling (Figure 5). During mid to late diastole, echo dense material returned to the right ventricle no longer remaining in the left ventricle when ventricular systole occurred. Thus, no echo dense material was visualized within the aorta in these patients. AT/RR ratio was from 0.60 to 0.69. All patients who possessed such a pattern had a right ventricular to left ventricular peak pressure ratio of from 0.6 to 0.8 and a Q_p/Q_s ratio of from 2.0 to 5.0. Again, this is the pattern to be anticipated based upon pressure–flow relationships shown to be present.

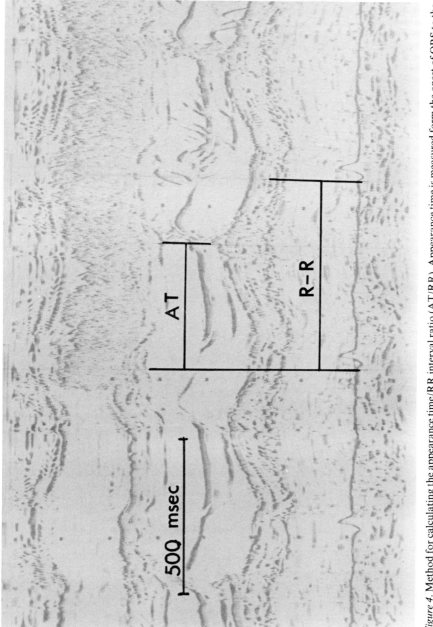

Figure 4. Method for calculating the appearance time/RR interval ratio (AT/RR). Appearance time is measured form the onset of QRS to the first appearance of dye in the left ventricle. This is divided by the RR interval. See text for details. By permission of the American Heart Association [7].

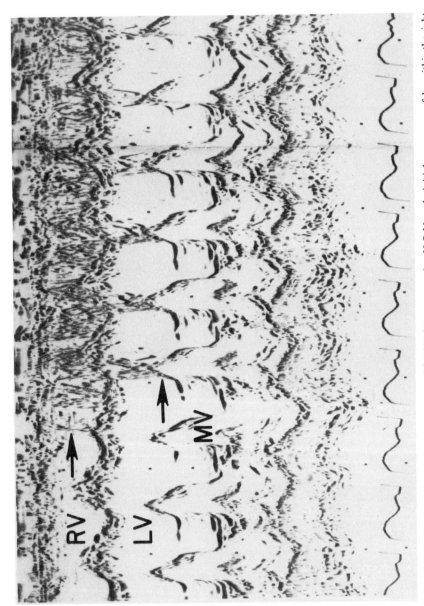

Figure 5. Echocardiographic study from a patient with RV/LV pressure ratio of 0.7. Note the initial appearance of dye within the right ventricle indicated by the arrow, followed by the appearance of dye anterior to the mitral valve in the left ventricle During late ventricular filling, dye returns completely to the right ventricle with none persisting in the left ventricle during ventricular systole. By permission of the American Heart Association [7].

Pattern three occurred in those patients who possessed systemic right ventricular pressure. All had left-to-right shunts greater than 3:1 and none had pulmonic stenosis or elevated pulmonary vascular resistance. Contrast material initially appeared in the left ventricle and, at the same time in the cardiac cycle as did the previous group (AT/RR 0.62–0.69); however, it remained in the left ventricle during ventricular systole and was ejected into the aorta (Figure 6). This again correlates well with the pressure–flow relationships discussed before with right-to-left flow during isovolumic relaxation and early ventricular diastole. Also the right-to-left-shunted blood remained in the left ventricle to be ejected into the aorta (Figure 6B). Thus, in patients with large ventricular septal defects there is a net right-to-left shunt present. This exists in the face of a large left-to-right shunt and normal pulmonary vascular resistance. In addition to the diagnostic implication that this has, it also points out the potential for paradoxical emboli in patients in whom the predominant intracardiac shunt is left-to-right.

The fourth pattern was found in patients in whom a significant degree of pulmonic stenosis was present. All patients had a significant right-to-left shunt with Q_p/Q_s ratio ranging from 0.40 to 0.80. Qualitatively, the echocardiographic picture was the same as for the third pattern with initial appearance of echo dense material during early ventricular diastole (Figure 7). Contrast again remained within the left ventricle during systole to be ejected into the aorta. However, appearance time of contrast within the left ventricle was earlier (compare Figures 6 and 7). AT/RR interval ratios for these patients ranged from 0.53 to 0.59. Again, this is the expected finding as the right-to-left pressure gradient develops earlier in patients with tetralogy of Fallot. Accurate determination of the AT/RR ratio permits easy and complete separation of those patients with pulmonic stenosis and a ventricular septal defect from those patients with an isolated VSD permitting clear distinction of those patients with systemic pulmonary artery pressure from those with low pulmonary artery pressure but systemic right ventricular pressure.

The final pattern was observed in three patients all of whom had an isolated ventricular septal defect and pulmonary vascular resistance greater than 15 units/m^2. In these patients, the appearance time of contrast in the left ventricle was even earlier than in those patients with pulmonic stenosis. This is reflected by the AT/RR ratio for these patients being 0.43, 0.46, and 0.47. While the patient numbers are small, such preliminary results would seem to indicate the sensitivity of this technique for distinguishing pulmonic stenosis from elevated pulmonary vascular resistance in the setting of a ventricular septal defect.

These echocardiographic patterns clearly reflect the pressure–flow patterns described using invasive techniques. One difference is the precise timing of contrast appearance within the left ventricle. Appearance of contrast within the left ventricle lagged slightly behind the development of the right-to-left gradient. Whether this is a reflection merely of a limited area being observed by the echo beam or whether it is a reflection of time necessary for flow to resume once the pressure gradient exists, we cannot say. Certainly inertial effects of the blood column need to be considered

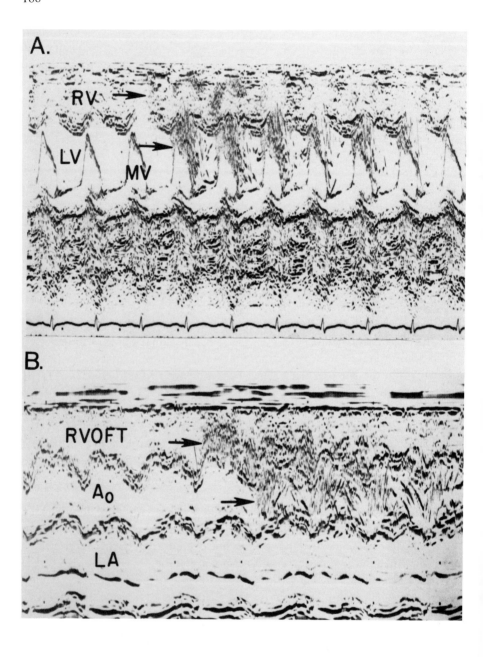

Figure 6. Echocardiographic study of a patient with a large left-to-right shunt and systemic right ventricular pressure. Panel A shows the initial appearance of dye in the right ventricle, indicated by the arrow, with subsequent appearance in the left ventricle anterior to the mitral valve. During ventricular ejection contrast remains in the left ventricle. Panel B shows the initial appearance of the dye in the right ventricular outflow tract followed by subsequent appearance in the aorta. Notice the absence of contrast material in the left atrium. By permission of the American Heart Association [7].

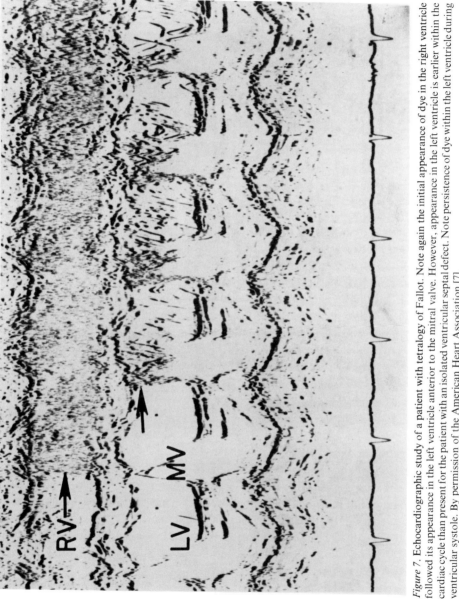

Figure 7. Echocardiographic study of a patient with tetralogy of Fallot. Note again the initial appearance of dye in the right ventricle followed its appearance in the left ventricle anterior to the mitral valve. However, appearance in the left ventricle is earlier within the cardiac cycle than present for the patient with an isolated ventricular septal defect. Note persistence of dye within the left ventricle during ventricular systole. By permission of the American Heart Association [7].

which may reflect the slightly delayed appearance of contrast beyond what would be anticipated if one evaluated pressure gradients alone.

SOURCES OF ERROR

As with any procedure, there are certain instances in which unreliable information is obtained. For accurate assessment of the patient with a ventricular septal defect by this technique, several factors must be fulfilled. From a technical standpoint, all injections must be of adequate quality to completely fill the right ventricle. Incomplete filling of the ventricle by contrast material may fail to show right-to-left flow which may be present. In addition, gain and reject controls must be set appropriately.

There are also several conditions which may exist in the patient negating the value of this technique. First, any atrial level right-to-left shunt creates confusion and makes the diagnosis of a ventricular septal defect and certainly the use of the AT/RR ratio suspect. Thus, any time contrast is visualized in the left ventricle, the left atrium must also be imaged and evaluated for the presence of any contrast material. While in isolated select cases, the diagnosis of both atrial and ventricular level shunting may be possible; in general, the presence of atrial level shunting prevents description of ventricular level shunting. We usually do not make a diagnosis of ventricular level shunting if atrial level shunting exists.

Second, the hemodynamic patterns described depend upon a normal sequence of cardiac activation. Factors which delay right ventricular activation such as right bundle branch block, Wolff-Parkinson-White syndrome with significant preexcitation, complete heart block, and certain ventricular and atrial arrhythmias may significantly alter pressure–flow relationships and invalidate the results presented in this chapter. Attempts to utilize these techniques in such patients should not be made.

The presence of a double-chambered right ventricle in which the ventricular septal defects enters the low pressure chamber obviously negates these results. The presence of ancillary tests that suggests elevation of right ventricular pressure, such as significant right ventricular hypertrophy on the electrocardiogram, coupled with a negative contrast echocardiographic study should alert one to the possibility of this entity being present. Also, the presence of low cardiac output may result in such dilution of the contrast agent that accurate visualization of such flow becomes impossible.

Finally, the position of the VSD itself within the ventricular septum may also alter these results. The presence of low muscular isolated defects results in the right-to-left shunt occurring in the apex of the left ventricle. Utilizing the routine echo positions this region is not visualized and the shunt may be missed. Two-dimensional techniques especially utilizing the subcostal four-chamber view are beneficial in this situation as apical shunts are visualized.

SUMMARY

The use of contrast echocardiography thus permits semiquantitative evaluation of right ventricular and pulmonary artery pressure in the patient with a ventricular septal defect. Coupled with relatively noninvasive techniques for estimating left-to-right shuntings such as radionuclide angiography, a very thorough evaluation of the patient with a ventricular septal defect can be obtained without the need for catheterization. Clearly catheterization is still indicated when surgery is being considered to evaluate the exact position of the defect and to exclude multiple defects. However, if only hemodynamic characterization of the defect is required, then noninvasive techniques are felt to be equally adequate and have the advantage of being performed serially to allow close following of the patient's course. As the natural history of many defects is to show progressive closure, this technique would be extremely beneficial and could potentially obviate the need for catheterization in certain situations. As with all techniques, limitations exist, but it is felt that with adequate knowledge of such limitations this is a very useful technique.

REFERENCES

1. Kerber RE, JM Kroschos, RM Lauer: Use of an ultrasonic contrast method in the diagnosis of valvular regurgitation and intracardiac shunts. Am J Cardiol 34:722, 1974.
2. Valdes-Cruz LM, DR Pieroni, JMA Roland, PJ Varghese: Echocardiographic detection of intracardiac right-to-left shunts following peripheral vein injections. Circulation 54: 558, 1977.
3. Fraker TD Jr, PJ Harris, VS Behar, JA Kisslo: Detection and exclusion of interatrial shunts by two-dimensional echocardiography and peripheral vein injections. Circulation 59:379, 1979.
4. Savard M, HJC Swan, JW Kirklin, EH Wood: Hemodynamics alterations associated with ventricular septal defect. In: Bass AD, GK Moe (eds) Symposium on Congenital Heart Disease, p 141. Am Assoc Adv Sci, Washington DC, 1960.
5. Levin AR, MS Spach, RV Canent Jr, JP Boeneau, MP Capp, V Jain, RC Barr: Intracardiac pressure-flow dynamics in isolated ventricular septal defects. Circulation 35:430, 1967.
6. Levin AR, JP Boineau, MS Spach, RV Canent Jr, MP Capp, PAW Anderson: Ventricular pressure-flow dynamics in tetralogy of Fallot. Circulation 34:1, 1966.
7. Serwer GA, BE Armstrong, PAW Anderson, D Sherman, DW Benson, SB Edwards: Use of contrast echocardiography for evaluation of right ventricular hemodynamics in the presence of ventricular septal defects. Circulation 58:327, 1978.

18. CONTRAST ECHOCARDIOGRAPHY IN VALVULAR REGURGITATION

R.S. MELTZER, P.W. SERRUYS, and J. ROELANDT

INTRODUCTION

Contrast echocardiography in aortic, mitral or pulmonic valvular regurgitation

For the first few years after the introduction of contrast echocardiography by Gramiak, its use was limited to structure identification and shunt detection. In 1974, Kerber reported the use of an ultrasonic contrast method in the diagnosis of valvular regurgitation and intracardiac shunts [1]. He noticed contrast appearing in the left atrium after left ventricular injection in 14 out of 16 patients with mitral regurgitation, and in the left ventricle after aortic root injections in 13 out of 16 patients with aortic regurgitation. Valvular regurgitation as low as 10%, according to angiographic calculations, was detected by this method. One false positive study due to catheter-induced mitral regurgitation was noted. The authors concluded that M-mode ultrasonic monitoring of catheter injections distal to a regurgitant valve is a sensitive and specific – though qualitative – technique for detecting valvular regurgitation. Other laboratories, including our own, have confirmed that intracardiac injections during catheterization can be monitored by echocardiography and that this is a sensitive method for the detection of valvular regurgitation. Little further work has been reported in this area, and this invasive technique probably has only limited applications in the occasional patient where there is a strong contraindication to the use of ionizing radiation, for example in early pregnancy [2].

This chapter will deal largely with a newer application of contrast echocardiography in the diagnosis of valvular regurgitation:

Contrast echocardiography for the diagnosis of tricuspid valvular regurgitation

In 1978, the group from Duke University reported on a contrast echocardiographic method for the diagnosis of tricuspid regurgitation [3]. Their subsequent experiences were detailed at the symposium in Rotterdam in 1979 [4], and at the American Heart Association meeting in late 1979 [5]. Their technique involved upper extremity injections of ultrasonic contrast material during two-dimensional echocardiographic imaging of the inferior vena cava, trying to detect retrograde flow of contrast agents into the inferior vena cava. They reported that the appearance of contrast during systole in the inferior vena cava was a sensitive and specific diagnostic sign for the presence of tricuspid regurgitation. We noticed the presence of systolic contrast in several patients without tricuspid regurgitation, and undertook the following study in order to: 1) examine sensitivity and specificity of peripheral contrast echocardiography in the diagnosis of tricuspid regurgitation, 2) attempt to ascertain the reason for false positive and false negative studies and 3) examine the utility of M-mode echocardiography in the diagnosis of tricuspid regurgitation [6].

METHODS

Patient population

We studied 62 patients with both M-mode and two-dimensional echocardiography of the inferior vena cava during upper extremity injections of 5% dextrose in water. Ten patients had a definite clinical diagnosis of tricuspid regurgitation, based on the jugular venous pulse, the holosystolic murmur increasing with respiration and, frequently, a pulsating liver.

Forty patients were studied because they had cardiac disorders frequently associated with tricuspid regurgitation, such as mitral stenosis, pulmonary hypertension, or former tricuspid valve surgery. Twelve further patients were included in the study because they were normal, as judged by history, physical examination and echocardiography.

Patients were divided into three groups on the basis of clinical and/or invasive evaluation of the tricuspid valve. Group A included 21 patients: 10 with clinically definite tricuspid regurgitation (5 also had the diagnosis confirmed by invasive studies) and 11 with clinically uncertain tricuspid regurgitation but positive invasive studies. Group B also comprised 21 patients: 12 normal subjects and 9 patients from the group with uncertain tricuspid regurgitation who had no tricuspid regurgitation at invasive studies. The remaining 20 patients with clinically uncertain tricuspid regurgitation and no invasive studies constituted group C.

Echocardiographic methods

All patients were studied in the supine position with the knees and hips slightly flexed to achieve maximal abdominal relaxation. The M-mode or two-dimensional echocardiographic transducer was placed in the subcostal position, just to the right of the midline, and the inferior vena cava was imaged in a sagittal plane by two-dimensional echocardiography [7]. A number 16 or 18 gauge intravenous cannula was introduced into an antecubital vein and a three-way stopcock was attached. Repeated, rapid, hand injections of 5-8 cc of 5% dextrose solution were made, using a 10 cc syringe. In some patients 1 cc to 3 cc of carbon dioxide were added to the 5% dextrose solution to insure adequate echocardiographic contrast [8]. M-mode echocardiograms were obtained with an EchocardioVisor SE (Organon Teknika) interfaced to a Honeywell LS6 stripchart recorder. Two-dimensional echocardiograms were recorded using a Toshiba SSH-10A phased-array sector-scanner or an Organon Teknika EchocardioVisor 03 multielement linear-array instrument. They were stored on videotape for subsequent analysis.

Diagnosis of tricuspid regurgitation

On right ventricular angiograms, tricuspid regurgitation was diagnosed if contrast appeared in the right atrium in the absence of premature beats. Intraoperative diagnosis of tricuspid regurgitation involved palpation of a thrill on the right atrium prior to cannulation for cardio-pulmonary bypass, making sure that there was no traction on the heart that might cause false tricuspid regurgitation [9].

RESULTS

Patterns of inferior vena cava contrast appearance

Using M-mode tracings of the inferior vena cava, we identified four different patterns of contrast appearance after upper extremity intravenous injections. The first is the pattern of tricuspid regurgitation, which we call the v-wave synchronous pattern. This is illustrated in Figure 1. The second pattern, the a-wave synchronous pattern, is characterized by the appearance of contrast in the inferior vena cava during the a-wave of the right atrial pressure tracing or jugular venous pulsation or even inferior vena cava "a" pulsation. The contrast reverses direction and, in the early part of systole, is seen returning to the right atrium, as illustrated in Figure 2. Both of these patterns give one pulsation per beat on the two-dimensional echocardiogram, and are very difficult to separate in real-time. Slow motion and stop frame analysis is necessary to analyze timing of inferior vena cava contrast appearance

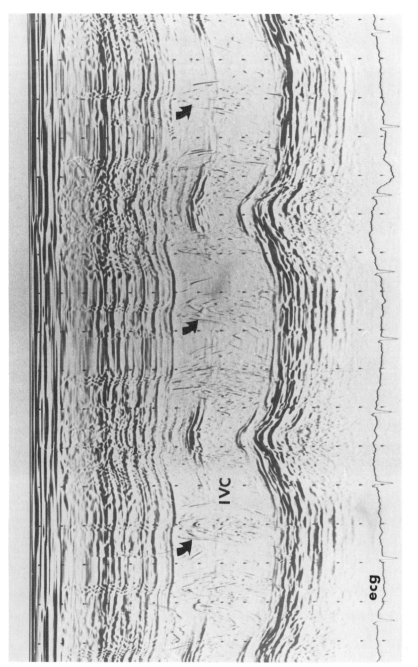

Figure 1. M-mode inferior vena cava (IVC) tracing after upper extremity intravenous injection of 5% dextrose solution in a patient with tricuspid regurgitation. Note appearance of v-wave synchronous contrast (arrows) in the IVC – a pattern diagnostic for tricuspid regurgitation.

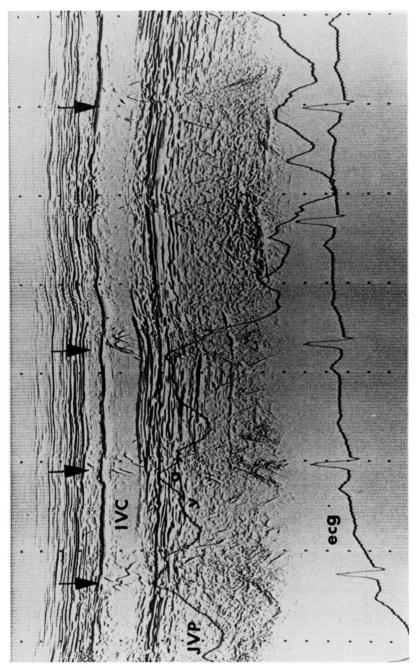

Figure 2. M-mode inferior vena cava (IVC) tracing after upper extremity intravenous injection of 5% dextrose solution in a patient without tricuspid regurgitation. Note contrast (arrows) in the IVC appearing during the "a" wave of the jugular venous pulse tracing (JVP). This a-wave synchronous pattern is not consistent with tricuspid regurgitation.

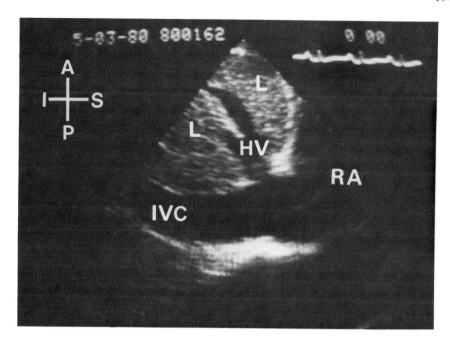

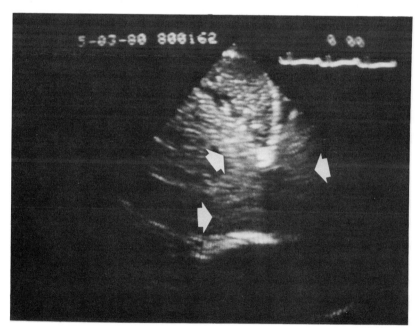

Figure 3. Upper panel: right parasagittal two-dimensional echocardiogram in a patient with tricuspid regurgitation, before upper extremity intravenous injection of 5% dextrose solution. Lower panel: 15 seconds later, with contrast (arrows) now filling the right atrium (RA), inferior vena cava (IVC) and hepatic vein (HV). Further abbreviations; L = liver; A = anterior; P = posterior; I = inferior; S = superior.

properly from two-dimensional echocardiograms (Figure 3). The initial appearance during normal respiration is the most important information for diagnosis. Timing analysis is considerably simplified using M-mode echocardiography. We have called the third pattern of contrast appearance in the inferior vena cava the "random" pattern. In this pattern, contrast is seen in the inferior vena cava with no definite relation to the cardiac cycle and mainly appears during deep inspiration. The "random" pattern is the false positive most frequently associated with atrial fibrillation, where an a-wave synchronous pattern is not possible. The last pattern identified was designated "no contrast appearance". That is, despite echocardiographic imaging of the inferior vena cava during and immediately after a peripheral contrast injection, no contrast is seen moving retrograde into the inferior vena cava at any time.

Relation of echocardiographic pattern to presence or absence of tricuspid regurgitation

The distribution of the four echocardiographic patterns among patient groups A, B and C is displayed in Table 1. It is clear from this table that the

Table 1. Distribution of patterns among patients groups (TR = tricuspid regurgitation).

Group	v-wave synch.	a-wave synch.	random	no contrast
A (n = 21) TR	19	0	0	2
B (n = 21) no TR	0	6	5	10
C (n = 20) ? TR	11	6	3	0

Table 2. Sensitivity and specificity of contrast echo in the diagnosis of tricuspid regurgitation.

		Presence of TR +	Presence of TR −
Contrast	+	19	0
Echo	−	2	21

Sensitivity   19/21 = 90%
Specificity   21/21 = 100%

v-wave synchronous pattern is the diagnostic pattern of tricuspid regurgitation, with a sensitivity of 90% and specificity of 100% in our patient
population (Table 2). However, group B patients frequently have contrast in
the inferior vena cava during systole, particularly in relation to deep
inspiration or at the end of a Valsalva maneuver, but its initial appearance is
always either an a-wave synchronous or a random pattern.

M-mode versus two-dimensional echocardiography in the diagnosis
of tricuspid regurgitation

The title of this section is misleading, since M-mode and two-dimensional
echocardiography are complementary and not inimical techniques. However,
we wished to examine the utility of M-mode echocardiography in the
diagnosis of tricuspid regurgitation, since the original report from Duke was
only concerned with two-dimensional echocardiography [3]. We had the
impression that M-mode echocardiography might be at least as good, and
perhaps preferable.

The 62 study subjects had both M-mode and two-dimensional contrast
echocardiograms. Each study was categorized as one of the four patterns
mentioned above (v-wave synchronous, a-wave synchronous, "random", or
no contrast appearance). Fifty-one patients had the same M-mode and
two-dimensional echocardiographic patterns of contrast appearance in the
inferior vena cava, divided as follows: 27 v-wave synchronous, 13 no
contrast, 8 a-wave synchronous, and 3 random. Within this group, timing
analysis was always easier by M-mode than by two-dimensional studies.
Eleven patients had contrast seen in the inferior vena cava on the M-mode
study but not during two-dimensional imaging after upper extremity contrast
injection. All 11 had verification of adequate right heart contrast during the
two-dimensional study. The distribution of M-mode patterns was as follows:
4 a-wave synchronous, 4 random, 3 v-wave synchronous. Only two of these
eleven patients had invasive diagnostic tests for tricuspid regurgitation. Both
of these were patients with no regurgitation; one had an M-mode a-wave
synchronous pattern. Two further clinically normal subjects had small
amounts of a-wave synchronous contrast in the inferior vena cava on the
M-mode study but not on the two-dimensional study.

Some signs of tricuspid regurgitation have been proposed that are unique
either to M-mode or to two-dimensional echocardiography. The "back-
and-forth motion" of contrast echo across the tricuspid valve during the
cardiac cycle on two-dimensional echocardiography has been proposed as a
sign of tricuspid regurgitation. It has also been proposed as a sign of
regurgitation of other cardiac valves. We found this to be an extremely
subjective sign, lacking either sensitivity or specificity. There is a normal

retrograde motion of contrast in both the right ventricle and right atrium as the tricuspid valve closes, and it was nearly impossible to differentiate reliably between where this normal retrograde movement ended and where abnormal "back-and-forth motion" began. A possibly more useful sign, but one which needs further study, is an M-mode sign: a large number of highly negatively-sloping contrast lines, seen in the right atrium just below the tricuspid valve during systole. We have noticed this sign in several patients, but have not systematically studied its sensitivity or specificity.

Studies after tricuspid valve surgery

Ten patients were studied more than one month after a De Vega tricuspid valvuloplasty for tricuspid regurgitation. Nine of these were in atrial fibrillation, and all nine had a "v-wave synchronous" pattern on echocardiography suggesting continued tricuspid regurgitation. Only 4 of these had tricuspid regurgitation clinically. Two patients were studied pre and postoperatively, and little change in their "v-wave synchronous" pattern could be detected. The patient in normal sinus rhythm had the "random" pattern suggesting the absence of significant tricuspid regurgitation.

Four patients were studied after tricuspid valve replacement with a porcine bioprosthesis. Three were in atrial fibrillation and demonstrated a "v-wave synchronous" pattern, with small amounts of inferior vena cava contrast, as assessed subjectively (one was positive only during end-inspiration, another had a positive M-mode but a negative two-dimensional study). The fourth, in normal sinus rhythm, had an "a-wave synchronous" pattern.

DISCUSSION

As indicated on Table 2, peripheral contrast echocardiography is a sensitive and specific test for the diagnosis of tricuspid insufficiency. However, this is the case only if the following precautions have been taken: studies must not be considered negative unless the echocardiographer is sure that adequate right heart opacification has been achieved on multiple injections, timing analysis has excluded v-wave synchronous inferior vena cava contrast appearance, and the operator is aware of the causes of false positive and false negative studies listed in Table 3.

Since timing analysis is improved when using M-mode, and we have encountered two-dimensional studies where contrast was not imaged in the inferior vena cava when it was seen by M-mode (but not vice versa), we feel that M-mode inferior vena cava imaging should always be used – either alone or in combination with two-dimensional studies.

Table 3. Contrast inferior vena cava echo for tricuspid regurgitation diagnosis.

False positive	False negative
— a-wave synchronous pattern	— Failure to achieve adequate central contrast
— Randon pattern	— Failure to use M-mode
— Deep inspiration	— M-mode beam too inferior
— M-mode beam too superior	

Our experience that tricuspid regurgitation in general does not completely resolve after tricuspid surgery is in line with other recently reported angiographic data [10]. We wish to emphasize, though, that contrast inferior vena cava echocardiography, as we report it, is not a quantitative technique. Perhaps Doppler echocardiography, either alone or possibly in combination with contrast, may help to further refine the noninvasive diagnosis and quantification of tricuspid regurgitation [11].

The role of contrast echocardiographic techniques in diagnosing non-tricuspid valvular regurgitation is at present minor, though it is conceivable that a large number of upward-sloping contrast trajectories during diastole may be an important M-mode diagnostic sign for pulmonary regurgitation [12]. Since, clinically, creation of left-sided contrast now requires cardiac catheterization, the use of contrast echocardiography to diagnose aortic or mitral regurgitation is rarely necessary. Even with transpulmonary transmission of contrast, the "back-and-forth" sign is unlikely to have sufficient sensitivity or specificity to aid considerably in the diagnosis of left-sided valvular regurgitation. It is conceivable that combined Doppler/contrast techniques may be useful in this setting in the future, if noninvasive trans-pulmonary transmission of echocardiographic contrast becomes available [13].

REFERENCES

1. Kerber RE, JM Kioschos, RM Lauer: Use of an ultrasonic contrast method in the diagnosis of valvular regurgitation and intracardiac shunts. Am J Cardiol 34:722, 1974.
2. Meltzer RS, PW Serruys, J McGhie, PG Hugenholtz, J Roelandt: Cardiac catheterization under echocardiographic control in a pregnant woman. Am J Med 71:481, 1981.
3. Lieppe W, VS Behar, R Scallion, JA Kisslo: Detection of tricuspid regurgitation with two-dimensional echocardiography and peripheral vein injections. Circulation 57:128, 1978.
4. Kisslo JA: Usefulness of M-mode and cross-sectional echocardiography for analysis of right-sided heart disease. In: Echocardiology (Lancée, CT, ed.), pp 37–47, Martinus Nijhoff, The Hague, 1979.

5. Wise NK, S Myers, JA Stewart, R Waugh, T Fraker, J Kisslo: Echo inferior venacavography: a technique for study of right sided heart disease. Circulation 59–60 (suppl II): II–202, 1979.
6. Meltzer RS, DCA van Hoogenhuyze, PW Serruys, MMP Haalebos, PG Hugenholtz, J Roelandt: The diagnosis of tricuspid regurgitation by contrast echocardiography. Circulation 63:1093, 1981.
7. Meltzer RS, C Meltzer, J Roelandt: Sector scanning views in echocardiography: a systematic approach. Europ Heart J 1:379, 1980.
8. Meltzer RS, PW Serruys, PG Hugenholtz, J Roelandt: Intravenous carbon dioxide as an echocardiographic contrast agent. J Clin Ultrasound 1:127, 1981.
9. Pepine CJ, WW Nichols, JH Selby: Diagnostic tests for tricuspid insufficiency: How good? Cath & Cardiovasc Diagnosis 5:1, 1979.
10. Simon R, H Oelert, HG Borst, PR Lichtlen: Influence of mitral valve surgery on tricuspid incompetence concomitant with mitral valve disease. Circulation 62 (suppl I):I–152, 1980.
11. Fantini F, A Magherini: Detection of tricuspid regurgitation with pulsed Doppler echocardiography. In: Echocardiology (Lancée CT, ed.), pp 233–235, Martinus Nijhoff, 1979.
12. Gullace G, M Savoia, V Locatelli, F Schubert, C Ranzi: Evaluation of linear contrast echo on pulmonary valve echogram. International Meeting on Bidimensional Echocardiography, Milan, 1980, pp 72–73 (abstract).
13. Meltzer RS, OEH Sartorius, CT Lancée, PW Serruys, PD Verdouw, C Essed, J Roelandt: Transmission of echocardiographic contrast through the lungs. Ultrasound in Medicine and Biology 7:377, 1981.

19. CONTRAST ECHOCARDIOGRAPHY IN PERSISTENT FETAL CIRCULATION

E. J. Meijboom, M. H. Gewitz, D. C. Wood, and W. W. Fox

INTRODUCTION

Echocardiography has an established role in the evaluation of the cyanotic newborn. Its value for the recognition of an abnormal intracardiac anatomy is well published and widely accepted.

Contrast echocardiography has less often been used to document and localize the exact level of right-to-left shunting. It can add substantially to the information about anatomic malformations already recognized by standard echocardiography, but it has unique features in cyanotic patients with normal intracardiac relations [9, 11, 12], for instance patients with persistent fetal circulation syndrome [1, 2, 3, 4, 5, 6, 7, 8]. This syndrome remains a complicated perinatal management problem and is associated with a high incidence of mortality, due to intractable hypoxemia. The right-to-left shunting in these patients is based on severely elevated pressures in the pulmonary artery system. An early diagnosis and initiation of therapy in these patients is important. The purpose of this paper is to describe our experience with contrast echocardiography as a tool for both, evaluation and management of such patients.

MATERIALS AND METHODS

The twenty-two newborns studied by contrast echocardiography were divided into two groups.

The control group of eleven newborns *without* persistent fetal circulation included four patients with congenital heart disease (three d-Transposition of the Great Arteries (d-TGA) and one cor triatriatum), three with mild meconium aspiration, three with transient cyanotic episodes without underlying cardiopulmonary disease and one with mild respiratory distress syndrome. Four of these patients required ventilatory assistance and five needed only supplemental oxygen. The three infants with d-TGA had contrast echocardiography performed before and after cardiac catheterization and balloon atrioseptostomy.

The eleven patients *with* persistent fetal circulation, all required extensive ventilatory support [1, 3, 7], ten of them at a very early stage. Five of the ten succumbed, four as a result of hypoxemia and one from a late complication (necrotizing enterocolitis).

Contrast studies were carried out according to previously described methods [9, 11, 12, 13]. The transducer (5.0 MHz) was positioned to view the right ventricular outflow tract, the aortic root at valvular level and the left atrium, from a standard M-mode transducer position, with the recorder set at a paper speed of either 100 mm per second or 50 mm per second [14]. A bolus of 5% dextrose/water was administered via an indwelling venous line in either the umbilical vein or a peripheral vein of a lower extremity. Approximately $\frac{1}{4}-\frac{1}{2}$ cc/kg of fluid was rapidly injected, the total never exceeding 2 cc. Each study was recorded at least twice and, for recording, the reject control was set to eliminate the overload phenomenon described by others [9]. If contrast was visualized in both the right ventricular outflow tract and the left atrium (and subsequently in the aortic root), the presence of a right-to-left intracardiac shunt was confirmed. In these patients, the time interval (in milliseconds) between the appearance of contrast in the right ventricular ourflow tract and its first appearance in the left atrium was measured and was recorded as the LA-RV difference. LA-RV difference measurements greater then zero milliseconds indicate that contrast was noted first in the left atrium and subsequantly in the right ventricular outflow tract, consistent with a large right-to-left shunt at the atrial level (Figure 1).

LA-RV difference measurements less than zero milliseconds indicate that contrast was noted first in the right ventricular outflow tract and later in the left atrium and was considered to be consistent with a relatively smaller degree of righ-to-left shunting (Figure 2).

On three occasions, the M-mode studies were confirmed using two-dimensional echocardiography, enabling more specific determination of the level of intracardiac shunting.

For this study, M-mode echocardiograms were obtained with an Irex Continuetrace System II echocardiograph and the two-dimensional echocar-diograms were performed using an ATL Mark V System.

RESULTS

Figure 3 shows an M-mode tracing of a control patient in which contrast is only seen in the right ventricular outflow tract while the left atrium and the aorta remain echo free. Figure 4 demonstrates a typical contrast echocardio-gram as obtained from a patient with persistent fetal circulation; contrast fills the left atrium, followed by the aortic root and the right ventricular outflow tract, indicating a marked degree of right-to-left shunting.

LA-RV differences were measured as previously described. For example in

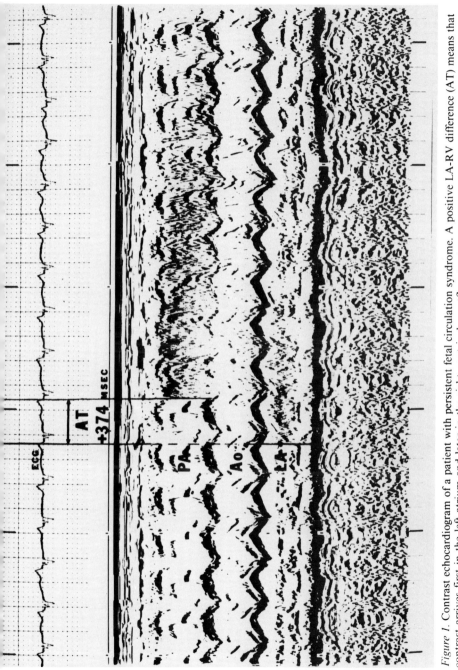

Figure 1. Contrast echocardiogram of a patient with persistent fetal circulation syndrome. A positive LA-RV difference (AT) means that contrast arrives first in the left atrium and later in the right ventricular outflow tract.

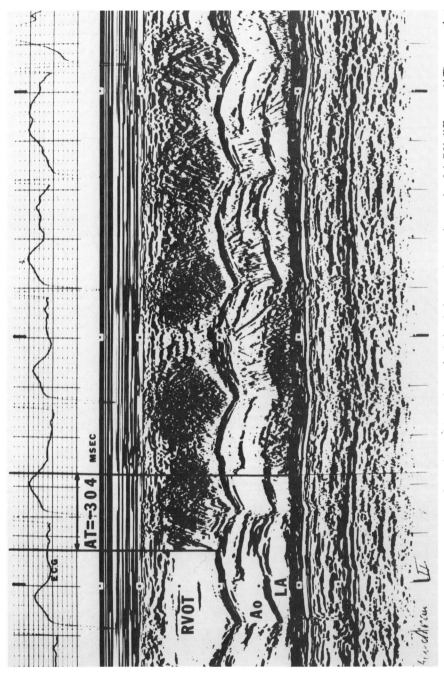

Figure 2. Contrast echocardiogram of a patient with persistent fetal circulation syndrome. A negative LA-RV difference (AT) means that contrast arrives first in the right ventricular outflow tract and later in the left atrium.

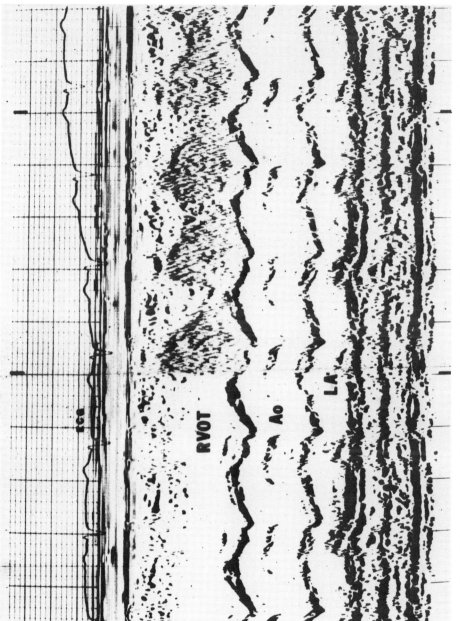

Figure 3. Contrast echocardiogram from a control patient in which no right-to-left intracardiac shunt is noted.

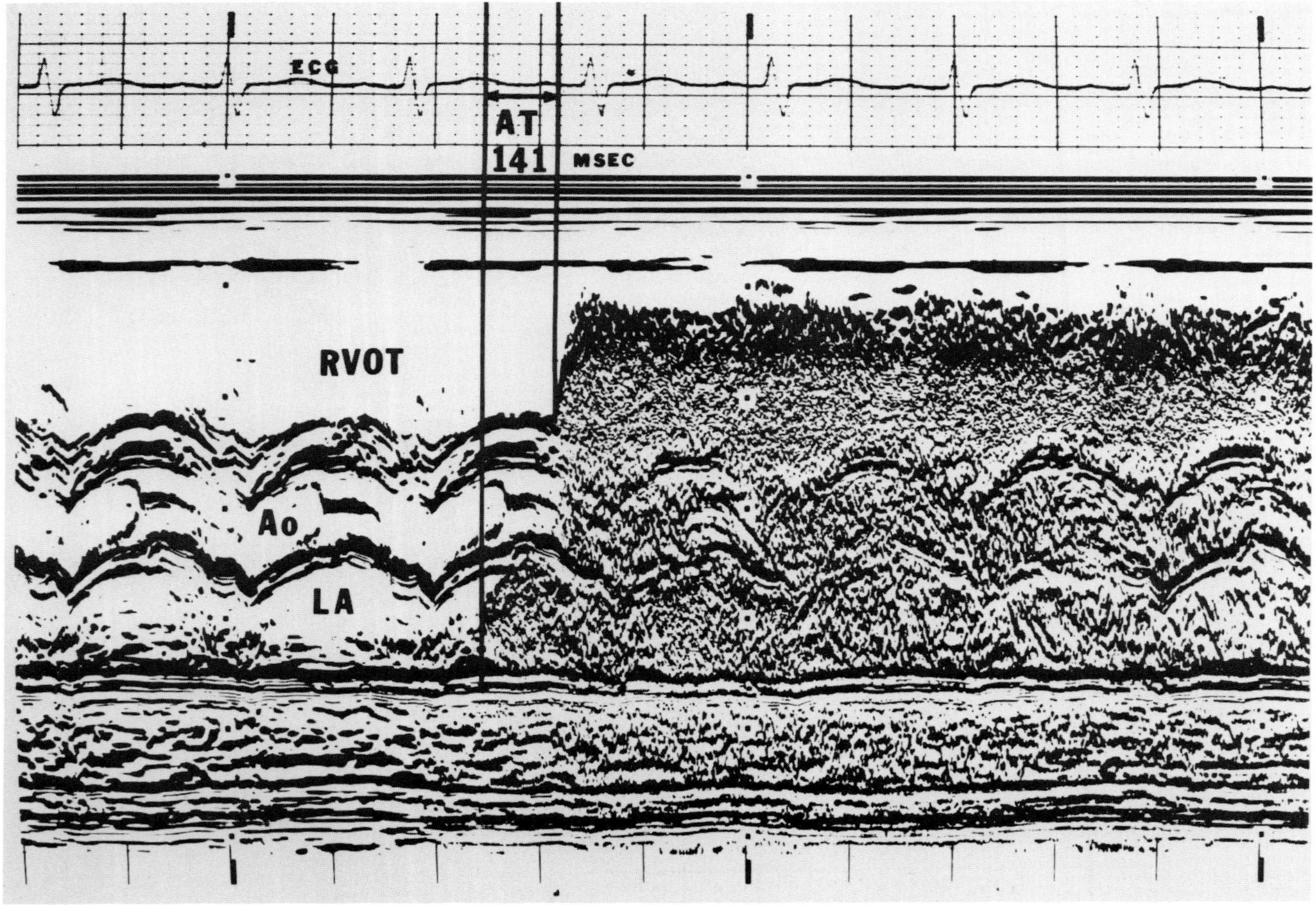

Figure 4. Initial contrast echocardiogram of a patient with persistent fetal circulation syndrome. Contrast is seen first in the left atrium

Figure 4, the time interval between the appearance of contrast in the left atrium and its first appearance in the right ventricular outflow tract is approximately 141 milliseconds.

In ten of the eleven control patients no right-to-left shunting was seen on the contrast echocardiogram, although contrast was clearly identified in the right ventricular outflow tract in all cases. In one control patient, later proven at cardiac catheterization to have cor triatriatum, contrast was apparent in the well defined inferior part of the left atrium. Thus this child did have right-to-left shunting at atrial level, but only in a part of the left atrial chamber below an atrial membrane, and this membrane had already been recognized as an anatomical abnormality.

In the three control patients with d-TGA, contrast echocardiography showed no right-to-left shunting before septostomy. After catheterization and balloon atrioseptostomy these contrast echocardiograms became positive, indicating that a satisfactory atrial communication had been established.

Ten of the eleven patients with persistent fetal circulation demonstrated right-to-left shunting on their initial contrast echocardiogram. In one patient no right-to-left shunting was present in the initial study, but was subsequently noted on the second contrast echocardiogram one day later. For the group, the LA-RV difference, on the inital contrast echocardiograms, varied from +755 milliseconds to −320 milliseconds, mean = +300 milliseconds. As indicated earlier, these values represented right-to-left shunting, with negative values being found in the smaller shunts.

Assessment of both highest (positive) and lowest (negative) LA-RV difference did not yield any specific correlation between either LA-RV difference and clinical indices of disease or LA-RV difference and prognosis.

As shown in Figure 5, the appearance times in eight of the eleven patients with persistent fetal circulation were followed serially over the first nine days of their illness. In the six surviving patients the pattern of LA-RV difference was seen to follow a consistently decreasing trend, which corresponded to an improving clinical picture. In one other infant a decresing LA-RV difference was recorded, which paralleled the patient's clinical course, but this infant ultimately succumbed to severe necrotizing enterocolitis despite improvement in the underlying persistent fetal circulation syndrome. Of the four infants who succumbed of intractable hypoxemia, three lived only long enough for one contrast echocardiogram and the fourth demonstrated an increasing LA-RV difference until he died.

Two-dimensional contrast echocardiography was performed in two patients with persistent fetal circulation and clearly localized the shunt to the atrial level while confirming the absence of other intracardiac abnormalities. A completely different picture was seen in the two-dimensional contrast study of the child with a cor triatriatum, where the membrane and the

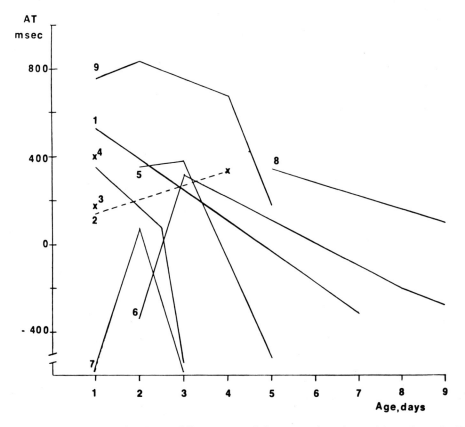

Figure 5. Serial changes in LA-RV difference over clinical course in patients with persistent fetal circulation.
AT = LA-RV difference, msec = milliseconds, x = expired.

contrast flow, which was confined to the lower left atrium, provided clear differentiation from the other patients.

DISCUSSION

These data demonstrate the usefulness of contrast echocardiography in establishing the diagnosis of intracardiac right-to-left shunting in newborns suspected of having persistent fetal circulation. In addition, serial evaluation of these patients with contrast echocardiography appears to verify objectively the changing magnitude of the intracardiac right-to-left shunt as the clinical course proceeds.

These results are consistent with previous publications which have demonstrated the ability of contrast echocardiography to evaluate intracardiac right-to-left shunting [9, 11, 12, 13]. Other noninvasive methods of estimating pulmonary artery pressure and pulmonary vascular resistance, such as the use of echocardiographic right ventricular systolic time intervals, have been proposed [15], but recent data have raised questions about the reliability of such techniques [16]. All but one of the persistent fetal circulation patients in this series showed right-to-left shunting on the first contrast echocardiography. In the patient whose contrast echocardiogram showed no intracardiac right-to-left shunting, a repeat study the following day did demonstrate a shunt. This patient followed a clinical course typical of some patients with persistent fetal circulation in whom pulmonary pressures may not be at their highest early in the disease but then gradually increase further over the first few days of life [1]. Thus, in such patients contrast echocardiography can be helpful for following the development of an intracardiac shunt.

The absence of right-to-left shunting on precatheterization contrast echocardiography in the three control patients with d-TGA is consistent with the severe clinical picture associated with negligible bidirectional flow at the atrial level. After successful balloon atrioseptostomy, mixing at the atrial level was demonstrated by contrast echocardiography.

Our findings underscore the point that if the diagnosis of persistent fetal circulation is suspected clinically, right-to-left shunting should be demonstrated on contrast echocardiography. If it is not seen, the diagnosis of persistent fetal circulation is suspect. Of course, right-to-left intracardiac shunting can occur in certain forms of congenital heart disease not necessarily associated with pulmonary hypertension, such as tricuspid or pulmonary atresia, Ebstein's anomaly or right ventricular dysfunction associated with myocardial ischemia. Similarly, the patient in our series with cor triatriatum exemplifies a situation in which congenital heart disease may be associated with pulmonary hypertension and intracardiac right-to-left shunting. In these instances, however, the total clinical picture, chest x-ray, electrocardiogram and standard echocardiogram usually point to a diagnosis other than persistent fetal circulation.

Finally, while the magnitude of the LA-RV difference was not correlated with any specific clinical factor such as blood gas data or ventilatory pressures, changes in the LA-RV difference in both degree and direction may be helpful for evaluation of therapy. Management of these patients often requires hyperventilation [1] which can be associated with serious complications, including pneumothorax and pneumopericardium. Since pCO_2 is often kept at low levels, and pO_2 may be variable, depending on several factors including parenchymal lung problems, measures of LA-RV difference offer a noninvasive means of evaluating changes in the intracardiac shunting

pattern. Although in these patients we did not use LA-RV difference for clinical management, our data suggest that a decreasing LA-RV difference would permit the clinician to reduce hyperventilation at a time when other measurements may not clearly suggest improvement. It should be noted, however, that the specific numerical value for LA-RV difference may be related to the timing of injection of contrast, as well as to the level of pulmonary arterial pressure. Thus, contrast arriving in the right atrium in. diastole may produce a shorter LA-RV difference than that produced by contrast reaching the right atrium in systole.

SUMMARY

Contrast echocardiography has been shown to be helpful in clarifying the diagnosis and in following the intracardiac shunting patterns in a group of infants with the clinical picture of persistent fetal circulation. In certain instances, contrast echocardiography can provide enough corroborating evidence to obviate the need for cardiac catheterization in these critically ill newborns. Serial evaluation of these children using contrast echocardiograms may be helpful in following their clinical course and in adjusting therapy.

REFERENCES

1. Peckham GJ, WW Fox: Physiologic factors affecting pulmonary artery pressure in infants with persistent pulmonary hypertension. J Pediatr 93:1005, 1978.
2. Gersony WM: Persistence of fetal circulation, a commentary. J Pediatr 82:1103, 1973.
3. Fox WW, MH Gewitz, R Dinwiddie, WH Drummond, GJ Peckman: Pulmonary hypertension in the perinatal aspiration syndromes. Pediatrics 59:205, 1977.
4. Haworth SG, L Reid: Persistent fetal circulation; newly recognized structural features. J Pediatr 88:614, 1976.
5. Burnell BH, MC Joseph, MH Lees: Progressive pulmonary hypertension in newborn infants. Amer J Dis Child 123:167, 1972.
6. Siassi B, SJ Goldberg, GC Emmanouilides, SM Higashino, L Elmore: Persistent pulmonary vascular obstruction in newborn infants. J Pediatr 78:610, 1971.
7. Drummond WH, GJ Peckman, WW Fox: The clinical profile of the newborn with persistent pulmonary hypertension: observations in 19 affected neonates. Clin Peds 16:335, 1977.
8. Rowe RD: Abnormal pulmonary vasoconstriction in the newborn. Peds 59:318, 1976.
9. Roelandt J, RS Meltzer, PW Serruys, J McGhie, W Gorissen, WB Vletter: Contrast Echocardiografie (preliminary information).
10. Levin DL, MA Heymann, JA Kitterman, GA Gregory, RH Phibbs, AM Rudolph: Persistent pulmonary hypertension of the newborn infant. J Pediatr 89:626, 1976.

11. Valdez-Cruz LM, DR Pieroni, A Roland, PJ Varghese: Echocardiographic detection of intracardiac right-to-left shunts following peripheral vein injections. Circulation 54:558, 1976.
12. Serwer GA, BE Armstrong, PAW Anderson, et al.: Use of contrast echocardiography for evaluation of right ventricular hemodynamics in the presence of ventricular septum defects. Circulation 58:327, 1978.
13. Serruys PW, M van den Brand, PG Hugenholtz, J Roelandt: Intracardiac right-to-left shunt demonstrated by two-dimensional echocardiography after peripheral vein injection. Br Heart J 42:429, 1979.
14. Meyer RA: Pediatric echocardiography. Lea and Febiger, Philadelphia, 1977.
15. Hirschfeld S, R Meyer, DC Schwartz, J Korfhagen, S Kaplan: Echocardiographic assessment of pulmonary artery pressure and pulmonary vascular resistance. Circulation 82:642, 1975.
16. Silverman MD, RA Snider, AM Rudolph: Evaluation of pulmonary hypertension by M-mode echocardiography in children with ventricular septal defect, Circulation 61:1125, 1980.

20. APPLICATIONS OF CONTRAST ECHOCARDIOGRAPHY FOR ANALYSIS OF COMPLEX CONGENITAL HEART DISEASE IN THE NEWBORN

DAVID J. SAHN, STANLEY J. GOLDBERG, HUGH D. ALLEN, and LILLIAM M. VALDES-CRUZ

INTRODUCTION

M-mode echocardiography, and subsequently two-dimensional echocardiography, have had a major impact in the evaluation of the critically ill neonate suspected of congenital heart disease. It is not uncommon for difficulties to arise in distinguishing cardiac from pulmonary disease in the newborn infant, as many forms of cyanotic heart disease and pulmonary disease have a similar physiology and symptomatology [1].

Echocardiography often provides such detailed anatomic information as to be of significant import in patient diagnosis and management. Nonetheless, it is not uncommon to wish to clarify certain aspects of the patient's condition by making a statement about cardiac flow. It is in this realm of clarification of cardiac flow patterns that M-mode and two-dimensional echo contrast studies are useful in the examination of infants [2].

Common to many forms of cyanotic heart disease in the newborn period are right-to-left shunts. These right-to-left shunts may occur at the atrial or ventricular level, or at the great artery level when complex malformations are present. As such, contrast echocardiography from the venous side of the heart provides important diagnostic information regarding the site and sometimes the magnitude of the right-to-left shunt. At the present time, experimental work continues into production of echo contrast agents which will traverse the lungs to the left ventricle, allowing diagnosis of left-to-right shunts on echocardiography. These agents are not, however, clinically applicable to humans at this time. In the critically ill neonate, the question of the presence of a right-to-left shunt is often a more important consideration. Venous echo contrast injections can supply this information.

There are several specific factors which appear to allow good venous echocardiographic contrast injections in the neonate, even with small amounts of relatively standard agents, such as saline, indocyanine, or the patient's own blood, without the need to progress to more sophisticated echocardiographic contrast agents. These factors include: 1) the prevalence of central venous lines in neonates (often umbilical lines) placed in the perinatal period; 2) the short distances involved between injection sites (even in peripheral veins) and the cardiac chambers; and 3) the small volume of the circulatory system and the rapid circulation time. These factors combine to produce good quality contrast venous injections, even from

1 cm^3 of contrast material injection [3]. Additionally, many sick neonates have an indwelling arterial line placed in the umbilical artery as well, allowing arterial contrast injections to define extracardiac communications at the aortic and pulmonary levels, such as patent ductus arteriosus. We had previously believed that these umbilical artery lines needed to lie above the diaphragm to allow adequate definition of patent ductus arteriosus and the thoracic aorta [4]. It has subsequently been our experience that placing the infant in a frog-legged position and applying a vigorous 1 cm^3 injection is often enough to produce contrast opacification of the aortic arch, even with an umbilical artery catheter placed below the diaphragm.

A cautionary note regarding the neonatal circulation in the transitional period is appropriate. The inferior vena caval return, which previously carried umbilical venous blood, appears to be significantly directed toward the left atrium, whereas superior vena caval return is directed toward the tricuspid valve. As such, if a right-to-left shunt exists at the atrial level, it is often significantly overestimated on inferior vena caval injections, and may be underestimated or even missed on superior vena caval injections. The site of injection is therefore important in evaluating the perinatal circulation, not only with regard to the aorta, as mentioned above, but also with regard to venous injection techniques as well.

This chapter will review the use of contrast M-mode echocardiography in the perinatal period and will summarize more recent observations involving two-dimensional echocardiography for elucidation of complex congenital heart disease. It should be pointed out, however, that the M-mode technique allowing a time–motion plot of contrast passage is often more adequate for defining small amounts of contrast within ventricular cavities or great arteries than replaying a real-time examination on videotape. Frame-by-frame review of videotapes of real-time examinations is of assistance in this matter, but the M-mode echocardiogram derived from a known location on a phased-array image appears to allow advantages of both spatial orientation and time–motion display. M-mode echocardiography will, therefore, continue to be useful for contrast evaluation despite the advent of the recent more dramatic two-dimensional techniques. Two-dimensional echocardiography, however, often shows the holes through which contrast passes and allows the possibility of surveying a larger area of the heart.

M-MODE VENOUS CONTRAST TECHNIQUES FOR ANALYSIS OF SHUNTING

Various forms of congenital heart disease present with cyanosis in the newborn infant. In addition, a number of types of lung disease may present with right-to-left shunts, either at atrial or ductal levels. Many normal newborn infants will have a right-to-left shunt at the atrial level, especially when they cry. Venous contrast injection techniques can demonstrate this right-to-left shunt, and two-dimensional echocardiography can also demonstrate that the foramen ovale in these infants is open when they cry. Figure 1 is an illustration from a newborn infant showing an

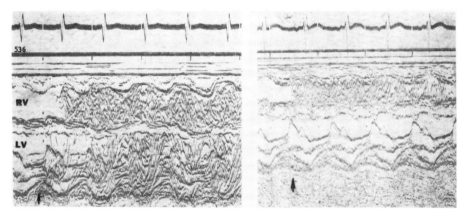

Figure 1. In the left panel, an inferior vena cava flush of an umbilical venous catheter in an infant undergoing exchange transfusion demonstrates a significant right-to-left atrial shunt which disappears by the time the infant is three days old, as shown in the right panel.

echocardiogram performed during an exchange transfusion for Rh disease. As can be seen in the left panel, when the infant is less than 24 hours of age, a significant right-to-left shunt exists, with contrast material passing through the mitral valve funnel into the left ventricle. The appearance of contrast in the mitral funnel actually seems to precede contrast appearing in the right ventricle. When the same infant was studied during a subsequent exchange transfusion 48 hours later, the right-to-left shunt disappeared. As such, a transient right-to-left atrial shunt is not uncommonly found in normal newborns who do not have any lung disease, and is even more commonly found in patients with cardiopulmonary disease. In infants with respiratory distress syndrome, pulmonary hypertension, and persistent fetal circulation, this right-to-left shunt may continue for a significant period of time beyond 48 hours and may be of significant magnitude. A right-to-left shunt may exist in these form of lung disease at the ductal level and is sometimes manifested as a difference in oxygen saturation between the ascending and descending aorta. This right-to-left shunt at the ductal level is difficult to demonstrate by M-mode echocardiography, but it can be demonstrated by two-dimensional echocardiography [5], and will be discussed briefly later in this chapter. In tetralogy of Fallot, forms of truncus arteriosus or pulmonary atresia with decreased blood flow, a significant right-to-left shunt may exist at the ventricular level. This right-to-left shunt may be visualized by contrast echoes traversing the ventricular septum in front of the mitral valve and is somewhat indistinguishable from the appearance of a hypertensive ventricular septal defect. The echo from an infant with ventricular septal defect and pulmonary hypertension is shown in Figure 2. In tetralogy of Fallot, however, the enlarged aorta overriding the septum and the filling of the aorta with contrast material with significant right-to-left shunting aids in distinguishing this abnormality. The suprasternal notch scan likewise gives important information regarding the relative distribution of flow to the pulmonary and systemic circulations after

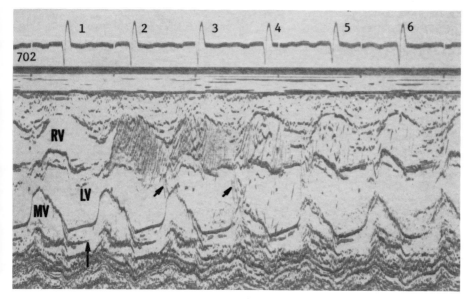

Figure 2. Right-to-left shunting through a large VSD in a neonate with hyperkinetic pulmonary hypertension is visualized by peripheral venous saline contrast appearing in front of the mitral valve.

venous contrast injection. When pulmonary blood flow is significantly decreased with poor communication between the right ventricle and the pulmonary artery, very little contrast material appears in the right pulmonary artery, with most of it appearing in the transverse aorta on echo contrast injection. This is true not only when there is significantly decreased flow because of tetralogy or forms of truncus arteriosus or pulmonary atresia, but also when there are significant intracardiac shunting and severe pulmonary hypertension (persistent fetal circulation). In forms of truncus arteriosus with increased pulmonary blood flow, delayed filling of the right pulmonary artery after venous contrast injection may be a clue to the diagnosis. The truncal override of the ventricular septum is visualized on the M-mode echo as well as the truncal root itself filling with contrast material after the venous injection. The suprasternal notch scan shows slightly delayed filling of the right pulmonary artery with contrast material.

Mortera et al. [6] suggested that infants with simple transposition have passage of more echo contrast material into the aorta on suprasternal notch scanning than into the pulmonary artery, and that this identification of aortic filling (since the aorta does not change its suprasternal notch position) suggests the diagnosis of transposition. We, in general, believe that this finding is true and an adjunct method for making the diagnosis of transposition of the great vessels, but believe that two-dimensional echocardiography is the method of choice for making this diagnosis [7]. We have found, as stated above, that it is not uncommon for extremely cyanotic infants, who have congenital heart disease or lung disease, to have significant aortic filling. These infants have massive right-to-left intracardiac shunts; as such, heavy

filling of the aorta with contrast material imaged on suprasternal notch scans is not specific for transposition.

Contrast echocardiography does have significant application in the diagnosis of transposition, however. As shown in Figure 3, venous injection of contrast material in transposition patients is a useful way of identifying a ventricular septal defect shunt, since the right ventricle is the systemic one at higher pressure. Contrast echoes pass into the lower pressure "pulmonary" ventricle traversing the ventricular septum if a ventricular septal defect is present. The illustration also suggests how the suprasternal notch approach in this particular case shows equal contrast effect in the transverse aorta and right pulmonary artery. Note, additionally, that this patient does not have very much contrast in the left atrium and appears to have very poor left atrial filling after venous contrast injection. We have applied contrast echocardiography extensively in transposition for evaluating the adequacy of interatrial mixing [1]. It has been our observation that, following balloon atrial septostomy and rise in pO_2, a significant increase in left atrial filling after venous injection can be observed. The venous contrast echocardiographic injection (Figure 4 left panel) from an infant with pO_2 of 18 Torr, shows filling of the right ventricular outflow tract but little filling of the pulmonary artery and left atrium, indicating a very poor interatrial mixing of arterial and venous blood. In the right panel after performance of a balloon atrial septostomy, contrast material is observed not only in the left atrium, but subsequently in the pulmonary artery, showing interatrial mixing in the face of transposition with intact ventricular septum.

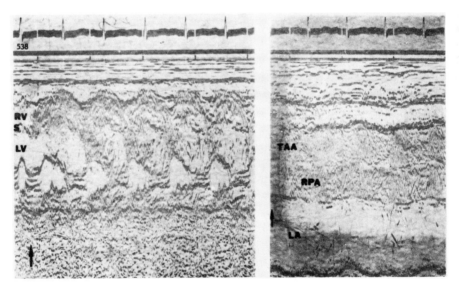

Figure 3. An infant with transposition: the left panel shows significant ventricular shunting with contrast appearing in front of the mitral valve. The right panel shows the suprasternal notch scan with equal filling of the transverse aorta and right pulmonary artery and scant filling of the left atrium. Reproduced by permission of the American Heart Association from Sahn et al., Circulation 56:6, 1977.

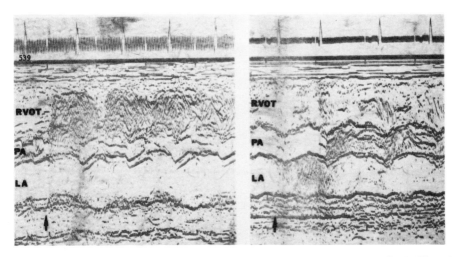

Figure 4. An infant with transposition of the great arteries. The left panel shows no significant filling of the left atrium an pulmonary artery, since there is no little interatrial mix. In the right panel after balloon septostomy significant filling of the left atrium and pulmonary artery is observed. Reproduced by permission of the American Heart Association from Sahn et al., as in Figure 3.

OBSERVATIONS IN NEONATES WITH COMPLEX FORMS OF CONGENITAL HEART DISEASE

Seward et al. [8] have published some elegant studies which suggest how contrast echo aids in evaluating atrioventricular valve morphology in single ventricle (i.e., univentricular heart). Figure 5 demonstrates an example of this utility. Two atrioventricular valves are visualized within one cavity. The majority of contrast filling, shown after the arrow, appears to come through the anterior atrioventricular valve. In this particular case, both atrioventricular valves were known to exist and there was no suggestion of ventricular septum. If one atrioventricular valve had been missed, the fact that contrast material would enter in front of the imaged atrioventricular valve gives a clue to the fact that there is a second atrioventricular valve within that single ventricular cavity. Seward and co-workers have also derived specific timing parameters which appear to allow distinction of single or double inlet left ventricle from large ventricular septal defects. We believe the latter anatomic distinctions are made more accurately using two-dimensional echocardiography.

Lesions in which pulmonary venous and systemic blood flows into one cavity and mixes before distribution to the body are commonly referred to as "admixture" lesions. The level of cyanosis in these patients is often proportional to the balance of pulmonary and systemic blood flow. Another example of a lesion like this is tricuspid atresia. Infants with tricuspid atresia have a significant right-to-left shunt at the atrial level and, usually, a left-to-right shunt at the ventricular level. As shown in Figure 6, injection of contrast in this infant with a small right ventricular outflow

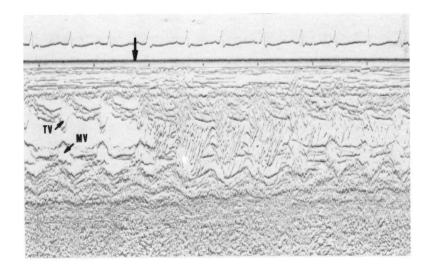

Figure 5. Two AV valves are visualized within a single ventricular cavity with contrast injection into a vein. Most of the contrast appears to enter this single ventricle through the anterior rightward AV valve. Reproduced by permission of Yearbook Medical Publishers from Goldberg et al., Pediatric and Adolescent Echocardiography, 2nd Ed, Chicago, Yearbook, 1980.

cavity initially shows right-to-left atrial passage with filling of the mitral funnel and left ventricle. Filling of the right ventricular outflow cavity occurs late after filling of the left side. This is also suggested in the lower left panel, which shows left atrial and, in fact, aortic filling preceding filling of the right ventricular outflow cavity. Early appearance of contrast in the left atrium followed by appearance of contrast in both the transverse aorta and right pulmonary artery is shown in the lower right panel. The contrast echocardiogram, therefore, shows a flow pattern consistent with late filling of the outflow cavity, a pattern which is not distinctive of tricuspid atresia, but is also seen in forms of single ventricle. Once again, the transverse aortic-right pulmonary artery image after contrast injection gives a suggestion of the distribution of flow between the aortic and pulmonary cirulations.

M-MODE ARTERIAL CONTRAST FOR IDENTIFYING PATENT DUCTUS ARTERIOSUS

The suprasternal notch view has been quite useful for contrast echocardiography not only in venous applications, as stated above, but in arterial or, most commonly, aortic injections performed through an umbilical artery catheter in infants. We have used these techniques for demonstrating left-to-right shunt in patients with patent ductus arteriosus not only when there is uncomplicated patent ductus arteriosus in premature infants, but also at times when patent ductus arteriosus coexists with

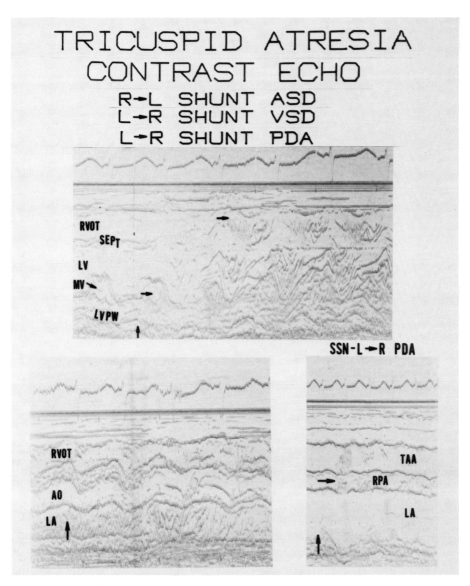

Figure 6. An M-mode contrast injection delineates the flow patterns in a patient with tricuspid atresia. Initial filling of the left ventricle occurs through the mitral valve funnel and there is late filling of the small right ventricular outflow cavity as shown in the upper panel. In the lower left panel again left atrial fill precedes filling of the aorta and the right ventricular outflow cavity. In the lower right panel left atrial fill precedes filling of both aorta and right pulmonary artery. Reproduced by permission of Yearbook Medical Publishers from Goldberg et al., as in Figure 5.

other forms of complex congenital heart disease [4]. As shown in Figure 7, the suprasternal notch view of a descending aortic injection demonstrates the left-to-right ductal shunt by filling of the right pulmonary artery. An example of one of these injections is shown in the echocardiogram displayed in Figure 8. We have used

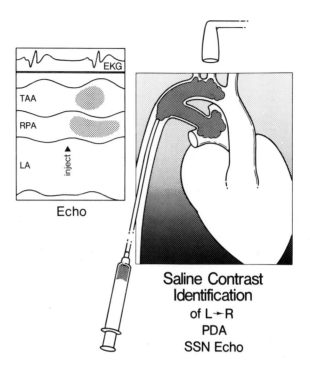

Figure 7. Diagrammatic illustration shows umbilical arterial contrast injection into the descending aorta and how it would show a left-to-right shunt through a patent ductus arteriosus during suprasternal notch echocardiography. Reproduced by permission of the American Heart Association from Sahn et al., as in Figure 3.

this technique serially to determine and follow ductal patency while the umbilical arterial catheter is in place.

In other infants in whom most pulmonary blood flow is derived from the transverse aorta, such as in tetralogy of Fallot or pulmonary atresia, the contrast echo is likewise useful when the small pulmonary artery can be identified. As shown in Figure 9 (left panel) the infant has truncus arteriosus with brisk, almost simultaneous, filling of the right pulmonary artery after an aortic flush. The right panel shows an infant with pulmonary atresia and small patent ductus arteriosus; the dotted area shows a small amount of contrast in the right pulmonary artery. The aortic injection shunt is not, however, specific for patent ductus arteriosus, but just demonstrates filling of the pulmonary artery from the aorta. In some infants, other injection sites for left-sided contrast can be used. Figure 10 shows an infant with a left-sided Blalock shunt placed for tetralogy of Fallot. In this illustration, the left radial arterial line is flushed, and filling of the right pulmonary artery documents the patency of the anastomosis.

The echocardiogram, therefore, assists in making some of these more complicated diagnoses and in following serially the physiology of these diseases through the perinatal and postoperative periods.

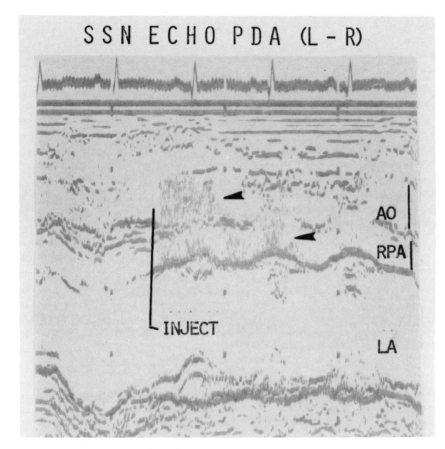

Figure 8. A suprasternal notch echocardiogram after aortic injection shows fill initially of the transverse aortic arch and significant and persistent fill of the right pulmonary artery in an infant with a left-to-right shunting patent ductus arteriosus.

TWO-DIMENSIONAL ECHOCARDIOGRAPHIC CONTRAST APPLICATIONS

Two-dimensional echocardiograms using contrast injections are often significantly more dramatic because contrast is visualized passing through the chambers on the two-dimensional image and the position of contrast and its passage can be more adequately localized. These techniques can be used to distinguish false "holes" caused by echo dropout from real holes, and can be used to assess the direction of shunting of defects that are visualized. The use of positive and negative contrasts in atrial septal defect and simple shunts is covered elsewhere in this book. We will emphasize techniques for using contrast in more complicated conditions specifically relevant to the newborn infant.

As stated above, silent patent ductus arteriosus, as a simple lesion, or ductus present in conjunction with other forms of congenital heart disease, may go un-

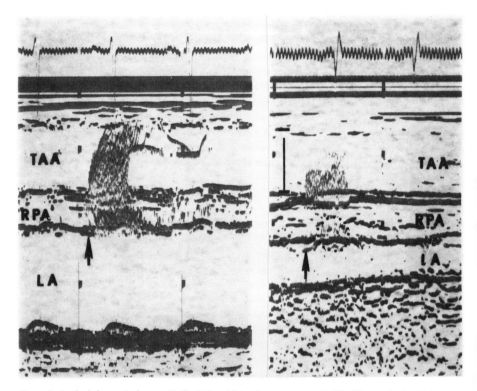

Figure 9. In the left panel after aortic flush the right pulmonary artery is filled in a patient with truncus arteriosus. Significant left-to-right shunting exists in this patient who really has an admixture lesion. In the right panel an infant with pulmonary atresia has a small ductus arteriosus and minimal contrast is visualized within the small right pulmonary artery after aortic injection.

detected in premature infants. Two-dimensional echocardiography can image the ductus as shown in Figure 11. As shown in Figure 12, injection of echo contrast material in the aorta often allows demonstration of contrast material passing into the pulmonary artery through the imaged patent ductus arteriosus. The same techniques can be used to demonstrate right-to-left shunting patent ductus arteriosus after venous contrast injection. Right-to-left shunting ductus arteriosus often accompanies significant pulmonary hypertension or left-sided inflow obstruction and is commonly seen in the hypoplastic left heart syndrome.

Shunting of blood across the atrial septal defect is often easy to demonstrate on two-dimensional echoes in four-chamber or subcostal views. Figure 13 shows a patient with an atrial septal defect which accompanied cyanotic congenital heart disease. In the lower panel, after venous injection, contrast appears not only in the left atrium just behind the mitral valve but also in the left ventricle. A significant right-to-left shunt through the atrial septal defect is shown. Ventricular septal defects can be imaged directly using two-dimensional echocardiography. Minimal right-to-left contrast passage across ventricular septal defects is quite frequent in

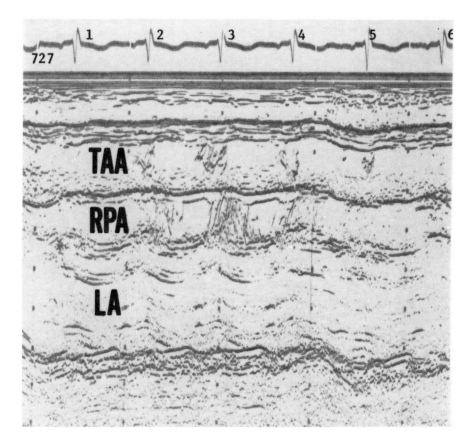

Figure 10. An infant with tetralogy of Fallot after a Blalock-Taussig shunt has a left radical line flushed. Significant fill of the right pulmonary artery through the left-sided Blalock-Taussig anastoms s is visualized by appearance of contrast in the right pulmonary artery.

the newborn period when pulmonary pressure is high. Therefore, when a question exists as to whether a ventricular septal defect as imaged is real or represents echo dropout, imaging of contrast passing across the ventricular septal defect is of help. We believe the positive passage of contrast across the ventricular septal defect from right ventricle to left ventricle is significanty of more use than the concept of negative contrast which we find difficult to apply in the newborn period.

We have also used contrast echocardiography for identification of additional ventricular septal defects in sick neonates undergoing heart surgery. Figure 14 shows a patient with a membranous ventricular septal defect who was studied during his surgery with the chest open and the sterilized ultrasound probe applied directly to the beating heart. This patient was found to have an additional muscular ventricular septal defect, demonstrated by contrast passing across the muscular ventricular septal defect from left to right after a saline injection into the left atrial appendage. These combinations of contrast echocardiography with intraoperative

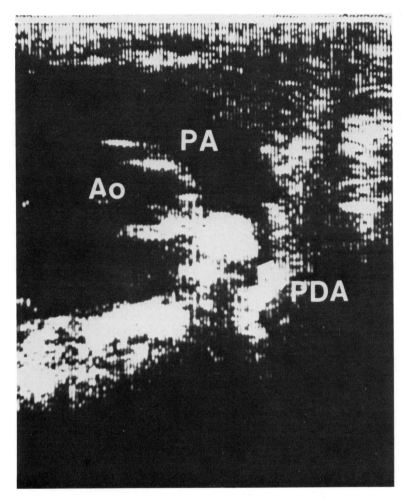

Figure 11. A short-axis view at the level of the great artery shows the technique for imaging a patent ductus arteriosus as the pulmonary artery wraps around the aorta and continues to the descending aorta as a tortuous ductus.

scanning appear to be quite useful for verifying surgical anatomy.

In infants with transposition of the great arteries, as stated in the section on M-mode contrast, the M-mode contrast injection technique is quite useful for verifying an adequate interatrial mix. As we have previously suggested [7], two-dimensional echocardiography is useful for imaging the atrial septal defect created by balloon atrial septostomy (Figure 15). The combination of contrast injection with sub-xiphoid imaging aids in defining the presence of right-to-left shunting and mixing of arterial and venous blood across this newly created atrial septal defect.

Other examples of the use of echocardiography in even more complicated lesions include definition of flow patterns through atrioventricular valves suspected of overriding the ventricular septum. As show in Figure 16, the diagnosis of a sus-

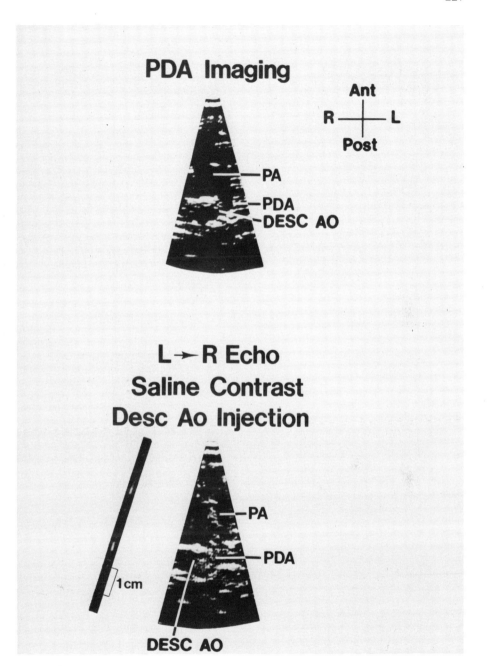

Figure 12. Shows descending aortic flush during ductal imaging. In the lower panel contrast passes left-to-right through the imaged ductus into the pulmonary artery.

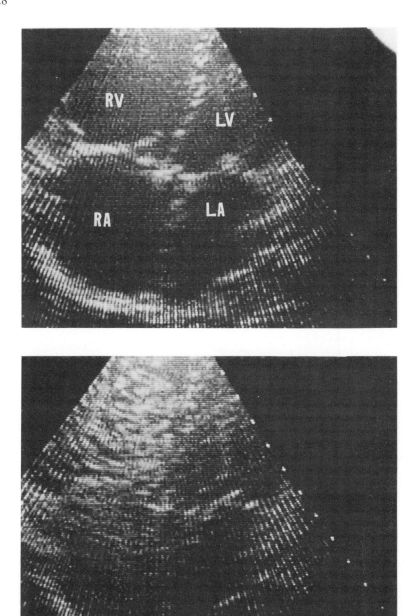

Figure 13. The upper panel shows a large right ventricle with a significant amount of atrial dropout. The lower panel verifies that there is a significant right-to-left shunt with filling of the left atrium and the left ventricle after venous contrast verifying the presence of a large atrial septal defect present in conjunction with cyanotic congenital heart disease.

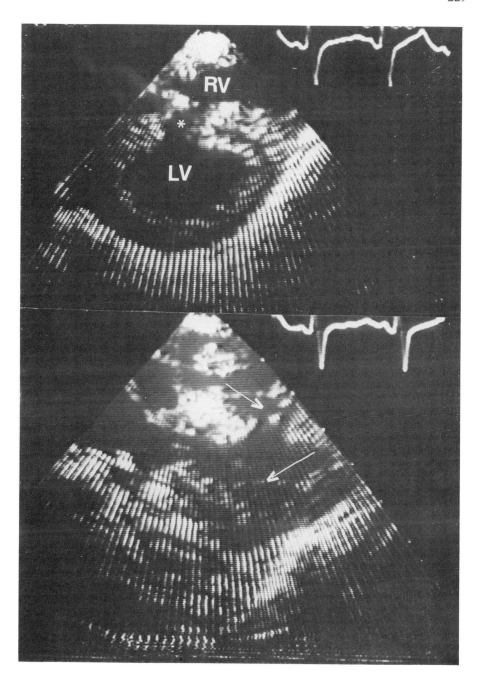

Figure 14. Intraoperative contrast study shows the filling of the right ventricle and contrast passage (arrows) through a muscular VSD (*) located low on the ventricular septum which was present in addition to the previously suspected membranous VSD in this patient.

230

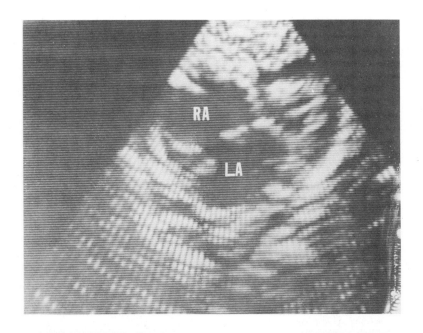

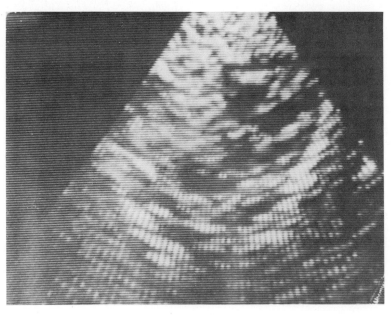

Figure 15. Subcostal echo shows the interatrial communication after balloon septostomy. The contrast injection shows contrast passing across the ASD into the left atrium.

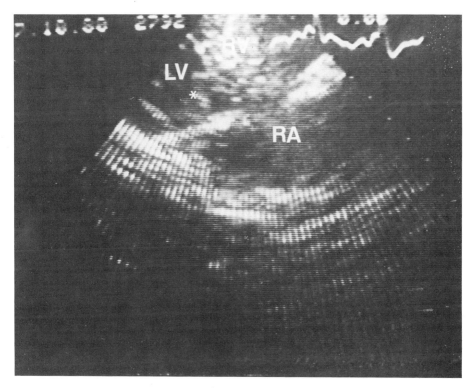

Figure 16. In this patient the tricuspid valve overrides a ventricular septal defect with tricuspid valve appearing to lie towards the left side of the septum (*). Filling of left ventricular inflow area along with the right ventricular cavity verifies the physiologic overriding of the tricuspid valve.

pected overriding tricuspid valve is verified when contrast is shown crossing the ventricular septal defect quite briskly through the tricuspid inflow, with small amounts of contrast passing just to the left of the ventricular septum into the left ventricle. A combination of contrast with two-dimensional echocardiography can define very complex atrioventricular valve relationships and complements angiography in defining the spatial relationships, since it is combined with positive structural imaging rather than a shadow technique. In these complicated cases, we commonly perform contrast echocardiography in the catheterization laboratory at the time of angiography to provide additional information without the osmotic load of additional radiographic contrast injection.

As another example, in neonates with univentricular hearts, two-dimensional echocardiography can help define flow patterns. Figure 17 shows a patient with univentricular heart after a venous contrast injection. The single ventricle fills completely with contrast as does the right atrium. Contrast, however, is not present in the left atrial cavity at all. In real-time, the separate washing out of the left atrioventricular valve inflow with unopacified blood with no contrast was visualized, as well as the complete mixing of contrast through the single ventricular cavity. In the

232

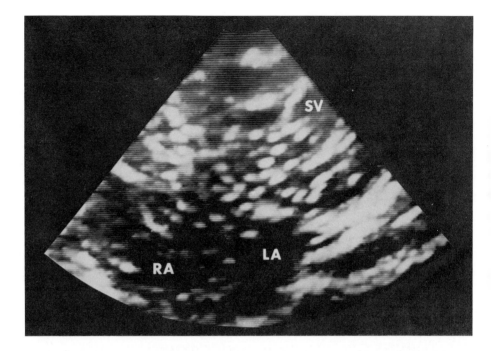

Figure 17. Venous contrast injection into a patient with single ventricle shows brisk filling and mixing of the entire single ventricular cavity, filling mainly with opacified contrast through the right AV valve. The atrial septum is intact and the left atrium remains free of contrast. In real-time the wash into the left AV valve was echo free. Reproduced by permission of Yearbook Medical Publishers from Goldberg et al., as in Figure 5.

patient shown in Figure 18, single ventricle exists in conjunction with what is suspected to be an atretic right-sided atrioventricular, or tricuspid, valve. In this patient, the injection of the contrast agent shows passage of the contrast material only across the left-sided valve (labeled mitral valve) with no contrast appearing to wash in through the atritic tricuspid bar.

As such, the contrast echo flow observations appear to validate and confirm the anatomical observations of two-dimensional echocardiography in defining the atrioventricular valve morphology of complex congenital cardiac malformations.

SUMMARY

The critically ill neonate is a fragile individual, who is difficult to move for diagnostic studies, and is particularly susceptible to the deleterious osmotic and other effects of radiographic contrast agents. Defining the anatomy and physiology with a combination of M-mode, two-dimensional, and contrast echocardiography is of significant assistance in diagnosing heart disease and following serially the

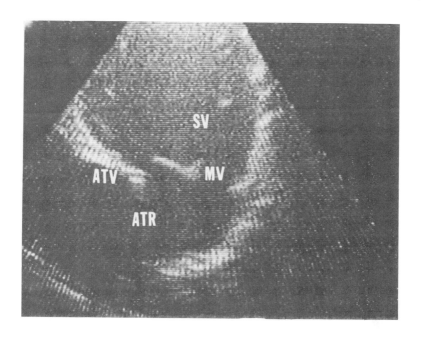

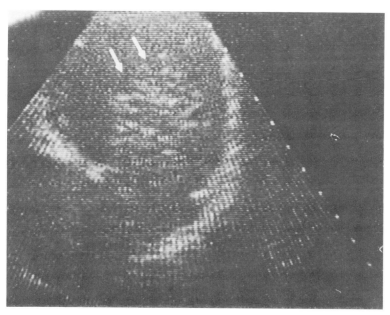

Figure 18. A patient with single ventricle appears to have one AV valve, a left-sided mitral valve and an atretic right-sided AV valve. Contrast injection verifies the passage of contrast into the single ventricular cavity only through the orifice of the patent left-sided AV valve.

dramatically changing cardiovascular physiology of these infants over the first few days of life. The large caliber umbilical arterial and venous lines, quite commonly placed in intensive care nurseries of monitoring purposes, aid in the performance of bedside contrast echocardiography. Two-dimensional echocardiography allows for accurate diagnosis and may be combined with contrast injection performed at cardiac catheterization or at surgery for defining additional lesions. Recent work in our laboratory suggests that Doppler echocardiography is even more sensitive for detecting contrast passage than M-mode or two-dimensional echo imaging. Additional work involving Doppler detection and evolution of contrast agents able to pass through the pulmonary capillary bed to produce opacification on the left side of the heart should add additional utility to contrast echocardiography for evaluation of the critically ill neonate.

REFERENCES

1. Sahn DJ, WF Friedman: Difficulties in distinguishing cardiac from pulmonary disease in the neonate. Pediatr Clin North Am 20:293–301, 1973.
2. Sahn DJ, HD Allen, W George, M Mason, SJ Goldberg: The utility of contrast echocardiographic techniques in the care of critically illl infants with cardiac and pulmonary disease. Circulation 56:959–603, 1977.
3. Valdes-Cruz LM, DR Pieroni, J-M Roland, PJ Varghese: Echocardiographic detection of intracardiac right-to-left shunts following peripheral vein injections. Circulation 54:558–562, 1976.
4. Allen HD, DJ Sahn, SJ Goldberg: New serial contrast technique for assessment of left-to-right shunting patent ductus arteriosus in the neonate. Am J Cardiol 41:288–294, 1978.
5. Sahn DJ, HD Allen: Real-time cross-sectional echocardiographic imaging and measurement of the patent ductus arteriosus in infants and children. Circulation 58:343–354, 1978.
6. Mortera C, S Hunter, M Tynan: Contrast echocardiography in the suprasternal notch approach in infants and children. Eur J Cardiol 9:437–454, 1979.
7. Lange LW, DJ Sahn, HD Allen, SJ Goldberg: Subxiphoid cross-sectional echocardiography in infants and children with congenital heart disease. Circulation 59:513–524, 1979.
8. Seward JB, AJ Tajik, DJ Hagler, DG Ritter: Contrast echocardiography in single or common ventricle. Circulation 53:513, 1977.

21. CONTRAST ECHOCARDIOGRAPHY IN THE ASSESSMENT OF CYANOTIC AND COMPLEX CONGENITAL HEART DISEASE: PERIPHERAL VENOUS, INVASIVE, AND UNIQUE APPLICATIONS

James B. Seward, Abdul J. Tajik, and Donald J. Hagler

Contrast echocardiography has become a well-established adjunct to the M-mode [1] and two-dimensional [2, 3] echocardiographic examinations. This statement is even more true when applied to congenital heart disease. In these situations, the echocardiographic anatomy and contrast echocardiographic blood-flow patterns are often such sensitive indicators and so diagnostic that the specific defect can be readily and confidently appreciated at the bedside [3, 4]. It can be stated that the more complex the defect, the more likely is the existence of lesion-specific echocardiographic anatomy and blood-flow patterns.

A few basic concepts regarding contrast echocardiography should be reemphasized. First, the contrast effect can be visualized not only at the site of injection but also downstream from that site. Second, all contrast effect is usually lost with a single transit through either the pulmonary or the systemic capillary bed. As implied in the cyanotic congenital lesion, there is right-to-left shunting at some level in the cardiopulmonary bed. This direct communication between the right and the left heart circulation can usually be appreciated and categorized by contrast echocardiography. If one takes into account the above physical characteristics of echo contrast agents, it is apparent that peripheral venous injections will usually suffice for the assessment of characteristic right-to-left shunting patterns in the majority of patients with a cyanotic heart defect. Blood flow within the heart, whether in association with normal or altered hemodynamics, usually follows predictable and reproducible patterns. By analyzing the sequential movement and timing of arrival of blood from chamber to chamber, one can make very specific observations.

Contrast echocardiography, when compared with conventional angiography, has the unique feature of eliminating potential interference from surrounding and overlying cardiac structures or chambers. The M-mode examination is an ice pick ("periscopic") view, unhampered by surrounding anatomy. This technique permits accurate timing of flow-related events in the chambers or vessels under examination [1]. Two-dimensional contrast echocardiography, on the other hand, is more comparable to a tomographic angiogram – that is, an echoangiogram [2]. This technique permits direct visualization of particular cardiac chambers and defects. The echoangiogram permits visualization of contrast-enhanced blood-flow patterns through or about these defects, free of interference from adjacent or overlying cardiac chambers. Timing of two-dimensional echocardiographic events is more difficult to analyze because of the videomatic recording medium. However, with slow motion analysis, recorded contrast patterns can be characterized and timed in a manner similar to conventional cineangiographic techniques.

Quantitation of the echo contrast effect is discussed elsewhere in this book. However, it should be noted that in spite of variable-contrast density from one injection to the next, the amount of contrast shunted with each injection remains relatively constant. This feature will permit accurate quantitation as well as visual appreciation of the degree of shunt [5]. However, in the case of the more complex congenital lesions, quantitation is usually not necessary and the examination more often emphasizes appreciation of "lesion-specific" contrast flow patterns (i.e., sequence of arrival, timing, and relative density).

Left-to-right shunt patterns are described under the topics of uncomplicated atrial and ventricular septal defects. This particular chapter deals primarily with right-to-left shunt patterns in the cyanotic or complex cardiac defect and contrast echocardiographic appreciation of frequently encountered associated anomalies. The chapter is divided into three sections on the basis of the means of utilizing contrast echocardiography for the assessment of cyanotic or complex congenital heart disease: (I) peripheral venous injections; (II) invasive contrast echocardiography performed during cardiac catheterization; and (III) unique applications.

PART I: DETECTION OF RIGHT-TO-LEFT SHUNT UTILIZING PERIPHERAL VENOUS INJECTIONS

The following lesions have distinctive patterns of right-to-left shunting which can be assessed by venous (peripheral or caval) injections of echo contrast medium.
1. Atrial septal defect
  a. Secundum, primum, and sinus venosus
2. Ventricular septal defect
  a. Eisenmenger's complex
3. Tetralogy of Fallot
  a. Includes: pulmonary atresia with ventricular septal defect; truncus arteriosus
4. Ebstein's anomaly
5. Tricuspid atresia and hypoplastic right heart
6. Univentricular heart
  a. With two atrioventricular valves
    — With outflow chamber
  b. With single (common) atrioventricular valve
    — With ventricular pouch
7. Complete transposition
8. Straddling/overriding atrioventricular valve
9. Crisscross heart

Atrial septal defect

The uncomplicated secundum atrial septal defect is usually associated with a small right-to-left shunt [6, 7]. This small right-to-left shunt is more commonly observed after lower-extremity venous or inferior vena caval injection in the presence of a secundum atrial septal defect [1] and upper-extremity injections with a sinus venosus atrial septal defect [8]. Blood will intermittently move from right atrium to left atrium during early ventricular systole. This shunting may be enhanced by various maneuvers, including the Valsalva maneuver [9], upright posture, and deep inspiration [7]. The following discussion will focus on the atrial septal defect associated with significant right-to-left shunt as a result of pulmonary hypertension or associated with certain predisposing anatomy or hemodynamics.

Secundum atrial septal defect

Large right-to-left shunt through a secundum atrial septal defect or patent foramen ovale will occur in the presence of pulmonary vascular obstructive disease of sufficient severity (Figure 1). The shunt at atrial level can be visualized directly by the two-dimensional contrast technique (Figure 2A), or it can be appreciated indirectly

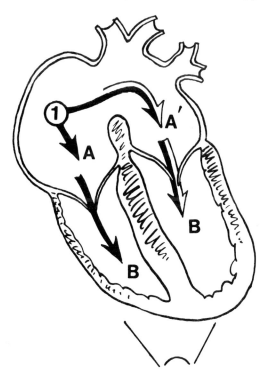

Figure 1. Atrial septal defect. Typical right-to-left shunt pattern in the presence of an atrial septal defect is shown. Contrast medium first arrives into the right atrium at 1. During ventricular systole, right-to-left shunt occurs at the atrial level (A to A'). With the next ventricular diastole, both ventricles opacify simultaneously, commencing with the rapid filling phase of ventricular diastole (B).

by the M-mode technique (Figure 2B). With milder degrees of pulmonary hypertension, right-to-left shunt at atrial level occurs predominantly during early ventricular systole. However, as pulmonary hypertension increases, the right-to-left atrial shunt will extend into ventricular diastole. In our institution, peripheral contrast echocardiography is used routinely to assess the presence and degree of shunting in patients suspected of having a secundum or sinus venosus atrial septal defect complicated by pulmonary hypertension.

Primum atrial septal defect (partial atrioventricular canal defect)

Invariably, all patients with primum atrial septal defect will show right-to-left shunt at atrial level with or without associated pulmonary hypertension. Because the primum defect is located posteriorly at the crest of the inflow ventricular septum, right-to-left shunt predictably occurs during the rapid filling phase of ventricular diastole. This pattern is easily demonstrated after upper-extremity contrast echocardiography.

Sinus venosus atrial septal defect [8]

This defect is found to lie just inferior to the orifice of the superior vena cava as it enters the right atrium. Upper-extremity contrast echo injection offers additional help, for there is invariably some right-to-left shunt. Direct visualization of dye crossing the high atrial septum is a further diagnostic observation.

Ventricular septal defect

It has been shown in earlier studies by us and others that right-to-left shunt through a ventricular septal defect occurs only when the right ventricular pressures approach one half to two thirds of systemic pressure. At this point, very specific right-to-left blood-flow patterns can be observed by the echo contrast technique [1, 3, 10] (Figures 3 and 4). At lower right ventricular pressures, direct appreciation of left-to-right shunt at ventricular level is made possible by visualization of a negative contrast effect (that is, undyed blood entering a bolus of dyed blood in the right heart chambers) [11]. (Refer to atrial septal defect and ventricular septal defect elsewhere in this book.)

Eisenmenger's complex

After opacification of the right atrium, blood empties into the right ventricle during diastole. With the next systole, blood is ejected directly and predominantly out of the pulmonary artery. Only with subsequent diastole will right-to-left shunting occur at ventricular level. This shunt commences at a very specific time during the cardiac cycle – that is, after closure of the aortic valve and before the opening of the mitral valve (i.e., isovolumic relaxation phase) [12]. Contrast will enter the left ventricular cavity anterior to the anterior leaflet of the mitral valve. With the next systole, contrast-containing blood is ejected out of both the aorta and the pul-

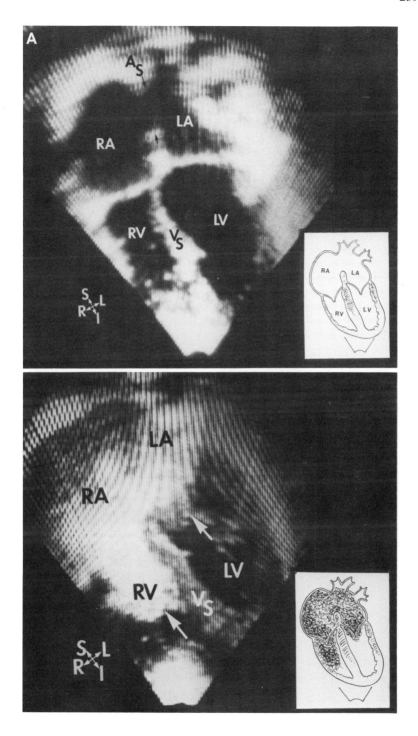

Figure 2A

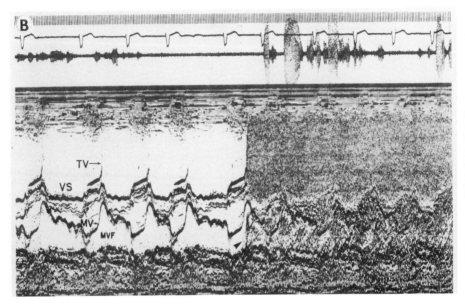

Figure 2B

Figure 2. Atrial septal defect. A—see p. 239) Two-dimensional echocardiograms illustrating right-to-left shunt at atrial level. Top panel: apical four-chamber view shows significant dropout in the midportion of the atrial septum (i.e., secundum atrial septal defect). Bottom panel: after the injection of contrast medium, both atria are opacified. Beginning with the rapid filling phase of ventricular diastole, both ventricles fill nearly simultaneously. Note that the right ventricle begins to opacify slightly ahead of the left ventricle (large arrows). This is consistent with the normal sequence of ventricular filling. AS = atrial septum; LA = left atrium; LV = left ventricle; VS = ventricular septum; RV = right ventricle; RA = right atrium; S = superior; L = left; I = inferior; R = right. (Top panel: modified from Seward JB, AJ Tajik: Two-dimensional echocardiography. Med Clin North Am 64:177–203, 1980 (March). By permission of WB Saunders Company). (Bottom panel: modified from ref. [39]. By permission). B) M-mode echocardiogram illustrating typical right-to-left flow pattern associated with atrial septal defect. After a hand vein injection of contrast medium, both ventricles are simultaneously opacified. Note that the right ventricle is opacified during the peak filling phase of diastole (use the anterior leaflet of the mitral valve and the electrocardiogram for timing). The diagnostic filling pattern of the left ventricle consists of initial opacification of the mitral valve funnel (MVF) and subsequent opacification of the left ventricle. TV = tricuspid valve; VS = ventricular septum; MV = mitral valve. (From ref. [4]. By permission of Technical Publishing Company).

monary artery. With increasing right ventricular hypertension, the diastolic right-to-left shunt will become more prolonged.

Tetralogy of Fallot

Pulmonary atresia with ventricular septal defect and truncus arteriosus

These three lesions have similar ventricular anatomy, characterized by a large great artery overriding a ventricular septal defect [13, 14]. The distinctive differential anatomy in the three defects is pulmonary outflow tract stenosis (tetralogy of Fallot), atresia (pulmonary atresia), or total absence (truncus arteriosus). An echo

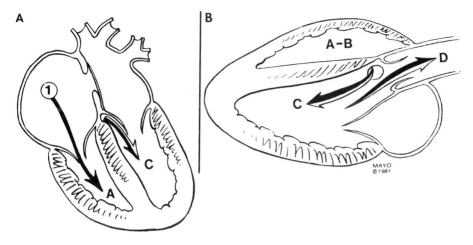

Figure 3. A and B: Ventricular septal defect. Illustrations (apical four-chamber and parasternal long axis) show the typical right-to-left flow pattern in the presence of a ventricular septal defect. After atrial opacification (1), the right ventricle is opacified (A) during the rapid filling phase of diastole. With the next systole, dye is ejected out the right ventricular outflow tract (B) to the pulmonary artery. Only with the subsequent diastole (isovolumic relaxation phase of early diastole) does contrast appear in the left ventricle (C). With the next systole, contrast is ejected out of both great arteries (D). Note: neither of these echocardiographic projections directly visualizes the typical paramembranous ventricular septum – (A) inflow septum (four-chamber view) and (B) outflow septum (parasternal long-axis view).

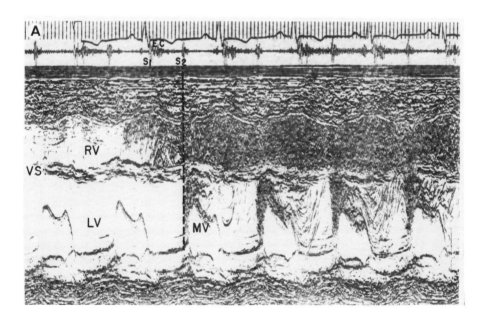

Figure 4A

242

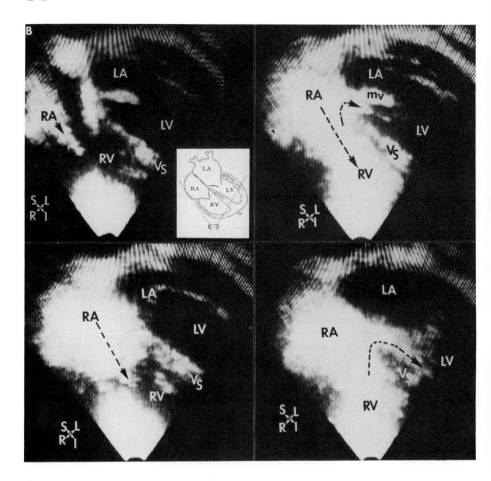

Figure 4B

Figure 4. Ventricular septal defect. A—see p. 242) Typical contrast M-mode features of right-to-left shunt at ventricular level. After diastolic opacification of the right ventricle, no dye appears in the left ventricle for one complete cardiac cycle. With subsequent diastole, a characteristic flow pattern is observed. Commencing with the isovolumic relaxation phase of early diastole, contrast material appears anterior to the mitral valve echo (MV); that is, it appears after the closure of the aortic valve (S_2, dashed line) and before the maximum opening of the mitral valve. This right-to-left shunt pattern is repetitive with each subsequent cardiac cycle. RV = right ventricle; VS = ventricular septum; LV = left ventricle; S_1 = first heart sound; EC = electrocardiogram. B) Two-dimensional echocardiographic frames illustrating the sequential flow pattern of right-to-left shunt across the ventricular septal defect (apical four-chamber view). Upper left: contrast initially appears in the right atrium. Lower left: with subsequent diastole a cloud of echoes opacifies the right ventricular cavity. There is no right-to-left shunt during the subsequent systole. Upper right: right-to-left shunt begins in early diastole (isovolumic relaxation phase) of the next cardiac cycle (curved-dashed arrow). Lower right: contrast material appears anterior to the anterior leaflet of mitral valve and subsequently opacifies the left ventricle. LA = left atrium; LV = left ventricle; VS = ventricular septum; RV = right ventricle; RA = right atrium; L = left; I = inferior; R = right; S = superior. (A from ref [13]. By permission of the American Heart Association).

contrast flow pattern somewhat different from that observed in the complicated ventricular septal defect (Figures 3 and 4) will be observed in this group of defects [3, 15] (Figure 5). After the diastolic opacification of the right ventricle, with the first systole, contrast material is ejected directly out of the overriding great artery. The echo contrast will tend to laminate along the anterior aspect of the aortic-truncal root. With the subsequent isovolumic relaxation phase of diastole, contrast is shunted from the right ventricle to the left ventricle across the ventricular septal defect. Dye appears anterior to the anterior leaflet of the mitral valve. With the next systole, echo dye is again ejected from both ventricles out of the great artery. (Note: blood ejected from the left ventricle tends to laminate along the posterior aspect of the aortic-truncal root.)

Ebstein's anomaly

Ebstein's anomaly is associated with variable cyanosis resulting from right-to-left shunt at the atrial level. The two-dimensional echocardiographic features of Ebstein's anomaly are diagnostic [16]. Peripheral echo contrast injections are utilized only to substantiate the right-to-left shunt at atrial level (see above). Secondly, tricuspid valve regurgitation, which usually accompanies Ebstein's anomaly, can be diagnosed and grossly quantitated by the contrast echocardiographic technique [17].

Tricuspid atresia

Although tricuspid atresia has recently been classified under the topic of univentricular heart by the pathologist, the M-mode and two-dimensional echocardiographic features of these anomalies are quite distinctive [3, 18]. Contrast echocardiographic blood-flow patterns are also uniquely different [3] (Figure 6).

After the arrival of contrast material into the right atrium, there is total and obligatory right-to-left shunting from right atrium to left atrium. With the next diastole, all blood enters the ventricle through the left (morphologic mitral) atrioventricular valve, to opacify the large, left ventricular chamber. With the subsequent systole, contrast-containing blood is shunted across the ventricular septal defect (if present) into the hypoplastic right ventricular chamber and simultaneously out of both great arteries (Figure 7). This flow pattern can easily be distinguished from the more frequently encountered forms of univentricular heart (see below).

If the tricuspid valve is hypoplastic but patent, the smaller, right-sided ventricular chamber will become opacified during diastole (Figures 8 and 9).

Univentricular heart

Univentricular heart is defined as a condition in which most of the atrial blood simul-

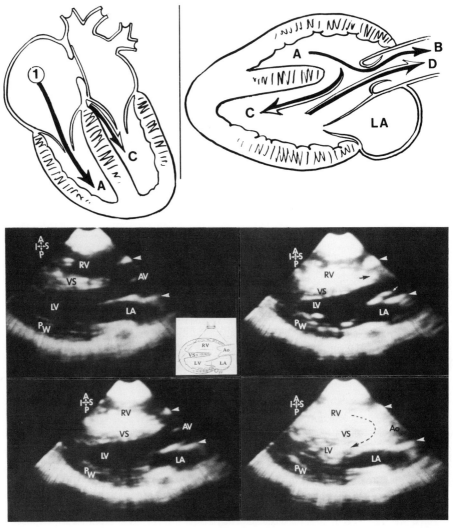

Figure 5. Aorta/truncus overriding ventricular septal defect. Top panels: drawings show the subtle differences in right-to-left shunt pattern from that of the isolated ventricular septal defect (Figure 3). The right-to-left shunt at ventricular level occurs during the isovolumic relaxation phase of diastole (C) identical to that of the ventricular septal defect. The difference is the initial systolic ejection of blood directly out of the overriding aorta (B). With the first systole, blood laminates along the anterior surface of the great artery. With subsequent systoles, when blood is ejected from the left ventricle, the left ventricular contrast material laminates along the posterior aspect of the aorta (D). LA = left atrium. Bottom panels: still frames of the two-dimensional echocardiogram illustrate, in a sequential flow pattern, right-to-left shunt in a patient with pulmonary atresia with ventricular septal defect. Upper left: the typical anatomy of great artery overriding a ventricular septal defect (arrowheads in all views) is illustrated. Lower left: after a venous injection, echoes initially opacify the right ventricle (RV). With the next systole (upper right), contrast is ejected directly out the aorta (black arrow) across the semilunar valve (small white arrow). Note that the blood tends to laminate along the superior surface of the great artery. With subsequent diastole (lower right), a right-to-left shunt occurs at ventricular level (curved arrow), appearing anterior to the anterior leaf of the mitral valve. RV = right ventricle; AV = aortic valve; LV = left ventricle; VS = ventricular septum; PW = posterior wall; LA = left atrium; Ao = aorta; A = anterior; S = superior; P = posterior; I = inferior. (Bottom from ref. [3]. By permission).

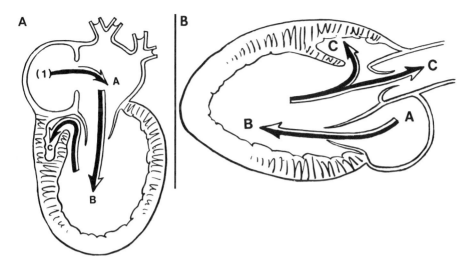

Figure 6. A and B: Tricuspid atresia. Illustrations (apical four-chamber view and parasternal long-axis view) show the typical flow pattern of tricuspid atresia. Immediately after the opacification of the right ventricle (1), contrast medium is shunted from right atrium to left atrium (A), and with subsequent ventricular diastole, the cloud of echoes opacifies the left ventricle (B). With the next systole, contrast is ejected through the ventricular septal defect and it opacifies the diminutive right ventricle and at the same time is ejected directly out of the great arteries (C). Note that all blood entering the left ventricle passes through the mitral valve orifice.

taneously empties directly into a single ventricular cavity through two atrioventricular valves or through a single (common) atrioventricular valve [19]. Various forms of the univentricular heart and associated anatomy have been recognized [20–22]. In this group of anomalies, typical blood-flow patterns have been described on the basis of peripheral contrast echocardiography [23, 24].

Univentricular heart with two atrioventricular valves

A very sensitive and reproducible blood-flow pattern is observed with this particular variant (Figures 10 and 11). After the initial arrival of contrast material into the right atrium, the ventricle is opacified via the right atrioventricular valve during the period of rapid diastolic filling. Even in the presence of an associated atrial septal defect, characteristic ventricular opacification is evident by contrast echocardiography [24]. The flow pattern is distinctly different from that in other complex lesions, including tricuspid atresia and ventricular septal defect with right-to-left shunt. Dye appears during the peak filling phase of diastole anterior to the posteriorly positioned atrioventricular valve (a pattern distinctly different from the appearance during the isovolumic phase of diastole as seen with a ventricular septal defect, or posterior to the left atrioventricular valve in patients with a single atrioventricular valve, e.g., tricuspid atresia).

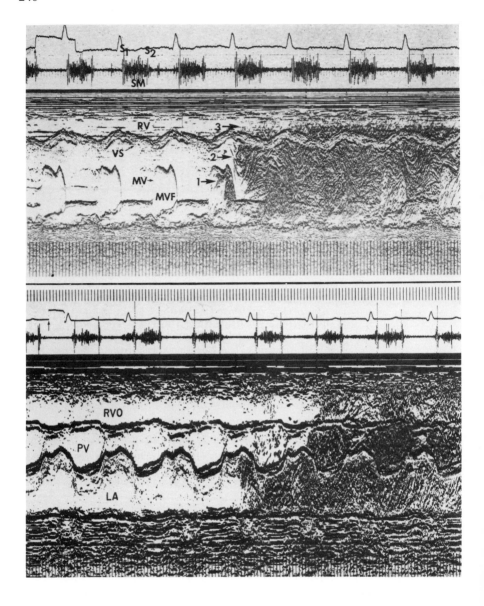

Figure 7. Tricuspid atresia. Contrast M-mode echocardiograms at ventricular (top panel) and pulmonary valve (bottom panel) levels are shown. Top panel: after contrast injection, echoes initially appear in the mitral valve funnel (MVF) (1) in diastole and subsequently opacify the left ventricle (2). Only with the next systole (3) does the diminutive right ventricle opacify.Bottom panel: this staggered flow pattern is better illustrated at pulmonary valve level in a patient with tricuspid atresia and transposed great arteries. The left atrium is initially opacified, and only with subsequent systole are the pulmonary valve orifice (PV) and lastly the right ventricular outflow tract (RVO) opacified. MV = mitral valve; VS = ventricular septum; RV = right ventricle; SM = systolic murmur; S$_1$ = first heart sound; S$_2$ = second heart sound; LA = left atrium. (Top panel from ref. [18]. By permission). (Bottom panel from ref. [4]. By permission of Technical Publishing Company).

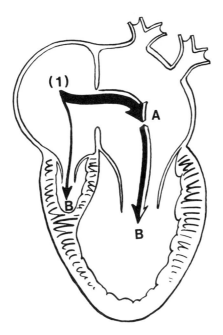

Figure 8. Hypoplastic tricuspid valve and right ventricle with intact ventricular septum and pulmonary atresia. After initial opacification of the right atrium (1), a right-to-left shunt occurs at atrial level during ventricular systole (A). With subsequent ventricular diastole, both the hypoplastic right ventricle and the larger, volume overloaded, left ventricle opacify simultaneously (B).

Univentricular heart with outflow chamber

This particular subgroup of univentricular heart is most commonly associated with two atrioventricular valves and transposition of the great arteries with the aorta committed to a small, anteriorly located outflow chamber [23]. The outflow chamber does not receive blood directly from either atrioventricular valve. The common ventricle is opacified during the peak filling phase of diastole, and with subsequent systole the outflow chamber is opacified as blood is simultaneously ejected out of both great arteries [24] (Figure 10).

Univentricular heart with single (common) atrioventricular valve

This form of univentricular heart rarely has an associated outflow chamber, and it has two-dimensional echocardiographic features that are distinctly different from those of tricuspid atresia or complete atrioventricular canal defect [23–25]. There is a single, large atrioventricular valve committed to a single, invariably heavily trabeculated common ventricular chamber. A large primum atrial septal defect or common atrium is usually present. After opacification of the atria, dye empties into the ventricle during the peak filling phase of diastole (Figure 12). The M-mode flow pattern would be similar to that observed in tricuspid atresia [18, 24]; however, associated two-dimensional echocardiographic anatomy is distinctly different between these two entities [23].

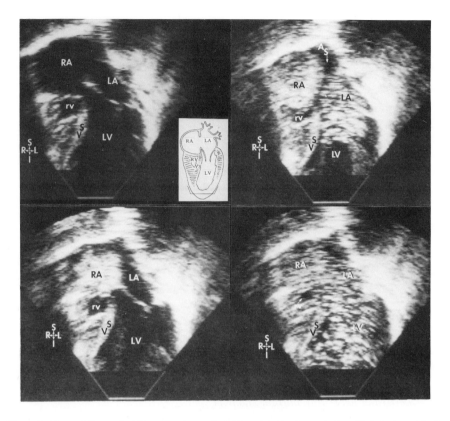

Figure 9. Upper left panel: tricuspid valve and right ventricular hypoplasia with intact ventricular septum and pulmonary valve atresia. Lower left panel: after peripheral venous injection of contrast medium, the right atrium initially opacifies. Upper right panel: During ventricular systole, the left atrium is opacified via a large atrial septal defect. Lower right panel: with subsequent systole, both the left ventricle (LV) and the diminutive right ventricle are opacified. Note: the difference between this flow pattern and true tricuspid atresia is diastolic opacification of the right ventricular remnant. The remainder of the flow pattern would be identical to that of tricuspid atresia. RA = right atrium; LA = left atrium; LV = left ventricle; VS = ventricular septum; rv = right ventricle; AS = atrial septum; S = superior; L = left; I = inferior; R = right. (Modified from ref. [3]. By permission).

Univentricular heart with ventricular pouch

A smaller subgroup of patients with univentricular heart will have a blind ventricular pouch, usually located laterally or posteriorly in the ventricular myocardium [26]. This is most commonly associated with univentricular heart and single atrioventricular valve. After diastolic opacification of the common ventricle, the ventricular pouch is opacified with subsequent systole [23]. Systolic opacification of a pouch is to be distinguished from diastolic opacification of ventricular recesses formed by trabeculation.

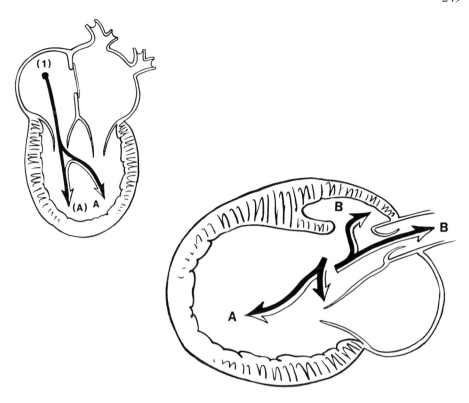

Figure 10. Univentricùlar heart. The more frequently encountered form of univentricular heart with two atrioventricular valves and transposed great arteries is illustrated. Top panel: apical "four"-chamber view. Bottom panel: parasternal long-axis view. After the venous injection of contrast material, the right atrium is initially opacified (1); with subsequent diastole, the entire ventricular chamber is opacified during the rapid filling phase of diastole ((A)A). Contrast material appears anterior to the left atrioventricular valve. (Note peak filling phase of diastole as opposed to the isovolumic relaxation phase as seen with a ventricular septal defect). With subsequent systole, contrast crosses the bulboventricular foramen into the outflow chamber and is ejected out of both great arteries (B). Note: the aorta is usually committed to the small outflow chamber.

Figure 11 (see next page). A) Univentricular heart with two atrioventricular valves. Upper left and lower left panels: typical anatomic features of univentricular heart; that is, two atrioventricular valves (rv and lv) totally committed to the common ventricle (CV). The upper left panel (systole) and the lower left panel (diastole) illustrate the "clapping" motion of the "septal" portions of the two atrioventricular valves. Upper right and lower right panels: Typical contrast pattern with opacification of the right atrium and subsequent diastolic opacification of the entire common ventricle. Note: the left atrium remains echo free. RA = right atrium; AS = atrial septum; LA = left atrium; CV = common ventricle; rv = right atrioventricular valve; lv = left atrioventricular valve; S = superior; L = left; I = inferior; R = right. (Upper left, lower left, and upper right modified from ref. [23]. By permission). B) M-mode contrast echocardiogram in a patient with univentricular heart and two atrioventricular valves. After a peripheral venous injection of contrast material, echoes appear initially anterior to the left atrioventricular valve (MV) during the peak filling phase of diastole. (Note: the speed of the paper at the left is slower and is then increased after the arrival of dye). With each subsequent cardiac cycle, contrast material is most dense anterior to the mitral valve during peak diastole. TV = right atrioventricular valve; MVF = funnel of the left atrioventricular valve. (From ref. [24]. By permission of the American Heart Association).

250

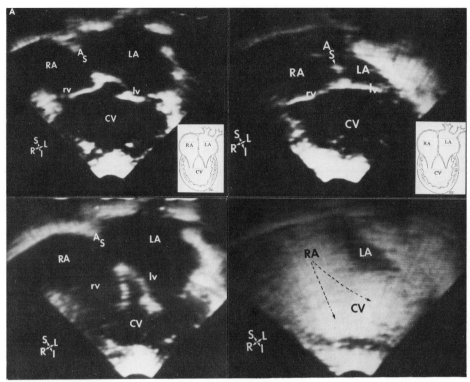

Figure 11A (Legend: see p. 249).

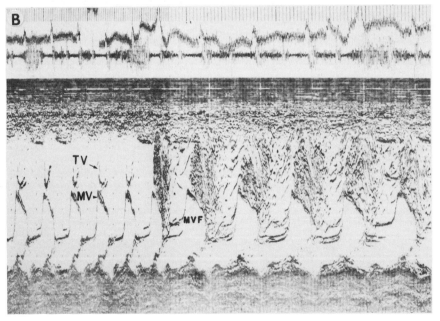

Figure 11B (Legend: see p. 249).

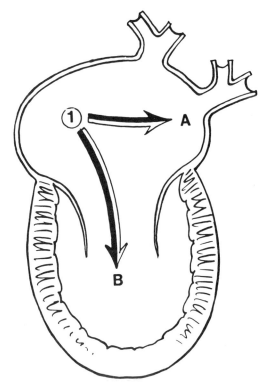

Figure 12. Univentricular heart with single (common) atrioventricular valve. Illustration shows the typical flow pattern. After arrival of contrast medium into the right portion of a common atrium (1), the entire atrial cavity is opacified (A), and with subsequent ventricular diastole the single ventricular chamber is opacified (B).

Complete transposition (ventricular-great artery discordance)

The M-mode and, more recently, two-dimensional echocardiographic features of complete transposition are usually more helpful in recognizing the anatomic derangement of complete transposition than are the reported contrast echocardiographic flow patterns [27, 28]. However, because of the commitment of the aorta to the right ventricular (systemic venous) chambers, a helpful, lesion-specific contrast flow pattern has been reported [29]. This pattern relies on visualization of an expected differential opacification of the great arteries in patients with transposition (i.e., prominent opacification of the aorta after injection into a systemic vein or the right ventricle). The suprasternal transducer position is utilized to image simultaneously the aorta and the right pulmonary artery (Figure 13). After a peripheral venous injection, the anterior-lying aorta will opacify more densely than the pulmonary artery in patients with transposed great arteries (see Chapter 22, Hunter and Sutherland). In our experience, direct two-dimensional echocardiographic features of transposition are more helpful. However, when M-mode echocardiography is more accessible, the above contrast flow pattern is an excellent and rapid

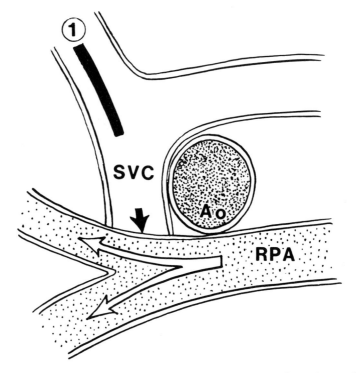

Figure 13. Complete transposition of the great arteries. The illustration shows the two-dimensional anatomy [2] that accounts for the reported M-mode [29] contrast flow pattern. After a venous injection (1), initial appearance of dye is in the superior vena cava (SVC). Subsequent opacification of the aorta and right pulmonary artery (RPA) results in a lesion-specific differential density. Because the aorta is committed to the right ventricle, the density will be greatest in the aorta (Ao).

means of indirectly establishing the diagnosis of transposed great arteries.

A second use of contrast echocardiography in patients with complete transposition of the great arteries is gross documentation of the degree of favorable right-to-left shunting at atrial level. This is particularly helpful in determining the adequacy of balloon septostomy.

Straddling/overriding atrioventricular valve

As with standard angiography, the simultaneous opacification of both ventricles after atrial injection is the typical contrast echocardiographic flow pattern seen in the straddling/overriding atrioventricular valve [3, 30] (Figures 14 and 15). As previously reported [31], there is a great echocardiographic spectrum of atrioventricular valve malalignment, all elements of which show this same flow pattern (i.e., simultaneous opacification of both ventricles).

"Straddling atrioventricular valve" is defined as the insertion of portions of the chordal support apparatus into the contralateral ventricle. Straddling atrioventricular valve need not be, although it usually is, associated with septal mal-

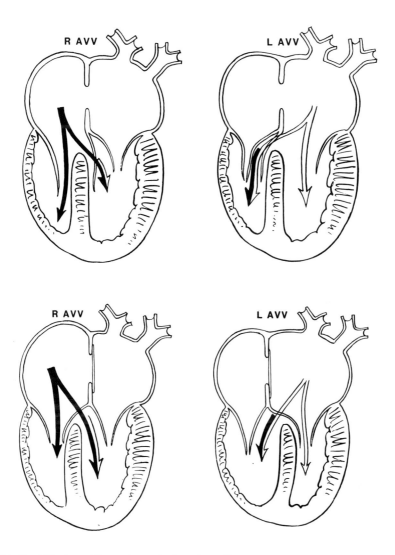

Figure 14. Straddling/overriding atrioventricular valves. Illustrations show the flow patterns encountered with straddling (top panel) and overriding (bottom panel) atrioventricular valve (AVV). All variations of this anomaly show simultaneous diastolic opacification of the ventricles. This results when there is either commitment of support apparatus to the contralateral ventricle (straddling, top panel) or septal malalignment (overriding, bottom panel).

alignment (override). The degree of straddling can also be quite variable, with insertions near the crest of the ventricular septum (type A), in the midportion of the contralateral ventricular septum (type B), or in the free wall of the contralateral ventricle (type C) [31]. Each variation of this anomaly is also typified by simultaneous opacification of both ventricles during the rapid filling phase of diastole [3, 30].

"Overriding atrioventricular valve" is defined as ventricular-atrial septal mal-

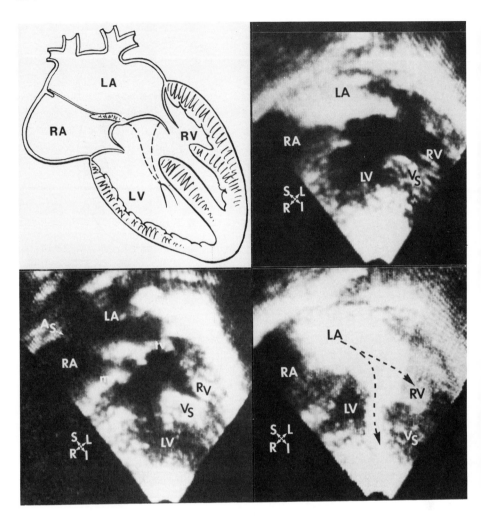

Figure 15. Straddling left atrioventricular valve in a patient with inverted ventricles. There is minor malalignment of the atrial and ventricular septa (override). Upper and lower left panel: support apparatus of the left atrioventricular valve (morphologic tricuspid) inserts into a papillary muscle in the contralateral ventricle (LV). A catheter is positioned in the left atrial cavity across a patent foramen ovale. Upper right panel: echo contrast material is injected into the left atrium (LA) (ventricular systole). Lower right panel: with ventricular diastole, contrast material simultaneously opacifies both ventricular cavities across the crest of the ventricular septum (VS) (curved-dashed arrows). RA = right atrium; LA = left atrium; RV = morphologic right ventricle; LV = morphologic left ventricle; VS = ventricular septum; AS = atrial septum; S = superior; L = left; I = inferior; R = right. (Lower left, upper right, and lower right panels modified from ref. [3]. By permission).

alignment (major commitment of the atrioventricular valve anulus to the contralateral ventricle) without straddling (chordal insertion into the contralateral ventricle). The annular displacement toward the contralateral ventricle can be quite variable. After injection of contrast medium above the atrioventricular valve, there is simultaneous diastolic opacification of both ventricles [3]. Overriding right atrioventricular valve can be assessed by peripheral venous injections, whereas over-riding left atrioventricular valve would require selective left atrial injections.

Thus, with either overriding or straddling atrioventricular valve, a similar blood-flow pattern will be observed. Direct visualization of the support apparatus or the degree of septal malalignment is more important than the observed blood-flow pattern. However, this pattern does substantiate altered hemodynamics consistent with atrioventricular valve malalignment. Assessment of an abnormally oriented left atrioventricular valve would require selective left atrial injections during an invasive procedure [31]. The malaligned right atrioventricular valve can be assessed from peripheral venous injections.

Crisscross heart

Crisscross heart is a rare anomaly [32] in which a right-sided atrium is committed to a left-sided ventricle and a left-sided atrium is committed to a right-sided ventricle. Ventricular inversion and varying degrees of atrioventricular valve malalignment are frequently associated lesions [33]. However, in spite of these associated anom-alies, a characteristic flow pattern is usually observed [30] (Figures 16A and 16B). After arrival of contrast into the right-sided atrium, contrast will predominantly be shunted to a left-sided ventricle. On the other hand, during an invasive study, selective injection of the contralateral atrium (left atrium) will result in diastolic opacification of the right-sided ventricle. This crisscross flow pattern is usually more easily assessed by the tomographic two-dimensional echocardiographic con-trast technique.

PART II: INVASIVE CONTRAST ECHOCARDIOGRAPHY –
      ECHO"ANGIOGRAPHY"

Although echocardiography is, for the most part, considered a noninvasive tool, it has been our experience that the simultaneous use of echocardiography during cardiac catheterization is very helpful in the elucidation of various congenital cardiac anomalies and associated defects [1, 3]. Simultaneous invasive contrast echo-cardiography – echoangiography [2] – has also proved to be an extremely useful adjunct to the catheterization procedure. Because of the tomographic presentation of the two-dimensional examination, contrast echoangiography can often supplant or greatly enhance standard angiographic techniques. All of the foregoing discus-sion concerning the use of venous contrast echocardiography would apply to the invasive environment. However, frequently a more central injection of contrast medium gives a superior echoangiographic effect. In addition to venous echo-angiography, there are certain diagnostic blood-flow patterns that can be appreci-ated only by selective chamber or vessel injections during cardiac catheterization (invasive echoangiography). Selective injection of contrast material into otherwise

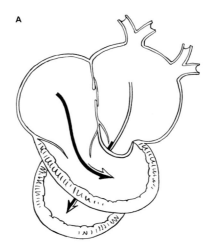

Figure 16A. Crisscross heart. Blood flow accounting for the diagnostic contrast two-dimensional and M-mode echocardiogram; that is, a right-sided atrium committed to a left-sided ventricle and a left-sided atrium committed to a right-sided ventricle.

inaccessible chambers not only permits localization of the catheter but can also result in the production of diagnostic blood-flow patterns.

The uses of invasive contrast echocardiography, which will not be discussed, include the selective injection of contrast material distal to an incompetent semilunar or atrioventricular valve. Recognition of the presence of valvular incompetence and gross estimation of a regurgitant fraction can be obtained with these techniques [1]. Left-sided abnormalities can be assessed better by the invasive echo contrast technique. An example would be selective left atrial injection of contrast material in a patient suspected of having straddling or overriding left atrioventricular valve (see above). The simultaneous opacification of both ventricles during the peak filling phase of diastole would be characteristic of atrioventricular valve malalignment.

The examples that follow illustrate some unique applications of the invasive echoangiogram in complex congenital heart disease. Certain anomalies disclose diagnostic flow patterns that complement or even supplant standard angiographic techniques. The unique tomographic presentation often eliminates interference of overlying chambers or confusing angiographic patterns caused by the mixing that is encountered with radiographic or isotope angiography. Lesions in which invasive echoangiography can demonstrate specific patterns include the following:

1. Atrioventricular canal defect (partial vs. complete)
2. Muscular ventricular septal defect (associated with a complex congenital lesion)
3. Anomalous pulmonary venous connection
   a. Partial
   b. Total
4. Patent ductus arteriosus
5. Aortopulmonary window

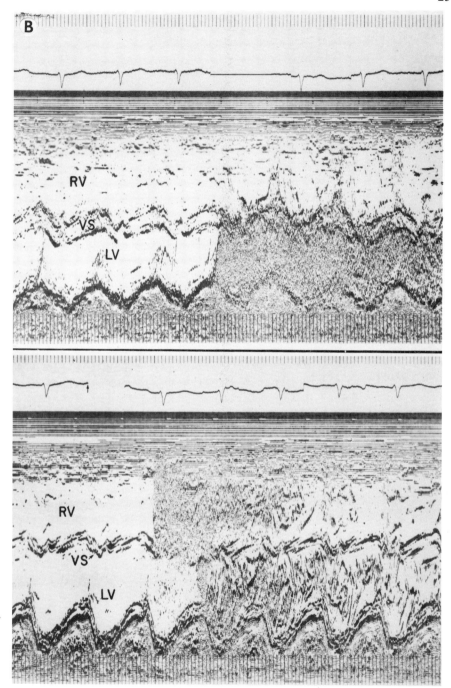

Figure 16B. Contrast M-mode echocardiogram illustrates the crossing pattern typical of this anomaly. Top panel: after a superior vena caval injection of contrast material, the left-sided ventricle is opacified. Bottom panel: conversely, when a selective injection is made into the left atrium, the right-sided ventricle is initially opacified. Note subsequent opacification of the left-sided ventricle. RV = right ventricle; VS = ventricular septum; LV = left ventricle. (B from ref. [33]. By permission).

258

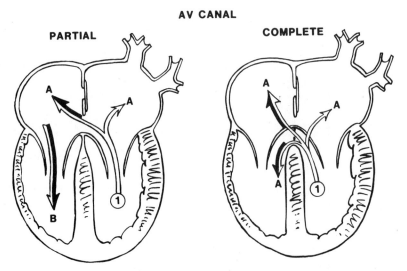

Figure 17. Partial versus complete atrioventricular canal. Illustrations (apical four-chamber projection) show the diagnostic flow patterns of partial versus complete atrioventricular canal. Left panel: partial atrioventricular canal. After the selective injection of contrast material into left ventricle (1), contrast is regurgitated to both atria (A), with the most predominant flow to the right atrium. Only with subsequent ventricular diastole does the cloud of echoes opacify the right ventricle (B). Right panel: complete atrioventricular canal. Conversely, in the presence of complete canal, after the injection of contrast medium into the left ventricle (1), echoes simultaneously opacify both atria and the right ventricle (denoting the presence of a ventricular septal defect – left-to-right shunt at ventricular level). Sensitive appreciation of even the smallest ventricular septal defect is possible by means of this technique (refer to references 25 and 34 for two-dimensional echocardiographic examples).

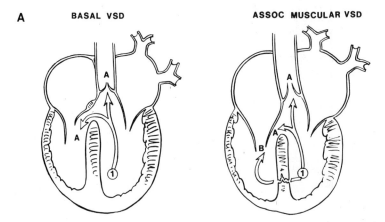

Figure 18. Muscular ventricular septal defect. A) Differential flow pattern of the "high" ventricular septal defect (left) versus that with associated muscular ventricular septal defect (right). Left panel: after selective injection of contrast material into the left ventricle (1), there is systolic opacification of the great artery (A) and left ventricle (A). Left ventricular opacification occurs over the ventricular septum (i.e., base to apex). Right panel: flow pattern with associated muscular ventricular septal defect is distinctively different. After the selective left ventricular injection of contrast material (1), contrast is injected into the great artery (A) and commences to cross over the crest of the ventricular septum (A). However, a dominant bolus of blood will arise out of the apex of the right ventricle (B), suggesting the presence of a lower (i.e., muscular) septal defect. This is an indirect means of appreciating associated defects.

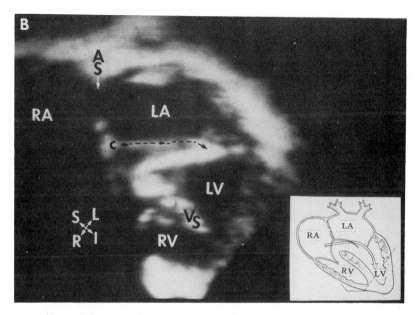

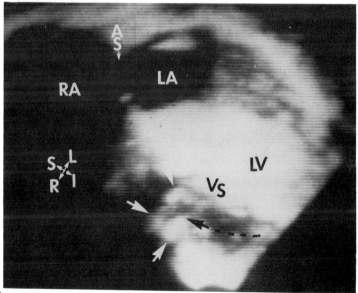

Figure 18B.

B) Representative still frames from a two-dimensional echocardiogram (modified subcostal four-chamber view) illustrating the flow pattern in a patient with a large paramembranous ventricular septal defect and associated muscular ventricular septal defect. Top panel: with a catheter (c) positioned in the left ventricular cavity, echo contrast material is selectively injected, with subsequent opacification of the entire left ventricle. Bottom panel: with systole, opacification of right ventricle occurs from the apex toward the base, suggesting an associated apical (i.e., muscular) ventricular septal defect (dashed arrow and white arrows). RA = right atrium; AS = atrial septum; LA = left atrium; LV = left ventricle; VS = ventricular septum; RV = right ventricle; S = superior; L = left; I = inferior; R = right. (B modified from ref. [3]. By permission).

6. Abnormal vascular communications
   a. Pulmonary valvular atresia with systemic-to-pulmonary collaterals
   b. Pulmonary arteriovenous fistula
   c. Peripheral or systemic arteriovenous fistula

Atrioventricular canal defect (partial versus complete)

Angiography has been utilized as the "gold standard" for the diagnosis of partial and complete atrioventricular canal. However, the differentiation of these two defects by angiographic means (i.e., recognition of the presence or absence of a canal ventricular septal defect) can be difficult, particularly when the ventricular septal defect is small or the streaming pattern is atypical [25]. Conversely, tomographic contrast echocardiography utilized during cardiac catheterization can confidently be used to visualize, and permits direct appreciation and localization of, very small amounts of shunted echo contrast material (Figure 17) [34]. Multiple tomographic views and contrast injections can be performed at virtually no added risk to the patient. The typical anatomy is directly visualized at the time of selective left ventricular echoangiography. We have found in our practice that, in most circumstances, two-dimensional echocardiography and invasive echoangiography are superior to standard angiography for the detailed assessment of the anatomic derangement of atrioventricular canals and for the differentiation of partial from complete forms. At this time, cardiac catheterization, in our laboratory, is utilized primarily for the assessment of hemodynamics, and angiography is used for the assessment of extracardiac anatomy, such as the pulmonary vascular tree. Invasive two-dimensional echoangiography is becoming a superior technique for the detailed assessment of ventricular anatomy and blood-flow patterns [25, 34].

Muscular ventricular septal defect

Occasionally associated with complex congenital cardiac defects, additional muscular septal defects have the potential of being easily overlooked. Selective left ventricular echoangiography is an excellent means of recognizing the presence of additional muscular septal defects [3]. Selective left ventricular echoangiography is utilized (Figure 18). In the presence of the usual paramembranous, inflow, or outflow ventricular septal defect, contrast medium will arise from the left ventricular cavity, cross the "high ventricular septal defect," and subsequently opacify the right ventricular cavity from base to apex. However, in the presence of a multiple muscular septal defect (Swiss cheese septum), left ventricular apical injection of contrast will opacify the right ventricle in a visibly different manner. Contrast will first appear in the apex or midright ventricle and then move toward the base. Two-dimensional echocardiography, in our experience, has a high likelihood of permitting direct visualization of a muscular ventricular septal defect; however, when combined with pulsed Doppler echocardiography and echoangiography, one can usually exclude or identify with confidence an associated muscular septal defect.

Anomalous pulmonary venous connection

Partial anomalous pulmonary venous connection
Echocardiography per se does not usually permit the direct visualization of anomalous pulmonary veins. However, with the catheter selectively positioned within the suspect pulmonary vein and with direct visualization of the atrial septum, the commitment of the pulmonary venous drainage can be confidently determined by echoangiography (Figure 19). With the use of the two-dimensional echocardiographic four-chamber view, the plane of the atrial septum can be visualized. After injection of echo contrast material into the pulmonary vein, dyed blood will initially opacify the atrium to which the pulmonary vein is connected (i.e., to the right of the atrial septum if the pulmonary vein is anomalous). This study can readily be performed, is highly sensitive, and does not require the injection of conventional radiographic contrast material.

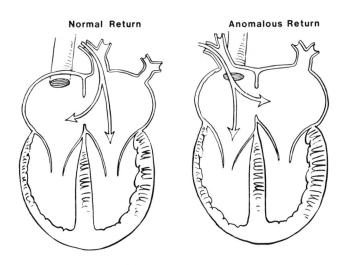

Figure 19. Partial anomalous pulmonary venous return. Illustrations show the differential flow pattern of normal pulmonary venous drainage (left panel) and anomalous venous return (right panel) as determined by invasive contrast echoangiography. Left panel: after the selective injection of contrast material into a suspect pulmonary vein, in the presence of normal venous drainage a cloud of echoes will appear to the left of the atrial septum (i.e., left atrium). There may be subsequent left-to-right shunt through an associated atrial septal defect; however, the initial appearance of dye in the left atrium is diagnostic of normal pulmonary venous return. Right panel: with a catheter positioned in an anomalous pulmonary vein, echo contrast material will initially opacify the right atrium and confirm the anomalous commitment to the right atrium.

Total anomalous pulmonary venous connection

Two-dimensional echocardiography can in most situations identify either the pulmonary confluence or the dilated structures that receive the anomalous pulmonary venous blood [35]. However, contrast echoangiography, with selective injection into the confluence or the receiving venous channels, can be very revealing, even if not diagnostic of the abnormal anatomy (Figures 20 and 21).

Patent ductus arteriosus

As opposed to the reported findings of others [36], we have only with great difficulty been able to achieve direct visualization of patent ductus arteriosus with either M-mode or two-dimensional echocardiography. Echocardiographic determination of the ratio of the left atrial/aortic root dimension has been utilized as a gross indicator of volume overload in the medical management of neonates with patent ductus arteriosus. Simultaneous use of pulsed Doppler echocardiography for detection of the presence of a continuous murmur in the left pulmonary artery appears to be the best noninvasive means of confirming patent ductus arteriosus [37]. However, reliable direct appreciation of a shunt is best obtained in the intensive care unit or at catheterization by selective injection of echo contrast material into the upper descending aorta while simultaneously visualizing the pulmonary arteries [38] (Figure 22).

Aortopulmonary window

Selective injection of echo contrast material into the aortic root while directly visualizing both the aorta and the pulmonary artery allows one to appreciate direct communication between the aorta and the pulmonary artery (aortopulmonary window) (Figure 23). However, care must be taken to determine accurately the exact

---

Figure 20. A) Total anomalous pulmonary venous connection via a vertical vein to the innominate vein ⟶ at the superior vena cava. The levophase pulmonary angiogram shows the typical pattern of total anomalous pulmonary venous drainage to a confluence (C), which drains via a vertical vein (V), innominate vein (IN), and superior vena cava (SVC). RA = right atrium. B) Suprasternal two-dimensional echocardiogram illustrating the same venous malformation of total anomalous connection (same patient as in A). Upper left panel: the typical upper portion of the venous malformation of total anomalous return including confluence (C), vertical vein (V), innominate vein (IN), and superior vena cava (SVC). Central to this venous structure is the aortic root (Ao) and proximal is the main pulmonary artery (PA). Lower left panel: after selective injection of contrast material into the venous confluence, there is opacification of the vertical vein, innominate vein, and superior vena cava. Upper right panel: further opacification better delineates the centrally located aortic root and pulmonary artery. Lower right panel: approximately two cardiac cycles later, there is simultaneous opacification of the aortic root and pulmonary artery. C = confluence; V = vertical vein; IN = innominate vein; SVC = superior vena cava; Ao = aortic root; PA = pulmonary artery; LPV = left pulmonary vein; S = superior; L = left; I = inferior; R = right.

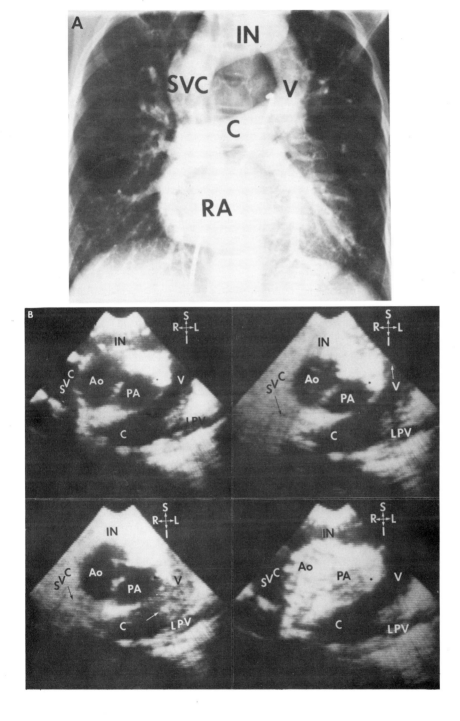

Figure 20. (Legend: see p. 262).

level of shunting and to exclude the more frequently encountered patent ductus arteriosus.

Abnormal vascular communications

Pulmonary valvular atresia with systemic-to-pulmonary collaterals

There is no direct communication between ventricle and pulmonary artery in this anomaly. However, in a high percentage of patients, surgically approachable true pulmonary arteries are supplied by systemic collaterals. These central pulmonary arteries can be visualized by suprasternal echocardiography [39–41]. During cardiac catheterization, selective injection of contrast material into the systemic collaterals can help determine which vessels communicate directly with the true pulmonary artery (direct visualization of the pulmonary artery while injecting a collateral vessel) (Figure 24) This aids in the selection of angiographic technique and in confirming the presence of a direct systemic-to-pulmonary communication.

Pulmonary arteriovenous fistula

Normally, the contrast echocardiographic effect is completely eliminated after transit through the pulmonary capillary bed. In the presence of a pulmonary arteriovenous fistula, the contrast effect will be transmitted directly from pulmonary artery to pulmonary vein and will appear in the left atrium [42]. Selective pulmonary contrast echocardiography or, actually, lobar echoangiography for isolation of the fistulous communication can be performed by the echo technique. These techniques are more sensitive than angiography and they permit localization and gross quantitation of the shunt.

Peripheral or systemic arteriovenous fistula

Echocardiography has been used occasionally in the detection of peripheral arteriovenous fistula [43]. However, in the cardiac catheterization laboratory, echocardiography has been more helpful in the detection of visceral and mediastinal arteriovenous fistula. These shunts can often be difficult to localize by conventional angiographic techniques. Injecting echo contrast material across a suspect capillary bed can confirm the presence or absence of a fistula. By observing the site and mechanism of contrast material returning to the heart, one can accurately localize the fistulous tract. These particular studies are best utilized to help select appropriate angiographic techniques for direct visualization of the fistulous communication.

PART III: UNIQUE APPLICATIONS OF CONTRAST ECHOCARDIOGRAPHY

There are certain applications of the contrast echocardiographic technique that are unique and best not discussed under the invasive or noninvasive angiographic application.

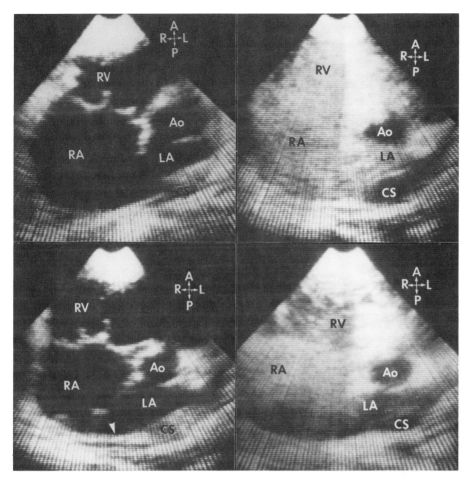

Figure 21. Total anomalous pulmonary venous connection to the coronary sinus. Still frames of two-dimensional contrast echocardiogram illustrate the sequential flow pattern after selective injection into a pulmonary vein entered via the coronary sinus. Upper left panel: after a pulmonary venous injection, the coronary sinus (CS) opacifies in the posterior aspect of the left atrium (LA). Lower left panel: contrast material exits from the coronary sinus and enters the inferior aspect of the right atrium (arrowhead). Upper right and lower right panels: there is subsequent opacification of the right atrium (RA), left atrium (LA), and right ventricle (RV). CS = coronary sinus; LA = left atrium; Ao = aorta; RA = right atrium; RV = right ventricle; A = anterior; L = left; P = posterior; R = right.

1. Orthodeoxia
2. Persistent left superior vena cava
   a. To coronary sinus
   b. To left atrium
3. Glenn anastomosis with acquired pulmonary arteriovenous fistula
4. Occluded superior vena cava
5. Blood-flow patterns after the Mustard procedure

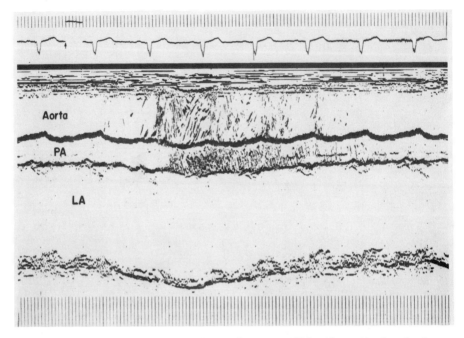

Figure 22. Patent ductus arteriosus. With the use of suprasternal M-mode examination, simultaneous visualization of the aortic arch and right pulmonary artery is shown. After the injection of contrast medium into the upper descending aorta there is subsequent opacification of the pulmonary artery consistent with the presence of a patent ductus arteriosus. LA = left atrium; PA = right pulmonary artery.

Orthodeoxia

This is a rare phenomenon in which the blood is predominantly desaturated (the patient is often cyanotic and symptomatically breathless) only when the patient is in the upright position [44]. The patient may have little or no right-to-left shunt when recumbent. This postural (i.e., dynamic) cyanotic condition has been reported most commonly in adult patients with various types of chronic lung disease or after pneumonectomy and is not associated with measurable pulmonary hypertension [45]. The mechanism for this interesting and often dramatic postural cyanosis is not known. Nevertheless, in the upright position these patients experience impressive right-to-left shunt at atrial level, usually across a patent foramen ovale. In our experience, recumbent and upright peripheral venous contrast echocardiography has been a most diagnostic and easily obtainable examination. With the use of a tilt table at the time of a contrast echocardiogram, minimal or no right-to-left shunt is observed in the recumbent position, whereas with a similar injection in the sitting or standing position, a pronounced increase in the amount of right-to-left shunt is visualized (Figure 25). In three such patients recently studied at our institution, simple closure of a patent foramen ovale has eliminated this unusual form of symptomatic cyanotic heart disease [46].

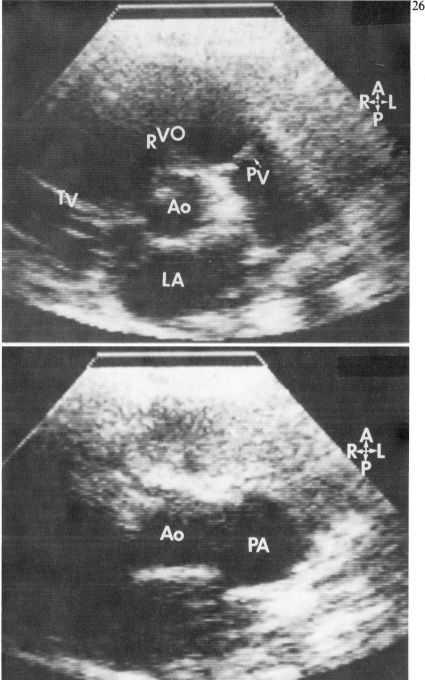

Figure 23. Aortopulmonary window. Two-dimensional echocardiographic features of aortopulmonary window include (top panel) the visualization of a pulmonary valve at aortic level. Bottom panel: with high parasternal short-axis scanning, direct communication between the aorta and the pulmonary artery can be visualized. This confirms the presence of an aortopulmonary communication. Aortic contrast injection was performed and showed simultaneous opacification of both aortic and pulmonary root (not shown). Ao = aorta; PA = pulmonary artery; PV = pulmonary valve; LA = left atrium; TV = tricuspid valve; RVO = right ventricular outflow tract; A = anterior; L = left; P = posterior; R = right.

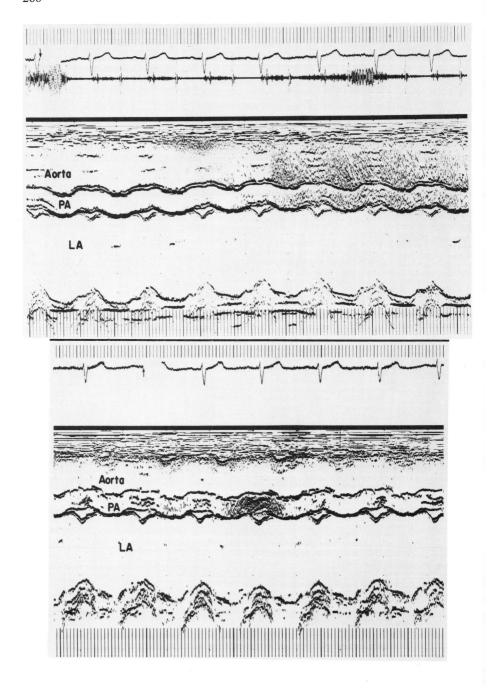

Figure 24. Pulmonary atresia with systemic-to-pulmonary collaterals shown on an M-mode suprasternal contrast echocardiogram. Top panel: a peripheral venous contrast injection shows a near-diagnostic pattern of initial opacification of the aorta with subsequent opacification of a visible right pulmonary artery (PA). This indicates that the only direct communication with the pulmonary artery is from the aorta or its branches. LA = left atrium. Bottom panel: at catheterization a selective injection into a systemic collateral shows opacification of the right pulmonary artery (PA) and designates the feeding collateral vessel. LA = left atrium.

Persistent left superior vena cava

Persistent left superior vena cava typically drains to the coronary sinus and thence to the right atrium. However, occasionally the left superior vena cava will enter the left or right atrium directly. Suprasternal echocardiography permits direct visualization of the persistent left superior vena cava (Figure 26). Peripheral venous injections of echo contrast material into the left upper extremity are utilized to confirm the left superior vena cava and its connections.

Persistent left superior vena cava to coronary sinus

This anomaly is usually best appreciated by the long-axis parasternal sector echocardiographic view [47]. In this particular projection, the dilated coronary sinus appears as an echo-free space just posterior to the left atrioventricular groove (Figure 27). After peripheral left upper-extremity injection of contrast material, the coronary sinus will be opacified first and then the right heart structures.

Persistent left superior vena cava to left atrium

The coronary sinus is not visibly dilated. After left upper-extremity injection of contrast material, the left atrium will be opacified initially (Figure 28). Two-dimensional echocardiographic suprasternal examination permits direct visualization of the left superior vena cava. Left upper-extremity contrast injections will confirm this identification, along with the anomalous return to the left atrium.

Glenn anastomosis with acquired pulmonary arteriovenous fistula

It has been our experience that in a high percentage of patients with a long-standing Glenn anastomosis, increasing numbers of pulmonary arteriovenous fistulas will develop in the lower lobes of the shunted lung [48]. Increasing cyanosis may result from arteriovenous fistula formation, as opposed to a deterioration of the complex anomaly for which the shunt was performed. The presence of these fistulas can be appreciated noninvasively by right upper-extremity peripheral venous injections of echo contrast material. In the presence of a pulmonary arteriovenous fistula, echo contrast material would be visualized in the left atrium. In the absence of such a fistula, no contrast material would be detected. If acquired venous collaterals are present, the contrast material would initially appear in the inferior vena cava and right atrium, as opposed to the left atrium. This second, often less important, collateral can usually be easily distinguished from the flow pattern observed with the acquired pulmonary arteriovenous fistula associated with increasing cyanosis.

Occluded superior vena cava

When caval obstruction is suspected, peripheral venous contrast echocardiography can be helpful in detecting the presence and, to some extent, degree of caval

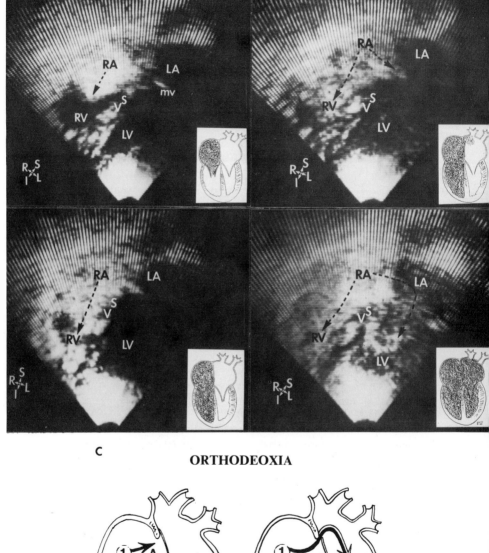

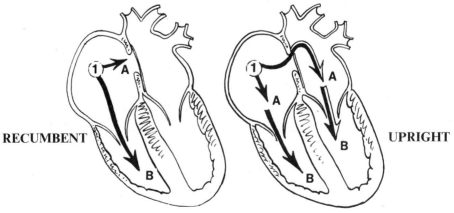

ORTHODEOXIA

RECUMBENT   UPRIGHT

Figure 25 (Legend: see p. 271).

interruption [49]. Collateral venous channels will develop, which will be appreciated as abnormal entry of contrast into the right heart chambers. An example would be total or partial occlusion of the superior vena cava after the Mustard procedure. In this example, upper-extremity injections of echo contrast material would produce variable opacification of the inferior vena cava via developing venous collaterals (i.e., the more contrast arriving from the inferior vena cava, the more will the superior vena cava be occluded).

←

Figure 25. Orthodeoxia. A) Recumbent peripheral venous contrast echocardiogram. After a peripheral venous injection of contrast medium, the right atrium is opacified (top panel) and with subsequent ventricular diastole (bottom panel) the contrast material empties into the right ventricle (arrow). There was no detectable right-to-left shunt in the recumbent position. B) Same patient in the upright position. After similar contrast injection, a cloud of echoes opacifies the right atrium and right ventricle. With one cardiac cycle delay, there is dense, near-equal opacification of the left atrium and left ventricle through an atrial septal defect (arrows). C) Illustration of characteristic flow pattern. No shunt is seen in the recumbent position (left), and an often dramatic right-to-left shunt occurs across a patent foramen ovale in the upright position (right). RA = right atrium; LA = left atrium; mv = mitral valve; LV = left ventricle; VS = ventricular septum; RV = right ventricle; S = superior; L = left; I = inferior; R = right.

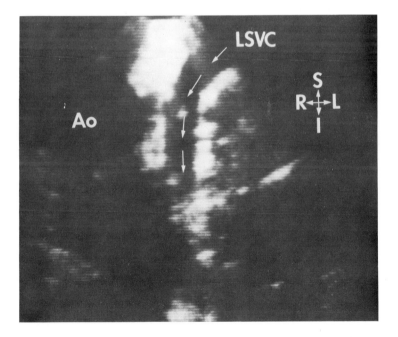

Figure 26. Suprasternal echocardiogram of persistent left superior vena cava. In the short-axis projection from the suprasternal notch, leftward tilt of the transducer permits direct visualization of a persistent left superior vena cava (LSVC). This structure can be confirmed by selective left upper-extremity echo contrast injection. Ao = aorta; S = superior; L = left; I = inferior; R = right.

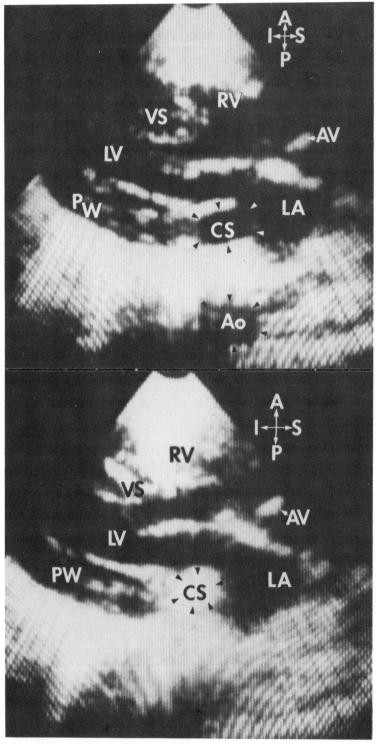

Figure 27 (Legend: see p. 273).

Blood-flow patterns after the Mustard procedure

The unique blood-flow patterns that occur after the Mustard operation have been well described [30]. Both peripheral echo contrast techniques and selective echo-angiography delineate the surgically altered venous return.

PART IV: CONCLUSION

Contrast echocardiography is an excellent means of enhancing the M-mode or two-dimensional echocardiographic examination. This examination can be utilized not

◄

Figure 27. Persistent left superior vena cava at a coronary sinus in a patient with double-outlet right ventricle. Top panel: a large echo-free structure is visualized in the left atrioventricular groove which represents a large dilated coronary sinus (CS). The aortic valve overrides the ventricular septum. A small portion of the right ventricle is visualized anterior to the ventricular septum. There is a large ventricular septal defect beneath the aortic valve. Bottom panel: after a left upper-extremity venous injection, the coronary sinus is opacified (CS) with subsequent opacification of the right ventricle (RV). This type of abnormal venous drainage by itself would not result in cyanosis. RV = right ventricle; AV = aortic valve; LA = left atrium; Ao = thoracic aorta; PW = posterior wall; LV = left ventricle; VS = ventricular septum; A = anterior; S = superior; P = posterior; I = inferior. (From ref. [3]. By permission).

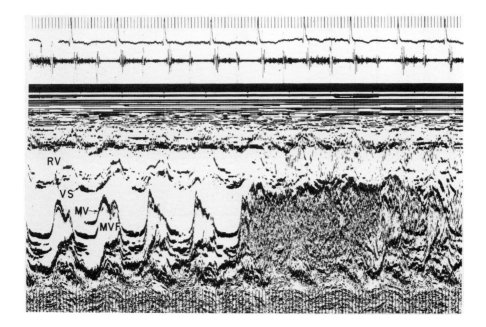

Figure 28. Persistent left superior vena cava to left atrium. After a left upper-extremity venous injection, contrast material initially appears at the mitral valve funnel (arrival from left atrium) and subsequently opacifies the left ventricle. MVF = mitral valve funnel; MV = mitral valve; VS = ventricular septum; RV = right ventricle. (From ref. [30]. By permission of FA Davis Company).

only at bedside with peripheral venous injections, but also in the cardiac catheterization laboratory as a complement to the invasive procedure. Many congenital anomalies have very specific blood-flow patterns that are pathognomonic for the entity in question. It can be stated that the more complex the cardiac lesion, the more likely one is to find a diagnostic echocardiographic contrast blood-flow pattern. Two-dimensional examination, with its lateral resolution and dynamic tomographic presentation, is superior to the M-mode contrast study; however, for the purposes of accurate timing of the arrival of the contrast material and of correlating the contrast effect with other cardiac events, M-mode is superior. The advantage of the two-dimensional contrast echocardiogram is its tomographic presentation. When used in conjunction with echo contrast material, it can provide unique documentation of the blood-flow pattern which at times is superior to that obtained with standard angiographic techniques. In most situations, contrast echoangiography can greatly enhance or eliminate standard ventriculography in the patient with complex congenital heart disease. In our laboratory, this has allowed the angiographer to concentrate more on cardiac hemodynamics and visualization of extracardiac vascular anatomy (pulmonary arterial distribution, venous anomalies, and systemic arterial anomalies).

M-mode and two-dimensional contrast echocardiography is a powerful tool when applied to congenital heart disease. Such techniques can greatly enhance or actually supplant the invasive examination. This technique has evolved into an essential part of the armamentarium of pediatric and adult cardiologists dealing with congenital heart disease.

REFERENCES

1. Seward JB, AJ Tajik, JG Spangler, DG Ritter: Echocardiographic contrast studies: initial experience. Mayo Clin Proc 50:163–192, 1975.
2. Tajik AJ, JB Seward, DJ Hagler, DD Mair: Experience with real-time two-dimensional sector angiography. Am J Cardiol 41:353, 1978 (abstract).
3. Seward JB, AJ Tajik, DJ Hagler: Two-dimensional contrast echoangiography. In: Lundström N-R (ed) Pediatric Echocardiography – Cross Sectional, M-mode and Doppler, p 239–255. Elsevier/North Holland Biomedical, Amsterdam, 1980.
4. Seward JB, AJ Tajik, DJ Hagler, DG Ritter: Peripheral venous contrast echocardiography. Am J Cardiol 39:202–212, 1977.
5. Hagler DJ, AJ Tajik, JB Seward, DD Mair, DG Ritter, EL Ritman: Videodensitometric quantitation of left-to-right shunts with contrast sector echocardiography. Circulation (Suppl II) 58:70, 1978 (abstract).
6. Swan HJC, HB Burchell, EH Wood: The presence of venoarterial shunts in patients with interatrial communications. Circulation 10:705–713, 1954.
7. Levin AR, MS Spach, JP Boineau, RV Canent Jr, MP Capp, PH Jewett: Atrial pressure–flow dynamics in atrial septal defects (secundum type). Circulation 37:476–488, 1968.
8. Nasser FN, AJ Tajik, JB Seward, DJ Hagler: Diagnosis of sinus venosus atrial septal defect by two-dimensional echocardiography. Mayo Clin Proc 56:568–572, 1981.
9. Kronik G, J Slany, H Moesslacher: Contrast M-mode echocardiography in diagnosis of

atrial septal defect in acyanotic patients. Circulation 59:372–378, 1979.

10. Serwer GA, BE Armstrong, PAW Anderson, D Sherman, DW Benson Jr, SB Edwards: Use of contrast echocardiography for evaluation of right ventricular hemodynamics in the presence of ventricular septal defects. Circulation 58:327–336, 1978.

11. Weyman AE, LS Wann, RA Hurwitz, JC Dillon, H Feigenbaum: Negative contrast echocardiography: a new technique for detecting left-to-right shunts. Circulation (Suppl III) 56:26, 1977 (abstract).

12. Levin AR, MS Spach, RV Canent Jr, JP Boineau, MP Capp, V Jain, RC Barr: Intra-cardiac pressure–flow dynamics in isolated ventricular septal defects. Circulation 35: 430–441, 1967.

13. Assad-Morell JL, JB Seward, AJ Tajik, DJ Hagler, ER Giuliani, DG Ritter: Echo-phonocardiographic and contrast studies in conditions associated with systemic arterial trunk overriding the ventricular septum: truncus arteriosus, tetralogy of Fallot, and pulmonary atresia with ventricular septal defect. Circulation 53:663–673, 1976.

14. Hagler DJ, AJ Tajik, JB Seward, DD Mair, DG Ritter: Wide-angle two-dimensional echocardiographic profiles of conotruncal abnormalities. Mayo Clin Proc 55:73–82, 1980.

15. Levin AR, JP Boineau, MS Spach, RV Canent Jr, MP Capp, PAW Anderson: Ven-tricular pressure–flow dynamics in tetralogy of Fallot. Circulation 34:4–13, 1966.

16. Ports TA, NH Silverman, NB Schiller: Two-dimensional echocardiographic assessment of Ebstein's anomaly. Circulation 58:336–343, 1978.

17. Lieppe WM, VS Behar, R Scallion, J Kisslo: Detection of tricuspid regurgitation with contrast two-dimensional echocardiography Am J Cardiol 41:371, 1978 (abstract).

18. Seward JB, AJ Tajik, DJ Hagler, DG Ritter: Echocardiographic spectrum of tricuspid atresia. Mayo Clin Proc 53:100–112, 1978.

19. Seward JB, AJ Tajik, DJ Hagler, ER Giuliani, GT Gau, DG Ritter: Echocardiogram in common (single) ventricle: angiographic–anatomic correlation. Am J Cardiol 39: 217–225, 1977.

20. Anderson RH, AE Becker, JL Wilkinson, LM Gerlis: Morphogenesis of univentricular hearts. Br Heart J 38:558–572, 1976.

21. Van Praagh R, PA Ongley, HJC Swan: Anatomic types of single or common ventricle in man: morphologic and geometric aspects of 60 necropsied cases. Am J Cardiol 13: 367–386, 1964.

22. Lev M, RR Liberthson, JR Kirkpatrick, FAO Eckner, RA Arcilla: Single (primitive) ventricle. Circulation 39:577–591, 1969.

23. Seward JB, AJ Tajik, DJ Hagler: Two-dimensional echocardiographic features of uni-ventricular heart. In: Lundström N-R (ed) Pediatric Echocardiography–Cross Sectional, M-mode and Doppler, p 157–169. Elsevier/North Holland Biomedical, Amsterdam, 1980.

24. Seward JB, AJ Tajik, DJ Hagler, DG Ritter: Contrast echocardiography in single or common ventricle. Circulation 55:513–519, 1977.

25. Hagler DJ, AJ Tajik, JB Seward, DD Mair, DG Ritter: Real-time wide-angle sector echocardiography: atrioventricular canal defects. Circulation 59:140–150, 1979.

26. Keeton BR, FJ Macartney, S Hunter, C Mortera, P Rees, EA Shinebourne, M Tynan, JL Wilkinson, RH Anderson: Univentricular heart of right ventricular type with double or common inlet. Circulation 59:403–411, 1979.

27. Bierman FZ, RG Williams: Prospective diagnosis of d-transposition of the great arteries in neonates by subxiphoid, two-dimensional echocardiography. Circulation 60:1496–1502, 1979.

28. Seward JB, AJ Tajik, DJ Hagler: Orientation of the great arteries: normal, complete transposition, corrected transposition. In: Lundström N-R (ed) Pediatric Echocardio-

graphy – Cross Sectional, M-mode and Doppler, p 105–120. Elsevier/North Holland Biomedical, Amsterdam, 1980.

29. Mortera C, S Hunter, M Tynan: Contrast echocardiography and the suprasternal approach in infants and children. Eur J Cardiol 9:437–454, 1979.
30. Tajik AJ, JB Seward: Contrast echocardiography. Cardiovasc Clin (2) 9:317–341, 1978.
31. Seward JB, AJ Tajik, DJ Hagler, DD Mair: Straddling atrioventricular valve: diagnostic two-dimensional echographic features. Am J Cardiol 41:354, 1978 (abstract).
32. Anderson RH, EA Shinebourne, LM Gerlis: Criss-cross atrioventricular relationships producing paradoxical atrioventricular concordance or discordance: their significance to nomenclature of congenital heart disease. Circulation 50:176–180, 1974.
33. Sieg K, DJ Hagler, DG Ritter, DC McGoon, JD Maloney, JB Seward, GD Davis: Straddling right atrioventricular valve in criss-cross atrioventricular relationship. Mayo Clin Proc 52:561–568, 1977.
34. Seward JB, AJ Tajik, DJ Hagler: Two-dimensional echocardiographic features of atrioventricular canal defect. In: Lundström N-R (ed) Pediatric Echocardiography–Cross Sectional, M-mode and Doppler, p 197–206. Elsevier/North Holland Biomedical, Amsterdam, 1980.
35. Sahn DJ, HD Allen, LW Lange, SJ Goldberg: Cross-sectional echocardiographic diagnosis of the sites of total anomalous pulmonary venous drainage. Circulation 60: 1317–1325, 1979.
36. Sahn DJ, HD Allen: Real-time cross-sectional echocardiographic imaging and measurement of the patent ductus arteriosus in infants and children. Circulation 58:343–354, 1978.
37. Goldberg SJ, J Areias, L Feldman, DJ Sahn, HD Allen: Lesions that cause aortic flow disturbance. Circulation 60:1539–1547, 1979.
38. Allen HD, DJ Sahn, SJ Goldberg: New serial contrast technique for assessment of left-to-right shunting patent ductus arteriosus in the neonate. Am J Cardiol 41:288–294, 1978.
39. Tajik AJ, JB Seward, DJ Hagler, DD Mair, JT Lie: Two-dimensional real-time ultrasonic imaging of the heart and great vessels: technique, image orientation, structure identification, and validation. Mayo Clin Proc 53:271–303, 1978.
40. Huhta JC, JM Piehler, AJ Tajik, JB Seward, DJ Hagler: Detection and measurement of the right pulmonary artery in pulmonary atresia-ventricular septal defect by two-dimensional echocardiography: angiographic and surgical correlation. Circulation (Suppl III) 62:333, 1980 (abstract).
41. Snider AR, NH Silverman: Suprasternal notch echocardiography: a two-dimensional technique for evaluating congenital heart disease. Circulation 63:165–173, 1981.
42. Shub C, AJ Tajik, JB Seward, DE Dines: Detecting intrapulmonary right-to-left shunt with contrast echocardiography: observations in a patient with diffuse pulmonary arteriovenous fistulas. Mayo Clin Proc 51:81–84, 1976.
43. Pritchard DA, JD Maloney, JB Seward, AJ Tajik, JF Fairbairn II, PC Pairolero: Peripheral arteriovenous fistula: detection by contrast echocardiography. Mayo Clin Proc 52:186–190, 1977.
44. Begin R: Platypnea after pneumonectomy. N Engl J Med 293:342–343, 1975.
45. Khan F, A Parekh: Reversible platypnea and orthodeoxia following recovery from adult respiratory distress syndrome. Chest 75:526–528, 1979.
46. Hayes DL, JB Seward, AJ Tajik, DE Williams, HC Smith, EC Rosenow III, GS Reeder: Platypnea-orthodeoxia: evaluation and management. Presented at the American College of Chest Physicians, San Francisco, October 25–29, 1981.
47. Snider AR, TA Ports, NH Silverman: Venous anomalies of the coronary sinus: detection by M-mode, two-dimensional and contrast echocardiography. Circulation 60:721–727, 1979.

48. McFaul RC, AJ Tajik, DD Mair, GK Danielson, JB Seward: Development of pulmonary arteriovenous shunt after superior vena cava-right pulmonary artery (Glenn) anastomosis: report of four cases. Circulation 55:212–216, 1977.
49. Coló J, R Snider, N Silverman: Echocardiographic detection of superior vena cava obstruction after Mustard's procedure. Circulation (Suppl III) 62:332, 1980 (abstract).

22. CONTRAST M-MODE ECHOCARDIOGRAPHY, THE SUPRASTERNAL NOTCH APPROACH

STEWART HUNTER and GEORGE R. SUTHERLAND

STEWART HUNTER and GEORGE R. SUTHERLAND

INTRODUCTION

The combination of contrast echocardiography and the suprasternal approach offers a very reliable method for the evaluation of right to left shunts and ventriculoarterial connections in infants and children with complex congenital heart disease to the clinician who does not have real-time two-dimensional echocardiography.

In our institution, contrast echocardiography was initially used at cardiac catheterisation to establish the origin of unidentified M-Mode echoes [1, 2]. Subsequently, we concentrated on peripheral vein contrast echocardiography with the suprasternal approach before catheterisation in infants and children with complex congenital heart disease. The combination of the two techniques has been invaluable in the assessment of the level of right to left shunts and of the ventriculoarterial connections in complex congenital heart disease.

Echocardiographic and anatomic considerations

Normally in the M-Mode echocardiogram cardiac structures are identified by characteristic patterns of movement associated with the varying phases of the cardiac cycle. The morphology of the individual cardiac structures has also to be inferred from their antero-posterior relationships, although there is some additional evidence from lateral relationships. It is thus assumed that anterior structures are part of the right heart and posterior structures part of the left. Of course, this is frequently very misleading in complex congenital lesions, because of changes in spacial orientation of the heart within the chest and in antero-posterior and lateral relationships of the cardiac structures. In particular, the semilunar valves in the neonate may be identical in appearance from the parasternal M-Mode approach.

The reliability of the underlying anatomical relationships of the aortic arch, right pulmonary artery and left atrium provides the suprasternal approach with an enormous advantage (Figure 1). The arch always lies closer to the transducer than the pulmonary artery, thus allowing the two individ-

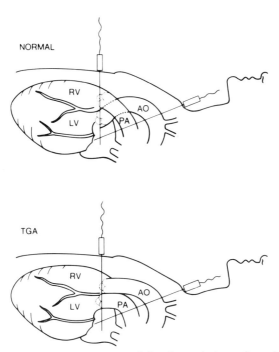

Figure 1. These diagrams illustrate the route of the ultrasonic beam from the parasternal and suprasternal approaches in the normal heart and in transposition of the great arteries. They demonstrate the constant relationship of aorta and pulmonary artery from the suprasternal approach.

AO = aorta;   PA = pulmonary   artery;   LV = left   ventricle;   RV = right   ventricle; TGA = transposition of the great arteries.

ual great arteries to be reliably differentiated. A bolus of ultrasonic indicator injected into the peripheral systemic venous system is observed suprasternally to provide the necessary diagnostic information.

METHODS

We usually place an intravenous cannula in the vein on the back of the hand or in the leg. It is preferable not to use a scalp vein as the injection tends to cause discomfort, making the child move and spoiling the echo. Babies are done shortly after feeding when they are quiet and settled, older children on the other hand may require sedation. The transducers used depend empirically on which gives the best definition.

The transducer is directed downwards through the suprasternal notch and slightly posteriorly to cut the underlying cardiac structures at right-angles to their walls. If parts of either semilunar valve are seen, then the beam is not angled through the appropriate part of the aortic arch and the right pulmonary artery. This is crucial, particularly in the diagnosis of ventriculo-arterial discordance. 5% dextrose is used as the contrast medium and is injected rapidly through a 1 ml syringe as a bolus. Quantities of gaseous microbubbles in the bolus reflect ultrasound intensely and the blood-filled cavities are opacified on the echocardiogram. In the normal heart, peripheral systemic venous injection is followed by opacification of the right ventricle and pulmonary artery in the parasternal and suprasternal views. The microbubbles are then filtered out in the lungs and none appear in the left heart. When a right to left shunt is present or an abnormality of ventriculoarterial connections, contrast also appears in the left heart. Several cardiac cycles are recorded before the injection so that the initial timing of opacification is clear. The recording is then continued until the contrast effect has disappeared. In the normal heart, contrast disappears within five to six cardiac cycles, but in the presence of right sided valvular regurgitation it may persist for as long as a minute. Such contrast injections are always made by hand and as a result there is a wide spread of intensity of opacification between individual injections and no attempt is made to compare the intensity and persistence of opacification in sequential injections. However, it is possible, as will be discussed later, to compare the relative opacification of two structures during the same injection.

RESULTS

Identification of the great arteries from the suprasternal approach

In the great majority of cases we have been able to identify the aortic arch and the right pulmonary artery. With increasing confidence in the technique, inability to record the right pulmonary artery strongly suggests that it is either abnormal in situation or absent. Although Allen et al. [3] have reported ranges of echo dimensions for the three structures in the suprasternal view in normal children, we confined ourselves to the relative size of the pulmonary artery and aorta. It is occasionally impossible to record the three cardiac structures in the presence of abnormalities of the aortic arch.

Detection of right to left atrial shunts

In our initial study we validated the detection of right to left atrial shunts by suprasternal contrast echocardiography in a large series of children who underwent cardiac catheterisation. We accepted only patients who at cardiac catheterisation had definite right to left shunts in the presence of full pulmonary venous saturation. In all of these contrast echocardiography

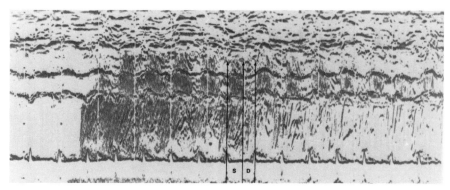

Figure 2. The aorta, pulmonary artery and left atrium are demonstrated in this suprasternal echocardiogram. Following peripheral venous injection of contrast the left atrium opacifies during diastole and subsequently both aorta and pulmonary artery opacify.
S = systole; D = diastole.

demonstrated opacification of the left atrium following peripheral venous injection, confirming a right to left atrial shunt.

Left atrial opacification was always associated with opacification of both great arteries (Figure 2). If a large amount of contrast appeared in the left atrium it was usually only possible to diagnose a right to left atrial shunt and not possible to infer the presence of an additional right to left ventricular shunt. However, on some occasions the great arteries opacified very intensely but the left atrium was barely opacified and in these we were able to demonstrate at catheterisation that the major right to left shunt was at the ventricular level and that there was a small atrial shunt.

Detection of right to left ventricular shunts

Again in the initial validatory study, the detection of right to left ventricular shunts was compared using catheterisation and contrast echocardiography. Again there was 100% correlation between the two methods. The left atrium remained unopacified while the great arteries opacified strongly (Figure 3).

Assessment of ventriculoarterial connections

In the normal heart, or in the absence of right to left shunting, contrast from the peripheral circulation will only appear in the right pulmonary artery in the suprasternal view. With the exception of the rare isolated ventricular inversion, it is possible for all clinical purposes to infer that the ventriculoar-terial connections are normal (Figure 4). In the presence of a right to left shunt at atrial or ventricular level, it is still usually possible to determine that

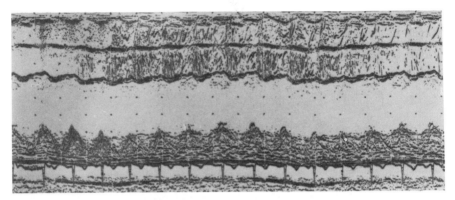

Figure 3. A suprasternal echocardiogram following selective peripheral venous injection of contrast. The left atrium does not opacify, but both great arteries do with about equal intensity. Only a right to left ventricular shunt was noted at cardiac catheterisation.

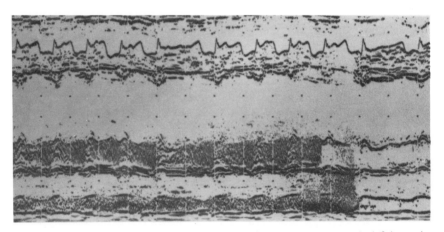

Figure 4. Selective peripheral venous injection in the left hand demonstrates the left innominate vein lying anterior to the aorta in the suprasternal view. Contrast appears first at this site and there is no constant relationship to ventricular systole, as judged on the ECG.

Later, the pulmonary artery, only, opacifies, establishing normal ventriculoarterial connections. At the start of opacification of the innominate vein, artefactual smearing of contrast occurs across the boundaries of the innominate vein and the aorta.

one great artery opacifies more persistently and more intensely, suggesting that it receives most of the systemic venous return (Figure 5). If this is the pulmonary artery, then, with the previously mentioned exception, it can be inferred that most of the systemic venous return goes to the pulmonary artery and hence ventriculoarterial connections are normal. In cases of ventriculoarterial discordance (Transposition of the Great Arteries), the pattern of opacification from the suprasternal approach is very different [4]. The aorta receives most of the systemic venous return and is thus opacified more intensely and persistently than the pulmonary artery. However, usually the left atrium and pulmonary artery will receive some opacification in view

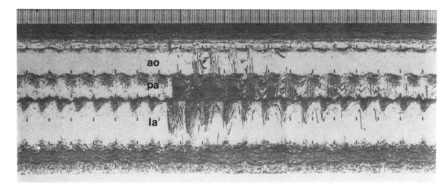

Figure 5. Selective peripheral venous injection into the right hand. The left atrium opacifies first in diastole and then the pulmonary artery and aorta also opacify. Both great arteries opacify most intensely in systole but the pulmonary artery receives most of the systemic venous return and opacifies most intensely and persistently.

of the obligatory intracardiac shunting which is required for the baby to survive.

Transposition differs from other cyanotic congenital heart disease in that the greater the right to left shunt at atrial or ventricular level, the higher the effective pulmonary blood flow will be and the higher the systemic arterial oxygen saturation. By comparing aortic percentage oxygen saturation in children with transposition to the relative opacification (at each injection) of

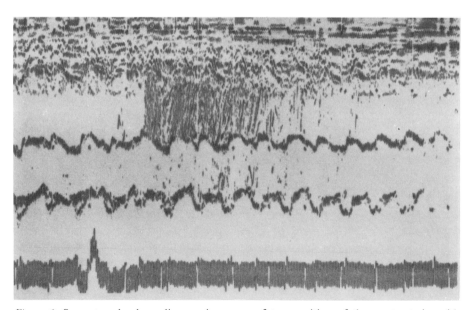

Figure 6. Suprasternal echocardiogram in a case of transposition of the great arteries with minimal interatrial shunting. Very little contrast appears in the pulmonary artery and most of the contrast is seen in the aorta.

284

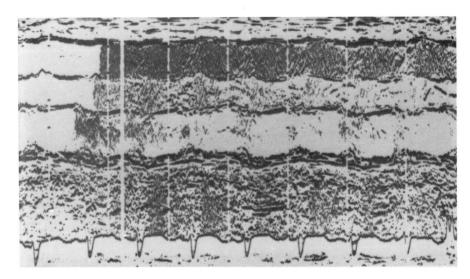

Figure 7. This suprasternal echocardiogram is from a patient with transposition of the great arteries. The left atrium opacifies followed by both great arteries. The aorta is more persistently and intensely opacified, suggesting that it receives most of the systemic venous return.

both great arteries, some comment can be made about the approximate effective pulmonary blood flow. When aortic saturation is less than 40%, the amount of contrast appearing in the left atrium on suprasternal echocardiogram is minimal and the aorta opacifies for more than twice as many cycles as the pulmonary artery (Figure 6). When the aortic saturation lies between 40% and 60%, the pulmonary artery opacifies more than half as many cycles as the aorta, although there is usually still sufficient differential opacification to make the diagnosis of ventriculoarterial discordance (Figure 7). When aortic saturation is greater than 60%, both great arteries opacify equally intensely and for the same number of cardiac cycles and accurate assessment of ventriculoarterial connections becomes impossible (Figure 8). Under these

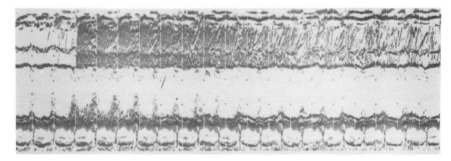

Figure 8. In this suprasternal echocardiogram both great arteries opacify with equal intensity and persistence, and it is not possible to assess accurately the ventriculoarterial connections, This patient had a very small right to left shunt which was not picked up on this echocardiogram. The major shunting occurred at ventricular level.

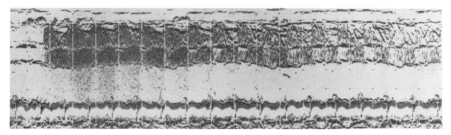

Figure 9. In this suprasternal echocardiogram the aorta and the pulmonary artery opacify in systole with similar intensity and little contrast reaches the left atrium. These findings suggest a right to left ventricular shunt which was present. In the later cardiac cycles the aorta opacifies more intensely in systole and the pulmonary artery in diastole. Indicating the presence of co-existing transposition of the great arteries and persistent ductus arteriosus.

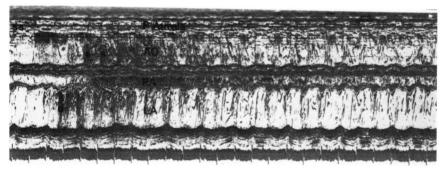

Figure 10. A suprasternal echocardiogram in a case of pulmonary atresia following systemic injection of contrast. The large aorta opacifies first, followed by left atrial opacification and finally by opacification of the pulmonary artery. The aorta is most intensely opacified in systole while the pulmonary artery initially shows a flat non-cyclical opacification, indicating that it is not connected to the heart directly by a semilunar valve but receives its blood supply from the aorta.

P. Atresia = pulmonary atresia; AO = aorta; PA = pulmonary artery; LA = left atrium.

circumstances, at cardiac catheterisation there is usually less than 10 % difference between aorta and pulmonary artery oxygen saturation.

In children with Transposition of the Great Arteries and persistent ductus arteriosus, a unique type of cyclical opacification of the pulmonary artery is seen. The aorta is cyclically opacified with each systole, but the pulmonary artery, even in the presence of a co-existing ventricular septal defect, shows mainly diastolic opacification (Figure 9). This suggests that most of the contrast reaches the pulmonary artery through an aortopulmonary communication in diastole and that blood with less contrast reaches the pulmonary artery in systole through the pulmonary valve, causing momentary clearing. This curious phenomenon disappears when the ductus is closed surgically or spontaneously.

In pulmonary valve atresia with ventricular septal defect and persistent ductus arteriosus, the aorta opacifies cyclically in systole. The pulmonary artery opacifies initially in diastole and later than the aorta. Thereafter, there is a flat, non-cyclical opacification of the pulmonary artery, suggesting that it is receiving none of its blood from the heart directly but rather through the persistent ductus arteriosus (Figure 10).

Visualisation of systemic veins

When contrast is injected into the left hand or arm, it is frequently possible to see an opacified space anterior to the aorta (Figure 4). This opacifies very early and without any cyclical change and almost certainly represents the left innominate vein. Again with increasing experience, the absence of this opacification following left hand or arm injection strongly suggests absence of the left innominate vein. Occasionally it is possible to diagnose a left superior vena cava draining to the coronary sinus, by suprasternal contrast echocardiography. In these circumstances, the left innominate vein does not opacify after a left hand injection, but the coronary sinus opacifies behind the left atrium.

CONCLUSION

Most infants admitted as emergencies to paediatric cardiological units undergo an extensive work-up, including clinical examination, chest X-ray blood/gas analysis and electrocardiography. It is now common practice to include in this pre-catheterisation diagnostic cascade M-Mode echocardiography. The use of the suprasternal technique and contrast echocardiography gives a great deal of diagnostic information, which is not only qualitative but can sometimes be semi-quantitative. The undoubted advantages of real-time two-dimensional echocardiography over M-Mode in such children is not available to all units because of cost. M-Mode contrast echocardiography from the suprasternal approach in our experience greatly enhances the diagnostic possibilities of the single probe technique.

REFERENCES

1. Goldberg BB: Ultrasonic measurement of aortic arch, right pulmonary artery and left atrium. Radiology 101:383, 1971.
2. Mortera C, M Tynan, A Goodwin, S Hunter: Infradiaphragmatic total anomalous pulmonary venous connection to the portal vein. Diagnostic implications of echocardiography. Brit Heart J 39:685, 1977.
3. Allen HD, SJ Goldberg, DJ Sahn, TW Ovitt, BB Goldberg: Suprasternal notch echocardiography. Assessment of its clinical utility in paediatric cardiology. Circulation 55:605, 1977.
4. Mortera C, S Hunter, M Tynan: Contrast echocardiography and the suprasternal approach in infants and children. European J of Cardiology 9/6:437–454, 1979. Elsevier/North-Holland Biomedical Press.

C. FUTURE PROSPECTS

23. DETERMINATION OF CARDIAC OUTPUT BY TWO-DIMENSIONAL CONTRAST ECHOCARDIOGRAPHY

ANTHONY N. DeMARIA, WILLIAM BOMMER, JULIA RASOR,
E. GLENN TICKNER, and DEAN T. MASON

Contrast echocardiography refers to the process of opacifying cardiac chambers and major vessels with dense "clouds" of reflected echoes by means of the intravascular injection of a variety of fluids [1]. Although the exact source of the contrast effect is not known, available evidence overwhelmingly points to the role of microscopic air bubbles in the genesis of the contrast effect [2]. Although indocyanine green, saline, and dextrose in water have been the solutions most routinely used to produce contrast echocardiograms, even intravascular injection of the patient's own blood can elicit similar phenomena. Recently a variety of gas containing substances have been utilized in the experimental laboratory to standardize the contrast recordings obtained [3].

Contrast echocardiography has found a variety of applications in clinical cardiology. Initially, contrast injections within the central circulation were utilized during echocardiography to verify ultrasonically determined cardiac anatomy [4]. Subsequently, contrast echocardiography has been utilized to evaluate blood flow patterns, especially in regard to intracardiac communications [5]: Since the contrast effect is removed by the transit of blood through the lungs, contrast is not normally seen in the left side cardiac chambers following intravenous injection, and the technique may therefore be of particular value in the recognition of right-to-left intracardiac shunting by either atrial or ventricular septal defects. In addition, a contrast free jet (negative contrast) may be observed during opacification of the right side chambers in patients with left-to-right shunting [6], and reflux of contrast into the inferior vena cava has proven to be of value in the detection of tricuspid regurgitation [7]. Unfortunately, none of these applications or approaches have yielded any quantitative data from contrast echocardiograms.

In the course of analysis of a number of two-dimensional contrast echocardiograms performed in our laboratory for clinical purposes, the qualitative observation was made that the time-course of appearance and disappearance of the contrast effect in an individual patient seemed to be related to the status of overall cardiac function at the time of the study. These initial qualitative observations were confirmed by the simple procedure of timing with a stopwatch the duration of the ultrasonic contrast effect in patients with varying levels of cardiac function. Stimulated by these findings, a series of projects were undertaken by which to obtain quantitative information from the appearance and disappearance characteristics of two-dimensional contrast echocardiograms.

PHOTOMETRIC AQUISITION OF INDICATOR DILUTION CURVES

The contrast effect obtained by two-dimensional echocardiography is presented as luminescence upon a video monitor or cathode ray oscilloscope. Further, the luminance may be readily recorded by means of a photometer (lightmeter) which is focused upon the screen of the monitor (Figure 1).

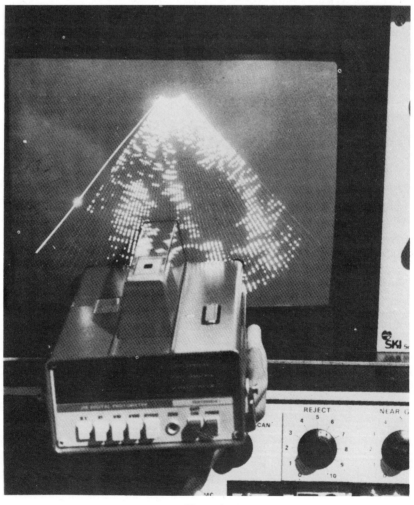

Figure 1

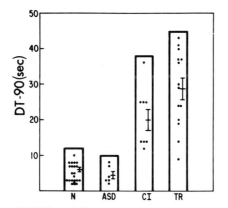

Figure 4. Measurements of DT/90 in different study groups.
N = normal, ASD = atrial septal defect, CI = reduced cardiac index, TR = tricuspid regurgitation.

seconds and 3.6 versus 23.0 seconds respectively, p<0.01). Thus, even simple measurements obtained from the disappearance phase of echocardiographic contrast curves showed good correlation with cardiac output measurements.

ADVANCES IN THE QUANTITATION OF ECHOCARDIOGRAPHIC INDICATOR DILUTION CURVES

Although the early experiments demonstrated that the disappearance characteristics of the indicator dilution curves from contrast echocardiography yielded information regarding cardiac output, a direct calculation of cardiac output was not possible from such recordings. The calculation of cardiac output (CO) from any indicator dilution curve is usually computed by means of the Hamilton equation as $CO = i/(\bar{c} \cdot t)$, where i is the mass of the indicator, $\bar{c}$ is the mean concentration of the indicator during its initial pass through the sampling area, and t is the total duration of the curve obtained. Accordingly, it was necessary to determine the mass of the contrast agent injected as well as to develop a method for the computation of the mean concentration of the agent during transit through the heart in order to calculate actual cardiac output from two-dimensional contrast echocardiograms.

In order to determine the mass of the injectate, it was necessary to utilize an agent which yielded a constant and predictable contrast effect. Since the contrast effect was predominantly referrable to microscopic air bubbles within the injected solution, an effort was undertaken to develop microbubbles of uniform size. Two agents were acquired: plastic microballoons whose size varied in a bell-shaped distribution about a mean of 30 microns in diameter and, secondly, gelatin-encapsulated microbubbles of precise size (each measuring exactly 10 microns), developed by Rasor Associates of Sunnyvale, California [10]. Initial studies indeed confirmed that the newer substances yielded contrast intensities which were both more reproducible and of consistantly higher amplitude when compared to commonly utilized contrast agents. Accordingly, utilizing these new contrast agents the mass of the contrast injected could be predicted.

In order to determine the mean concentration of contrast during a recording it was necessary to develop a system in which the analog signal obtained from the luminance of opacification was linear with respect to the concentration of the contrast present. To accomplish this, a videodensitometer was constructed which sensed the voltage peaks from a video signal over a triangular sample volume and expressed its output as the sum of the products of voltage and time. The ultrasound/videodensitometer system was tested by examining a series of plastic bags containing 30 micron microballoons suspended at various concentrations by volume, ranging from 1.7 to 6.3×10^{-5} in a viscous medium. The system was found to yield a linear signal throughout the concentrations evaluated. The final requirement was, of course, a calibration factor representing the analog signal which would be obtained by a known amount of contrast diluted in a known amount of blood from within the patient. Unfortunately, at present a calibration factor from which to determine absolute concentration of the contrast agent has not been developed.

IN VITRO EVALUATION OF VIDEODENSITOMETRIC CONTRAST INDICATOR DILUTION CURVES

The availability of an injectate of uniform and predictable mass, and ultrasonic videodensitometer system capable of yielding linear analog signals with regard to contrast amplitude enabled the evaluation of contrast curves to indicate directional changes in cardiac output. Therefore, a series of studies were undertaken to determine whether indicator dilution curves obtained by this method of contrast echocardiography could be correlated with measurements of flow and cardiac output.

Initially, in vitro studies were performed in a mechanical simulated heart and lung system in which pump flow could be adjusted to any rate. Gelatin encapsulated precision 10 micron microbubbles were utilized as the contrast agent for these studies.

A fixed concentration of gelatin microballoons dissolved in a vehicle was injected into the right atrial port of the heart-lung simulator while echocardiograms were performed from a water bath surrounding the pulmonary artery segment of the model. Multiple contrast injections were performed at simulated cardiac output flow rates varying from 4 to 12 liters per minute, and indicator dilution curves were obtained by videodensitometry of these ultrasonic recordings. The area under these curves was then determined by simple planimetry. Analysis of this data yielded a correlation coefficient of r = 0.99 between the inverse planed area under the curve and model flow rate [11]. Accordingly, it was documented that indicator dilution curves obtained by contrast echocardiography in vitro were capable of yielding estimates of cardiac output which correlated extremely closely with actual measurements.

IN VIVO EVALUATION OF VIDEODENSITOMETRIC INDICATOR DILUTION CURVES

Subsequently, a series of studies were performed to determine if indicator dilution curves obtained by two-dimensional contrast echocardiography were capable of yielding estimates of cardiac output in vivo [12]. Studies were carried out in a group of open-chested mongrel dogs in whom cardiac output was measured by thermodilution techniques with the thermister positioned in the pulmonary artery and in whom alterations of cardiac output were induced by the administration of either isoproterenol, propranolol, or blood withdrawal. Contrast was produced by the left atrial injection of 10 cc of 1:100,000 concentration by volume of 30 micron plastic microballoons. Echocardiograms were performed in the long-axis plane of the left ventricle by means of the direct epicardial positioning of a wide-angle, rotatory, mechanical sector-scanner. The two-dimensional contrast echocardiograms were recorded on videotape, and subsequently analyzed by ultrasonic videodensitometry with the sample volume in the left ventricle to yield indicator dilution curves (Figure 5). Five injections were carried out at each cardiac output in every animal, and a total of 60 cardiac outputs were

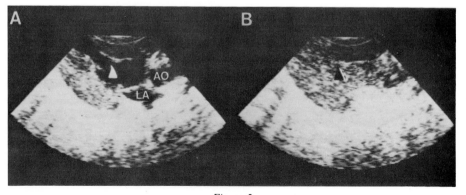

Figure 5

obtained in the group of animals studied. The indicator dilution curves obtained were quantified by means of planimetry to obtain the total area under the curve, as well as the extrapolated area under the curve using the forward triangle method.

When the area measurements of the indicator dilution curves were compared to actual measurements of cardiac output by thermodilution, an extremely close correlation was obtained in each of the individual animals studied. However, the number of cardiac output levels in individual animals were limited, and ranged from 4 to 7, with the mean of 5.2 per·experiment. Nevertheless, it was clear that the indicator dilution curves obtained by two-dimensional contrast echocardiograms in vivo correlated extremely closely with thermodilution cardiac output in individual animals. Further, when the data for all cardiac outputs in all animals was evaluated, a general correlation was observed between the area under the curve, expressed as either total area or extrapolated by the forward triangle method, and thermodilution cardiac output, with correlation coefficients being $r = 0.65$ and 0.61, respectively.

Although these data indicating good correlation between the contrast indicator dilution curves and thermodilution cardiac output are most encouraging, several important limitations to this technique must be kept in mind. Firstly, no method of obtaining a calibration factor has yet been devised for this procedure. Accordingly, at the present time this method is capable of yielding estimates of cardiac output which are of value only in terms of directional changes within an individual subject. Secondly, despite utilizing a closed system in all studies, it was never possible to totally eliminate the extraneous introduction of micro quantities of air into the animal, thereby resulting in the inclusion of a contrast effect unrelated to the injectate itself. However, the intensity of such extraneous contrast was small in comparison to that introduced by the actual agent, and was constant after the initial 1 to 2 injections. Finally, in utilizing this methodology it is necessary to avoid producing a quantity of contrast which is so great that it saturates the ultrasonic videodensitometry system. Although studies in our laboratory determined a suitable concentration for this animal model, similar data will have to be accumulated in a clinical setting, and may vary from patient to patient.

CONCLUSION

Contrast echocardiography offers exciting new potentials for the application of ultrasonic methods in the diagnosis and management of patients with heart disease. However, in order to realize the full potential of contrast echocardiography it will be necessary to apply quantitative methods to the analysis of these recordings. Studies in our laboratory in association with Rasor Associates have demonstrated that biodegradeable contrast agents of uniform size can be utilized to yield indicator dilution curves from the videodensitometric analysis of two-dimensional echocardiograms. Further, such indicator dilution curves have been demonstrated to correlate well with cardiac flow and cardiac output measurements both in vitro and in vivo. It is fully anticipated that further developments in this area will enable the determination of cardiac output in man by means of two-dimensional contrast echocardiography.

REFERENCES

1. Seward JB, AJ Tajik, DJ Hagler, DG Ritter: Peripheral venous contrast echocardiography. Am J Cardiol 39:202–209, 1977.
2. Meltzer RS, EG Tickner, RL Popp: The source of ultrasound contrast effect. J Clin Ultrasound 8:121, 1980.
3. Bommer WJ, DT Mason, AN DeMaria: Studies in contrast echocardiography: Development of new agents with superior reproducibility and transmission through lungs. Circulation 60 (Suppl II):II–17, 1979.
4. Gramiak R, PM Shaw, DH Kramer: Ultrasound cardiology: Contrast studies in anatomy and function. Radiology 92:939–946, 1969.
5. Kerber RE, JM Kioschos, RM Lauer: Use of an ultrasonic contrast method in the diagnosis of valvular regurgitation and intracardiac shunts. Am J Cardiol 34:722–730, 1974.
6. Weyman AE, LS Wann, RA Hurwitz, et al.: Negative contrast echocardiography: A new technique for detecting left-to-right shunts. Circulation 56 (Suppl III):III–26, 1977.
7. Lieppe W, VS Behar, R Scallion, JA Kisslo: Detection of tricuspid regurgitation with two-dimensional echocardiography and peripheral vein injections. Circulation 57:128–32, 1978.
8. Bommer WJ, J Neef, A Neumann, L Weinert G Lee, DT Mason, AN DeMaria: Indicator-dilution curves obtained by photometric analysis of two-dimensional echo-contrast studies. Am J Cardiol 41:370, 1978 (abstract).
9. DeMaria AN, W Bommer, L George, Neumann, L Weinert, DT Mason: Combined peripheral venous injection and cross-sectional echocardiography in the evaluation of cardiac disease. Am J Cardiol 41:370, 1978 (abstract).
10. Bommer WJ, G Tickner, J Rasor, T Grehl, DT Mason, AN DeMaria: Development of a new echocardiographic contrast agent capable of pulmonary transmission and left heart opacification following peripheral venous injection. Circulation 62 (Supp III):III, 1980 (abstract).
11. Bommer W, Lantz Bo, Miller, Larry, Naifeh, Jerome, Riggs, Kay, Kwan, Oi Ling, DT Mason, AN DeMaria: Advances in Quantitative contrast echocardiography: Recording and calibration of linear time-concentration curves by videodensitometry. Circulation 60 (Part II-18), 1979 (abstract).
12. DeMaria AN, W Bommer, K Riggs, A Dajje, L Miller, DT Mason: In vivo correlation of cardiac output and densitometric dilution curves obtained by contrast two-dimensional echocardiography Circulation (Supp III):III–101, 1980 (abstract).

24. VIDEODENSITOMETRIC QUANTITATION OF LEFT-TO-RIGHT SHUNTS WITH CONTRAST ECHOCARDIOGRAPHY

DONALD J. HAGLER, ABDUL J. TAJIK, JAMES B. SEWARD, and ERIK L. RITMAN

Contrast echocardiography is a sensitive indicator of intracardiac shunts. It has allowed the precise definition of the site of intracardiac shunts and visual, subjective assessment of shunt size [1, 2]. A photometric analysis of two-dimensional echocardiography has demonstrated indicator–dilution type curves for assessment of appearance and disappearance with time [3]. Previously, our group [4] reported an attempt to quantitatively assess shunt size. We applied computer-based roentgen videodensitometric techniques to video recordings of contrast two-dimensional echocardiography to quantitate left-to-right shunts. For this preliminary study, patients with ventricular septal defect were selected for assessment of shunt size, because comparative data would be available during cardiac catheterization [4]. For contrast two-dimensional echocardiography, indocyanine green dye (1 ml) with a saline flush was selectively injected by catheter into the left ventricular cavity. Parasternal long-axis and short-axis scans, as well as subxiphoid and suprasternal scans, were recorded with sequential dye injections. Two-inch videotape recordings were obtained and subsequently transferred to video disc for replay.

Twelve patients with left-to-right ventricular shunts were studied. Two patients had previous surgery for more complex congenital heart disease but had small ventricular septal defects remaining. Two patients had ventricular septal defects with associated pulmonary stenosis, and the remaining eight patients had only a simple ventricular septal defect. The ages of the 12 patients ranged from 9 months to 52 years, with an average of 10.8 years. During cardiac catheterization, the magnitudes of the left-to-right shunts were estimated by the Fick technique in all 12 patients and by indicator–dilution techniques in eight. Double-sampling dye curves were obtained in four patients, and single-sampling dye curves in the remaining eight.

By means of a videodensitometric system [5] developed by our biodynamic research unit, but currently commercially available (Chapman Engineers, Chicago, IL, USA), a sampling window was placed over the respective right and left heart sites in order to determine the density of the echo contrast effect (Figure 1). Care was taken to allow for window placement if possible over the right and left ventricular outflow tracts and to avoid catheter artifact or areas of uneven flow and inadequate dye mixing. The videodensitometry provides a time-gated sample of the video signal which is proportional to an integrated amount of reflected ultrasound. In this study, we assessed this ability to quantitate left-to-right shunts on the basis of the density

292

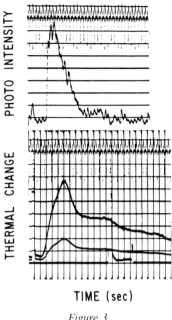

TIME (sec)

Figure 3

shunts. A series of studies was performed to assess the reproducibility of photometric indicator dilution curves in patients. Utilizing the methodology described, a variability of approximately plus or minus fifteen percent was found in consecutive curves. Further central circulatory injections yielded data which was only slightly superior to those from injections in peripheral veins. Accordingly, a method was developed which was capable of yielding reasonably reproducible indicator dilution curves from two-dimensional contrast echocardiograms.

The initial quantitative analysis of the photometric indicator dilution curves was confined to the disappearance phase of the tracing. Two parameters were defined for each contrast curve, the time from peak contrast effect (peak of the curve) to the point of 50% decrease in amplitude (DT/50) and the time from the peak of the curve to 90% reduction in amplitude (DT/90). Application of the measurement of either DT/50 or DT/90 immediately revealed a striking separation between groups of normal subjects or patients with atrial septal defect and patients with either markedly reduced cardiac indices or tricuspid regurgitation [9] (Figure 4). In addition, when either DT/50 or DT/90 were subjected to linear regression analysis in comparison with thermodilution measurements of cardiac output, good correlations were obtained with the correlation coefficient ranging from r = 0.70 to 0.92. Importantly, when patients were divided into two groups, one with reduced cardiac index (below 2.5 liters/minute/m^2) and one having normal cardiac index, striking differences existed for both DT/50 and DT/90 (1.3 versus 8.9

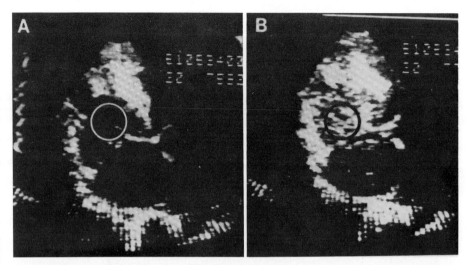

Figure 2

Accordingly, a system was developed whereby the luminescence emitted by a video monitor during a two-dimensional contrast echocardiogram was continuously recorded by a photometer focused upon the screen, and the analog signal was transferred to a stripchart recorder for a paper printout [8]. The photometer utilized was a Tektronics model J6503 with a light-sensitive area one centimeter in diameter which yielded readings expressed in foot-lamberts. The signal from the photometer was recorded by means of a standard fiberoptic Honeywell model 1856 stripchart recorder.

Indicator dilution curves were obtained from two-dimensional echocardiograms performed from the cardiac apex in the four-chamber view, with the transducer manipulated to maximize the size of the right ventricular and right atrial chambers. The contrast agent utilized for the initial studies was 10 cc of normal saline, which was delivered into an indwelling 19 gauge plastic cannula inserted in the brachial vein. Contrast visualization was recorded onto video tape for subsequent playback, during which the photometer was focused upon an area of interest centered in the right ventricular cavity (Figure 2) and the analog signal was continuously recorded on paper.

The result of photometric analysis of two-dimensional contrast echocardiograms was to yield an indicator dilution type curve whose upstroke was related to luminescence created by the appearance of contrast on the video screen and whose downslope was created by the disappearance or washout of the contrast agent (Figure 3). Although contrast indicator dilution curves appeared similar to those produced by indocyanine green or thermodilution, the ultrasonic opacification was removed in the lungs and therefore a break in the downslope was not observed in patients with left-to-right cardiac in patients with varying levels of cardiac function. Stimulated by these findings, a series of projects were undertaken by which to obtain quantitative information from the appearance and disappearance characteristics of two-dimensional contrast echocardiograms.

PHOTOMETRIC AQUISITION OF INDICATOR DILUTION CURVES

The contrast effect obtained by two-dimensional echocardiography is presented as luminescence upon a video monitor or cathode ray oscilloscope. Further, the luminance may be readily recorded by means of a photometer (lightmeter) which is focused upon the screen of the monitor (Figure 1).

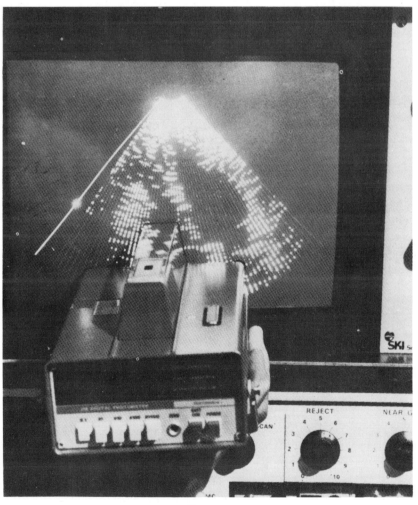

Figure 1

23. DETERMINATION OF CARDIAC OUTPUT BY TWO-DIMENSIONAL CONTRAST ECHOCARDIOGRAPHY

Anthony N. DeMaria, William Bommer, Julia Rasor, E. Glenn Tickner, and Dean T. Mason

Contrast echocardiography refers to the process of opacifying cardiac chambers and major vessels with dense "clouds" of reflected echoes by means of the intravascular injection of a variety of fluids [1]. Although the exact source of the contrast effect is not known, available evidence overwhelmingly points to the role of microscopic air bubbles in the genesis of the contrast effect [2]. Although indocyanine green, saline, and dextrose in water have been the solutions most routinely used to produce contrast echocardiograms, even intravascular injection of the patient's own blood can elicit similar phenomena. Recently a variety of gas containing substances have been utilized in the experimental laboratory to standardize the contrast recordings obtained [3].

Contrast echocardiography has found a variety of applications in clinical cardiology. Initially, contrast injections within the central circulation were utilized during echocardiography to verify ultrasonically determined cardiac anatomy [4]. Subsequently, contrast echocardiography has been utilized to evaluate blood flow patterns, especially in regard to intracardiac communications [5]: Since the contrast effect is removed by the transit of blood through the lungs, contrast is not normally seen in the left side cardiac chambers following intravenous injection, and the technique may therefore be of particular value in the recognition of right-to-left intracardiac shunting by either atrial or ventricular septal defects. In addition, a contrast free jet (negative contrast) may be observed during opacification of the right side chambers in patients with left-to-right shunting [6], and reflux of contrast into the inferior vena cava has proven to be of value in the detection of tricuspid regurgitation [7]. Unfortunately, none of these applications or approaches have yielded any quantitative data from contrast echocardiograms.

In the course of analysis of a number of two-dimensional contrast echocardiograms performed in our laboratory for clinical purposes, the qualitative observation was made that the time-course of appearance and disappearance of the contrast effect in an individual patient seemed to be related to the status of overall cardiac function at the time of the study. These initial qualitative observations were confirmed by the simple procedure of timing with a stopwatch the duration of the ultrasonic contrast effect

C. FUTURE PROSPECTS

artery opacifies initially in diastole and later than the aorta. Thereafter, there is a flat, non-cyclical opacification of the pulmonary artery, suggesting that it is receiving none of its blood from the heart directly but rather through the persistent ductus arteriosus (Figure 10).

Visualisation of systemic veins

When contrast is injected into the left hand or arm, it is frequently possible to see an opacified space anterior to the aorta (Figure 4). This opacifies very early and without any cyclical change and almost certainly represents the left innominate vein. Again with increasing experience, the absence of this opacification following left hand or arm injection strongly suggests absence of the left innominate vein. Occasionally it is possible to diagnose a left superior vena cava draining to the coronary sinus, by suprasternal contrast echocardiography. In these circumstances, the left innominate vein does not opacify after a left hand injection, but the coronary sinus opacifies behind the left atrium.

CONCLUSION

Most infants admitted as emergencies to paediatric cardiological units undergo an extensive work-up, including clinical examination, chest X-ray blood/gas analysis and electrocardiography. It is now common practice to include in this pre-catheterisation diagnostic cascade M-Mode echocardiography. The use of the suprasternal technique and contrast echocardiography gives a great deal of diagnostic information, which is not only qualitative but can sometimes be semi-quantitative. The undoubted advantages of real-time two-dimensional echocardiography over M-Mode in such children is not available to all units because of cost. M-Mode contrast echocardiography from the suprasternal approach in our experience greatly enhances the diagnostic possibilities of the single probe technique.

REFERENCES

1. Goldberg BB: Ultrasonic measurement of aortic arch, right pulmonary artery and left atrium. Radiology 101:383, 1971.
2. Mortera C, M Tynan, A Goodwin, S Hunter: Infradiaphragmatic total anomalous pulmonary venous connection to the portal vein. Diagnostic implications of echocardiography. Brit Heart J 39:685, 1977.
3. Allen HD, SJ Goldberg, DJ Sahn, TW Ovitt, BB Goldberg: Suprasternal notch echocardiography. Assessment of its clinical utility in paediatric cardiology. Circulation 55:605, 1977.
4. Mortera C, S Hunter, M Tynan: Contrast echocardiography and the suprasternal approach in infants and children. European J of Cardiology 9/6:437–454, 1979. Elsevier/North-Holland Biomedical Press.

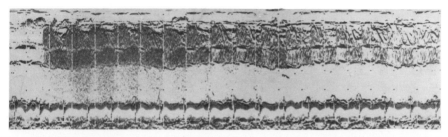

Figure 9. In this suprasternal echocardiogram the aorta and the pulmonary artery opacify in systole with similar intensity and little contrast reaches the left atrium. These findings suggest a right to left ventricular shunt which was present. In the later cardiac cycles the aorta opacifies more intensely in systole and the pulmonary artery in diastole. Indicating the presence of co-existing transposition of the great arteries and persistent ductus arteriosus.

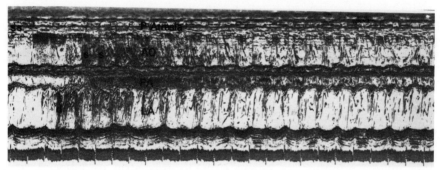

Figure 10. A suprasternal echocardiogram in a case of pulmonary atresia following systemic injection of contrast. The large aorta opacifies first, followed by left atrial opacification and finally by opacification of the pulmonary artery. The aorta is most intensely opacified in systole while the pulmonary artery initially shows a flat non-cyclical opacification, indicating that it is not connected to the heart directly by a semilunar valve but receives its blood supply from the aorta.

P. Atresia = pulmonary atresia; AO = aorta; PA = pulmonary artery; LA = left atrium.

circumstances, at cardiac catheterisation there is usually less than 10% difference between aorta and pulmonary artery oxygen saturation.

In children with Transposition of the Great Arteries and persistent ductus arteriosus, a unique type of cyclical opacification of the pulmonary artery is seen. The aorta is cyclically opacified with each systole, but the pulmonary artery, even in the presence of a co-existing ventricular septal defect, shows mainly diastolic opacification (Figure 9). This suggests that most of the contrast reaches the pulmonary artery through an aortopulmonary communication in diastole and that blood with less contrast reaches the pulmonary artery in systole through the pulmonary valve, causing momentary clearing. This curious phenomenon disappears when the ductus is closed surgically or spontaneously.

In pulmonary valve atresia with ventricular septal defect and persistent ductus arteriosus, the aorta opacifies cyclically in systole. The pulmonary

284

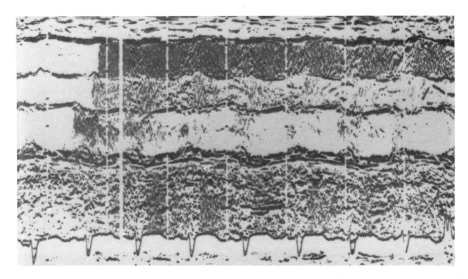

Figure 7. This suprasternal echocardiogram is from a patient with transposition of the great arteries. The left atrium opacifies followed by both great arteries. The aorta is more persistently and intensely opacified, suggesting that it receives most of the systemic venous return.

both great arteries, some comment can be made about the approximate effective pulmonary blood flow. When aortic saturation is less than 40%, the amount of contrast appearing in the left atrium on suprasternal echocardiogram is minimal and the aorta opacifies for more than twice as many cycles as the pulmonary artery (Figure 6). When the aortic saturation lies between 40% and 60%, the pulmonary artery opacifies more than half as many cycles as the aorta, although there is usually still sufficient differential opacification to make the diagnosis of ventriculoarterial discordance (Figure 7). When aortic saturation is greater than 60%, both great arteries opacify equally intensely and for the same number of cardiac cycles and accurate assessment of ventriculoarterial connections becomes impossible (Figure 8). Under these

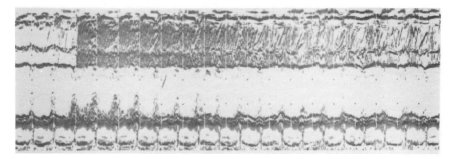

Figure 8. In this suprasternal echocardiogram both great arteries opacify with equal intensity and persistence, and it is not possible to assess accurately the ventriculoarterial connections, This patient had a very small right to left shunt which was not picked up on this echocardiogram. The major shunting occurred at ventricular level.

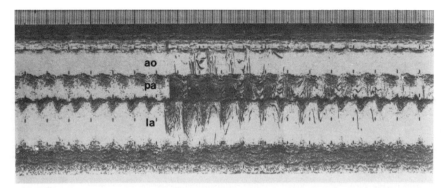

Figure 5. Selective peripheral venous injection into the right hand. The left atrium opacifies first in diastole and then the pulmonary artery and aorta also opacify. Both great arteries opacify most intensely in systole but the pulmonary artery receives most of the systemic venous return and opacifies most intensely and persistently.

of the obligatory intracardiac shunting which is required for the baby to survive.

Transposition differs from other cyanotic congenital heart disease in that the greater the right to left shunt at atrial or ventricular level, the higher the effective pulmonary blood flow will be and the higher the systemic arterial oxygen saturation. By comparing aortic percentage oxygen saturation in children with transposition to the relative opacification (at each injection) of

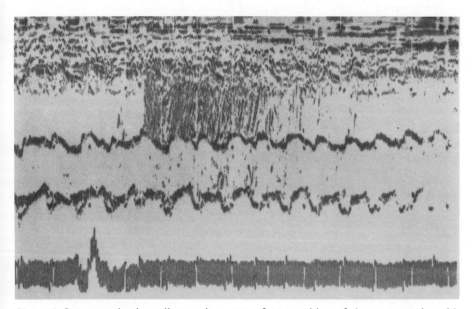

Figure 6. Suprasternal echocardiogram in a case of transposition of the great arteries with minimal interatrial shunting. Very little contrast appears in the pulmonary artery and most of the contrast is seen in the aorta.

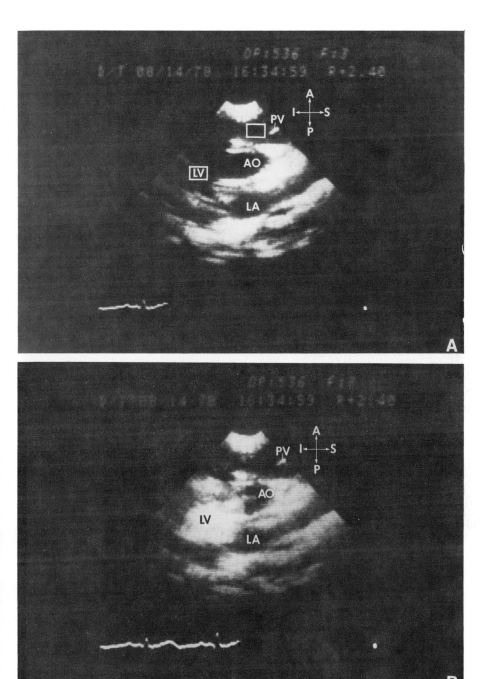

Figure 1. A) Parasternal right ventricular long-axis scan shows both right ventricular and left ventricular outflow tracts. Squares schematically represent placement of videodensitometric windows for shunt assessment. B) Selective left ventricular echocontrast (indocyanine green dye) injection with opacification of left ventricle. C — see following page) Later frame shows subsequent opacification of right and left ventricular outflow tracts by echo contrast, demonstrating left-to-right ventricular shunt. Videodensitometric windows as placed in panel A would detect the density of dye in both right and left ventricular outflow outflow tracts.

300

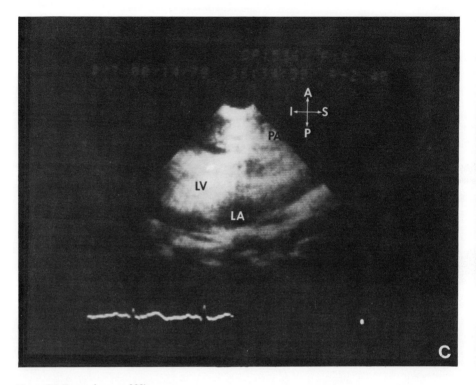

Figure 3C (Legend: see p. 299).

of shunted contrast effect as observed with two-dimensional echocardiography and compared this estimate with values estimated by the standard Fick and dye-dilution techniques.

In this manner, time–density histograms of right and left heart sampling sites were generated. In order to correct for artifactual densities relative to cardiac motion, background videodensity was subtracted and the corrected area under the resultant curves determined, using an electrocardiographic-gated computer program. The percentage of left-to-right shunt was calculated by dividing the right heart curve area by the left heart curve area and multiplying by 100. A typical time–density histogram from right and left heart sampling sites is shown in Figure 2. The corrected curve areas are indicated, yielding an estimate of 48% for the left-to-right shunt. The estimates of left-to-right shunts using contrast echocardiography and Fick and dye-dilution techniques were computed (Figure 3). The average left-to-right shunt estimates were 32% by Fick, 39% by dye, and 41% by contrast echocardiography, utilizing all of the views obtained. Left-to-right shunt estimates from all three methods were highly associated (Table 1). Rank correlation between Fick and echocardiographic estimates yielded r values of 0.914 and between dye and echocardiographic estimates, an r value of 0.929.

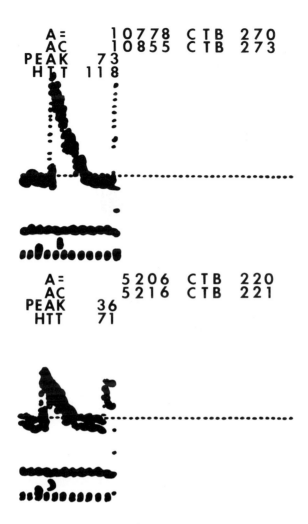

Figure 2. Time–density histogram generated from computer-based videodensitometric windows in patient with ventricular septal defect. After selective left ventricular dye injection, the appearance of dye in right and left ventricular outflow tracts is simultaneously recorded, yielding histograms closely resembling indicator–dilution curves.

DISCUSSION

These preliminary results demonstrate a positive correlation among the three methods. However, moderate-sized shunts were not well represented in this preliminary study. Only large and small shunts were present; however, one would assume that moderate-sized shunts also could be accurately predicted. These techniques seem to provide accurate estimates of shunt size, although strict attention to proper placement of the sampling window was important. Gain controls could

Table 1. Comparisons among three methods of quantitation of left-to-right shunts in patients with ventricular septal defect.

Comparison	Spearman's rank–order correlation			Wilcoxon signed–rank correlation	
	N	r	P value	N	P value
Fick vs. dye	8	0.917	0.003	8	0.008
Fick vs. echo	12	0.914	<0.001	12	0.018
Dye vs. echo	8	0.929	0.002	8	>0.10

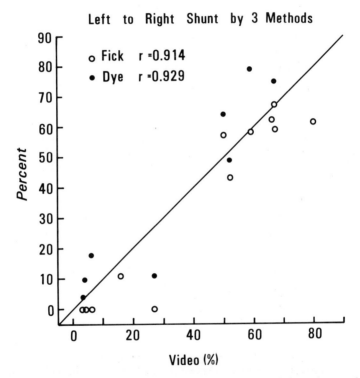

Figure 3. Graph demonstration comparison of echo (video), Fick, and dye estimates of left-to-right shunt. Fick values are indicated by open circles, and the dye values are indicated by closed circles. Note the line of identity.

potentially affect estimates of density; however, care taken to ensure a uniform good quality image was essential to obtain consistent results. Because all of the contrast effect is cleared with one passage through a capillary bed, selective indocyanine green dye injection into the left heart is necessary for the assessment of shunt size in ventricular septal defect. However, because of the lack of toxicity of the contrast agent (indocyanine green dye), the technique allows repeated injections utilizing multiple scanning sites [6].

Upon individual review of the curves obtained, it was noted that with a standard long-axis view, placement of the sampling window over the right and left ventricular outflow tracts occasionally overestimated the left-to-right shunt. Also, the inflow area of the ventricle had to be avoided because of the uneven distribution of dye. The short-axis scans of the aorta and the pulmonary artery provided a more consistent site for sampling, thus allowing more complete mixing of contrast dye. However, cardiac motion in small infants often made it difficult to place the sampling window completely within the great arteries. The suprasternal views allowed the most stable sites for sampling windows but were more difficult to obtain and often provided less contrast effect. Our group currently employs all views available, recognizing that sampling error can occur with ventricular sampling sites.

Present results suggest that accurate quantitation of left-to-right shunts can be achieved with these techniques. In addition, the assessment of valvular regurgitation with selective great-vessel or ventricular dye injections may be possible, as well as quantitative assessment of right-to-left shunting, utilizing peripheral venous dye injections. In summary, contrast echocardiography can provide precise definition of the site of an intracardiac shunt. Quantitation of left-to-right shunt in ventricular septal defect, utilizing videodensitometric techniques, has correlated well with standard Fick and dye-dilution methods. These encouraging initial results suggest that accurate quantitation of shunts or valvular regurgitation may be possible using these techniques.

REFERENCES

1. Seward JB, AJ Tajik, JG Spangler, DG Ritter: Echocardiographic contrast studies: initial experience. Mayo Clin Proc 50:163–192, 1975.
2. Tajik AJ, JB Seward, DJ Hagler, DD Mair: Experience with real-time two-dimensional sector angiography. Am J Cardiol 41:353, 1978 (abstract).
3. Bommer W, J Neef, A Neumann, L Weinert, G Lee, DT Mason, AN DeMaria: Indicator-dilution curves obtained by photometric analysis of two-dimensional echo-contrast studies. Am J Cardiol 41:370, 1978 (abstract).
4. Hagler DJ, AJ Tajik, JB Seward, DD Mair, DG Ritter, EL Ritman: Videodensitometric quantitation of left-to-right shunts with contrast sector echocardiography. Circulation Suppl II 58:70, 1978 (abstract).
5. Bürsch JH, EL Ritman, RE Strum, EH Wood: Videodensitometric determination of left ventricular ejection and filling characteristics. Ann Biomed Eng 3:62–71, 1975.
6. Tajik AJ, JB Seward, DJ Hagler, DD Mair, JT Lie: Two-dimensional real-time ultrasonic imaging of the heart and great vessels: technique, image orientation, structure identification, and validation. Mayo Clin Proc 53:271–303, 1978.

25. TRANSMISSION OF ECHOCARDIOGRAPHIC CONTRAST THROUGH THE LUNGS

RICHARD S. MELTZER, CHARLES T. LANCÉE, and JOS ROELANDT

INTRODUCTION

Potential utility

At present echocardiographic contrast can only be obtained on the left side of the heart with the aid of direct left heart catheterization. Chapters 10 and 11 are devoted to the as yet experimental technique of causing left heart contrast by performing injections through catheters in the pulmonary wedge position, thus only necessitating right heart catheterization. Though this is preferable to left heart catheterization, the ability to create left heart contrast noninvasively (we include peripheral venous injections) would be still better.

The left heart can be imaged echocardiographically without contrast, though contrast occasionally will enhance contours or structures not seen on the pre-contrast study (Chapter 11, Figure 5). Thus, the main reason for wanting contrast on the left side of the heart is fundamentally different from that for angiography or nuclear medicine, where contrast is necessary to see the outlines of the left atrium and left ventricle. Rather, contrast will help identify and analyze transvalvular or intracavitary flow disturbances or left-to-right shunts. Unlike the dense contrast intensity necessary to adequately define contours, flow phenomena may often be diagnosed in the presence of only a few imaged microbubbles of contrast – this is especially true of shunt detection, and is also illustrated by inferior vena cava contrast echocardiography (Chapter 18). Turbulence, vortices, and local flow phenomena in the left heart (the flow around the mitral valve in IHSS with and without SAM, jets of aortic or mitral insufficiency) may be studied with contrast echocardiography in a unique way, unavailable by any other technique.

Another potential application of left heart contrast is in the echocardiographic diagnosis of proximal coronary artery disease. The authors do not feel that currently available two-dimensional echocardiographic techniques allow accurate diagnosis of proximal coronary artery stenosis. However, we are optimistic that the combination of improved resolution, computer-assisted tracking of structures such as the aortic root, and Doppler echocardiography, combined with contrast in the left heart, may allow such noninvasive diagnosis. We do not believe that distal coronary disease will ever be accessible to echocardiographic diagnosis. It is possible that carotid or systemic arterial imaging by ultrasound will also be aided by an ability to transmit contrast through the lungs to arterial circulation.

Toxicity

A vital and unanswered question is whether transmission of contrast (i.e. micro-bubbles) through the lungs is safe. There is one major argument to suggest that this is indeed the case: routine injections during cardiac catheterization cause echo-cardiographic contrast. This applies not only to the angiographic contrast dye injections, but also to the catheter flushing by hand using dextrose or saline so-lutions. Indeed, the phenomenon of ultrasonic contrast was serendipitously dis-covered in this setting – performing echocardiograms in the catheterization labora-tory during indocyanine green dye injections. We are unaware of any reported toxicity of these left heart injections in the absence of gross air bubbles, despite the extensive world experience with cardiac catheterization. Thus we feel that left heart echocardiographic contrast need not be toxic, even though it contains micro-bubbles. Also, the total amount of gas necessary for a strong contrast effect is fortunately quite small and can be less than 0.05% of total volume [1]. However, introducing a gas phase into the systemic circulation raises the possibility of toxicity due to air embolism. This cannot be taken lightly, and the safety of any proposed technique will need meticulous scrutiny before it can be introduced into clinical practice. We did not find any published work on the toxicity of attempted trans-mission of echocardiographic contrast through the lungs, with the exception of the very preliminary work done in our own laboratory [2, 3]. We were aware of animal [4] and human [5, 6] work showing that wedge injections can yield left heart echocardiographic contrast. We therefore decided to test for toxicity by direct pathological examination of animals subjected to wedge injections. In order to increase the risk of toxicity, we deliberately allowed a small amount of air to be injected along with the physiologic saline.

THEORETIC CONSIDERATIONS

Microbubbles are the source of ultrasonic contrast (Chapter 2) and are removed by the pulmonary capillaries after intravenous injection due to the mechanical "sieve" effect which stops larger bubbles, or surface tension effects leading to rapid and complete dissolution of bubbles small enough to pass these capillaries (Chapter 4) [6]. This understanding of bubble dynamics in the circulation is necessary to pro-pose several possible methods for changing conditions so that microbubbles will be able to pass the lungs and survive in the circulation until the left heart is reached:

1. A very active surfactant might be able to stabilize bubbles small enough to pass pulmonary capillaries so they would survive until they reached the left heart before dissolving.
2. A solid coat might protect a "mini-microbubble" so it can traverse the pul-monary capillary bed without dissolution due to diffusion or surface tension

effects. There is preliminary work suggesting that such a method, using a saccharide coating, can be successful [7].

3. A liquid, such as diethyl ether, could be administrated intravenously and pass through the pulmonary capillary bed in a liquid state, but then boil on the left side of the heart, yielding a gas phase and therefore ultrasonic contrast.

4. A liquid or combination of substances could be administered intravenously which would pass through the lungs and undergo a chemical reaction on the left side of the heart, yielding a gas. The most likely candidate would be carbon dioxide, because it is relatively nontoxic and many chemical reactions liberate large quantitities of carbon dioxide.

5. Bubbles of gas can be forced through the capillary bed by the increased local pressure that could be applied by an injection through a catheter firmly in the pulmonary wedge position. This is discussed in chapters 10 and 11.

6. An inhaled gas might, due to its composition and pressure, sufficiently alter the local partial pressures in the alveoli and capillaries that intravenously injected microbubbles would grow rather than decay during their transit through the lungs.

7. High energy ultrasound can be focused on a point within the left heart to cause cavitation.

8. Lower energy ultrasound than that necessary to cause cavitation could be employed to cause growth rather than decay of peripherally injected microbubbles, using the mechanism of "rectified diffusion" [8].

9. A liquid of sufficient acoustic impedance difference from blood to yield ultrasonic contrast could pass through the pulmonary capillary bed without the difficulties faced by gas bubbles. It is possible that suspensions of specially treated collagen or gelatin may fit into this category [9].

10. A combination of two or more of these methods.

METHODS

Right Heart Injections (ether and H_2O_2)

Twenty-two pigs were anesthetized with barbiturates and placed on respirators. The thorax was opened by midline sternotomy and a 3.5 Mhz Krautkramer-Branson transducer was sutured directly to the epicardium of the left ventricular free wall. This was used to monitor the left ventricular cavity for the appearance of echocardiographic contrast. A catheter was inserted into the right atrium, right ventricle or pulmonary artery. Control injections of 5 – 8 cm^3 physiologic saline were monitored to insure that no left heart echocardiographic contrast resulted. Three pids had contrast and were excluded from further analysis due to presumed arteriovenous shunting in the lungs. Nine of the remaining 19 pigs received injections of diethyl ether (one or more of the following volumes: 0.5 ml, 1 ml, 1.5 ml,

2 ml, or 3 ml) followed by a 3 ml "flush" of physiologic saline. After each injection the left ventricular echocardiogram was monitored for between 30 and 60 s for the appearance of contrast. The other ten of 19 pigs without intrapulmonary shunting received right heart injections of hydrogen peroxide (0.75 to 30% concentration) followed by a 3 ml physiologic saline flush.

Pulmonary Wedge Injections (saline with small amounts of air)

Seven rabbits were anesthetized with intramuscular fluanison. In each a number 6 French Swan-Ganz balloon-tipped catheter was advanced to the pulmonary wedge position under pressure and fluoroscopic monitoring, and the balloon was inflated with 0.5 – 0.75 ml of air. Three to ten repeated hand injections of normal saline were then performed. We allowed between 0.1 and 1 cm^3 of air to be injected along with the physiologic saline solution on each injection. This is not our technique in human injections, but we wanted to examine the potential toxicity of small amounts of air injected in the pulmonary wedge position in this animal model.

Twenty-four hours later the animals were sacrificed by rapid intravenous barbiturate overdose and the heart, lungs, and kidneys were removed for gross and microscopic pathological examination.

Intravenous saccharide-coated "mini-microbubbles"

Seventeen pigs had injections of saccharide-coated "mini-microbubbles" in a peripheral vein. "Mini-microbubbles" are microbubbles of a diameter small enough to pass a capillary bed: since capillary diameters are about 10 μm, "mini-microbubbles" have diameter of 10 μm or less. The "mini-microbubbles" used were provided by Ultra Med, Inc., Sunnyvale, California.

The pigs were open-chested and echocardiography was performed using a Toshiba SSH-10A phased-array sector-scanner with the transducer applied directly to the ventricular epicardium. A four-chamber view was obtained, and control injections of saline were performed to exclude intracardiac or intrapulmonary shunts.

RESULTS

Right Heart Injections of Ether and Hydrogen Peroxide

Seven of the nine pigs with ether injections in the right heart and left heart echocardiographic contrast (Figure 1). Two had no detectable contrast effect in the left heart despite at least two injections.

Eight of the ten pigs receiving hydrogen peroxide injections had echocardiographic contrast in the left heart (Figure 2). There was a threshold concentration in one pig such that all injections above a concentration of 1.5% H$_2$O$_2$ yielded contrast

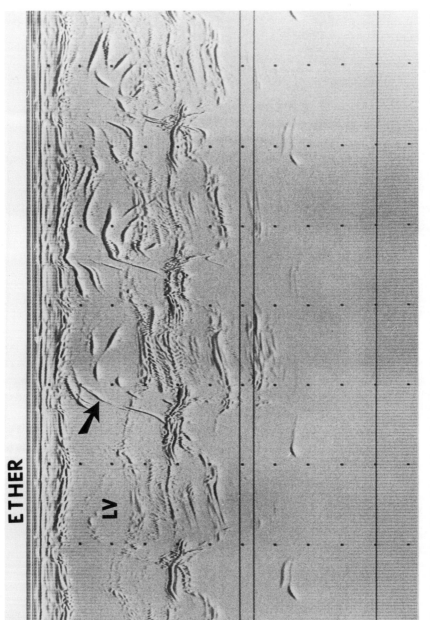

Figure 1. M-mode echocardiographic tracing during right heart injection of diethyl ether. Transducer is sutured directly to the left ventricular epicardium. LV: left ventricular lumen. Note appearance of contrast (arrow) in the LV.

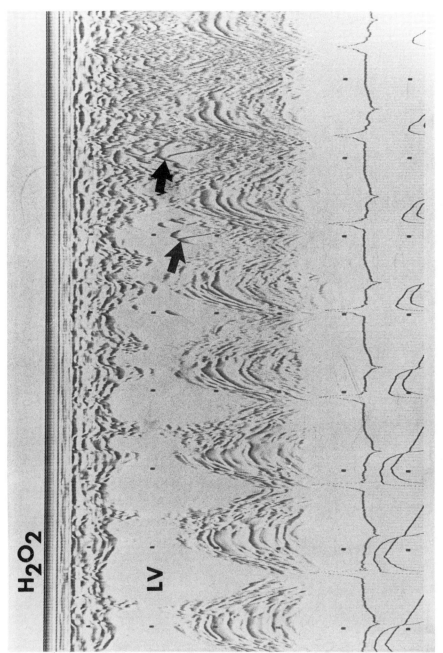

Figure 2. M-mode echocardiographic tracing during right heart injection of hydrogen peroxide (H$_2$O$_2$). Transducer is sutured directly to the left ventricular epicardium. Note appearance of contrast (arrows) in the left ventricular lumen (LV).

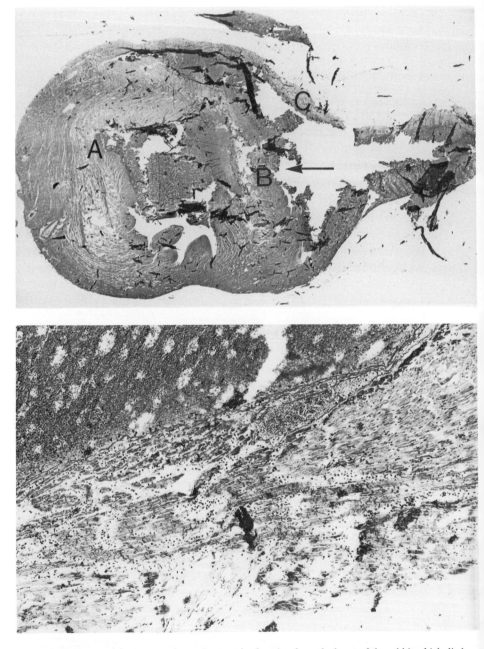

Figure 3. Upper panel: low power photomicrograph of section from the heart of the rabbit which died prior to scheduled sacrifice, showing an extensive area of coagulation necrosis. The left ventricle is to the left and the right ventricle is to the right. There is a subendocardial infarct at area A in the left ventricle, an extensive area of necrosis in the interventricalar septum at area B, and a rupture of the interventricular septum (arrow). Infarct extends to area C. Lower panel: higher power magnification (× 100) of area B above, from the interventricular septum. Note the granulocyte infiltrate, suggesting an infarct approximately one day old.

and no injections below this concentration did so. This was not carefully searched for in other animals, though there were four others where lower concentrations failed and higher concentrations succeeded in causing left heart echocardiographic contrast.

Pulmonary Wedge Injections

Of the seven rabbits subjected to wedge injections, one died during the night after the injection. At autopsy, it had a large myocardial infarction (Figure 3) and pulmonary congestion. All of the remaining six rabbits survived until sacrifice 24 h after injection. None of the rabbits had definite lesions in the pulmonary arterial tree which could be related to the balloon inflation or wedge injection. Three of the six rabbits had small myocardial infarctions, however. There were no coronary narrowing or thrombi to explain the presence of infarctions in any of the rabbits. There were signs of acute tubular necrosis in the renal tubules of the rabbit that died prematurely with the large infarction; no other rabbit had signs of renal damage.

Intravenous saccharide-coated "mini-microbubbles"

Contrast was seen in all pigs in the right heart after both saline and saccharide coated "mini-microbubbles". No pig had intracardiac or intrapulmonary shunting (i.e., contrast was never seen in the left heart). Nine of the 17 pigs receiving "mini-microbubbles" had contrast in the left heart apparent several heartbeats after right heart opacification. There were no hemodynamic or electrocardiographic changes associated with "mini-microbubble" injections.

DISCUSSION

The feasibility of transmission of echocardiographic contrast through the lungs has been demonstrated and multiple methods are theoretically possible. Wedge injections (Chapters 10 and 11), sugar covered gas microbubbles [7], and liquids yielding contrast by physical (ether) or chemical (peroxide decomposition) means have all now been shown to yield left heart echocardiographic contrast. This has been aided by the more basic understanding of microbubble dynamics developed recently [1, 6].

The problem is therefore toxicity. Few data on toxicity are available. The ultimate method of left heart echo contrast creation will probably be the one shown to be safe. Neither ether nor hydrogen peroxide can be injected intravenously in sufficient quantities to cause contrast on the left side of the heart without prohibitive toxicity – though hydrogen peroxide has been used in lower concentration to obtain right heart echocardiographic contrast in hundreds of patients in China with no adverse effects [10]. Our rabbit experiments suggest caution before accepting any

312

method as safe, and reemphasize that at present pulmonary wedge injections should be considered experimental even though no toxicity has been reported in the initial two series [5, 6].

ACKNOWLEDGMENTS

The authors wish to thank Pieter D. Verdouw, Marita Rutteman, Rob van Bremen, and Catharina Essed for assistance with this work, and Machtelt Brussé for help in manuscript preparation.

REFERENCES

1. Meltzer RS, EG Tickner, TP Sahines, RL Popp: The source of ultrasound contrast effect. J Clin Ultrasound 8:121, 1980.
2. Meltzer RS, OEH Sartorius, CT Lancée, PW Serruys, PD Verdouw, CE Essed, J Roelandt: Transmission of ultrasonic contrast through the lungs. Ultrasound Med Biol 7: 377, 1981.
3. Meltzer RS, PW Serruys, J McGhie, N Verbaan, J Roelandt: Pulmonary wedge injections yielding left-sided echocardiographic contrast. Br Heart J 44:390, 1980.
4. Bommer WJ, DT Mason, AN DeMaria: Studies in contrast echocardiography: development of new agents with superior reproducibility and transmission through lungs. Circulation (Suppl II) 60:II–17, 1979.
5. Reale A, F Pizzuto, PA Gioffrè, A Nigri, F Romeo, E Martuscelli, E Mangieri, G Scibilia G: Contrast echocardiography: transmission of echoes to the left heart across the pulmonary vascular bed. Eur Heart J 1:101, 1980.
6. Meltzer RS, EG Tickner, RL Popp: Why do the lungs clear ultrasonic contrast? Ultrasound Med Biol 6:263, 1980.
7. Bommer WJ, EG Tickner, J Rason, T Grehl, DT Mason, AN DeMaria: Development of a new echocardiographic contrast agent capable of pulmonary transmission and left heart opacification following peripheral venous injection. Circulation (Suppl III) 62: III–34, 1980.
8. Higashiizumi T, H Tashiro, K Sakamoto, F Kanai: The new ultrasonic method for the elimination of the microairbubbles in the extracorporeal circulation. Proc of the 2nd Meeting of the World Federation of Ultrasound in Med Biol, p 372. Japan, 1979.
9. Ophir J, Gobuty, RE McWhirt, NF Maklad: Ultrasonic backscatter from contrast producing collagen microspheres. Ultrasonic Imaging 2:67, 1980.
10. Wang X, J Wang, H Chen, C Lu: Contrast echocardiography with hydrogen peroxide. II. Clinical application. Chin Med J 92:693, 1979.

26. PRECISION MICROBUBBLES FOR RIGHT SIDE INTRA-CARDIAC PRESSURE AND FLOW MEASUREMENTS

E. GLENN TICKNER

INTRODUCTION

A noninvasive "cath-lab" has long been a dream in the medical community. Two parameters often measured by employing catheters are cardiac pressures and flow. Now the potential for both measurements to be performed noninvasively or minimally invasively exists with the use of precision gas microbubble agents, developed by Ultra Med Inc.*, Sunnyvale California. Microbubbles injected into a convenient vein, such as the median cubital, flow into the heart. These bubbles, in conjunction with specialized ultrasonic equipment, can be used to measure both these cardiac parameters. The purpose of this text is to discuss these methods which have been made possible by the establishment of microbubble technology. Microbubbles are defined as gas bubbles generally smaller than 100 microns in diameter. In some cases, these microbubbles are encapsulated in rigid substances.

PRESSURE MEASUREMENTS

Background

Bubbles exhibit in their purest form a simple, one-degree-of-freedom, damped oscillatory behavior [1, 2, 3]. Their dynamic characteristics are comparable to a simple spring/mass system. The spring constant is represented by the compression of the bubble gas, and the mass is equivalent to some effective mass of the liquid surrounding the bubble. Damping is caused by thermal and viscous effects of the gas and the surrounding liquid.

The free ringing frequency f_r of a bubble which oscillates as a sphere is given by

$$f_r = (3\gamma p/\rho)^{\frac{1}{2}}/\pi d, \tag{1}$$

where p is the absolute pressure of gas in the bubble, γ is the specific heat ratio of the gas, ρ is the density of the liquid, and d is the bubble diameter.

* Formerly Rasor Associates, Inc.

Spherical oscillations or volume oscillations create compression waves which readily propagate through body tissue. The oscillatory frequency for a given gas bubble depends solely on the bubble diameter and its absolute pressure. Hence, if the physical properties and diameter are known, then the free ringing oscillation uniquely indicates the absolute local blood pressure.

In order to better appreciate the significance of Eq. (1), let us assume that a bubble of carbon dioxide is near a pressure of one atmosphere. The ringing frequency in kHz when d is in microns is approximately given by

$$f_r = 6500/d. \tag{2}$$

Hence, a 100 micron bubble oscillates at an ultrasonic frequency of 65 kHz. Any bubble smaller than 325 microns will ring ultrasonically, i.e. $f_r > 20$ kHz. Conversely, bubbles larger than 325 microns ring sonically. For this reason, we have taken 325 microns as the break point between microbubbles and bubbles. Sounds of babbling brooks, sizzling ocean surf, or champagne bubbles are examples of sonic oscillations of bubbles. We intend to use microbubbles and the relationship of Eq. (1) to measure cardiac pressures.

Since the bubble diameter $d = \sqrt[3]{6V/\pi}$ depends upon its volume V, the pressure and volume are related by the compressibility equation ($pV^n = $ constant), Eq. (1) yields

$$p = p_0(f/f_0)^c, \tag{3}$$

where the zero subscripts refer to the reference condition (e.g. atmospheric pressure) and c is a gas constant which depends solely upon the polytropic coefficient at the excitation frequency. The constant c is determined experimentally. Differentiating Eq. (3) gives

$$\Delta p/p_0 = c\Delta f_r/f_0. \tag{4}$$

It can be seen, therefore, that local changes in blood pressure Δp can be directly determined by measurement of the change in ringing frequency Δf_r of bubbles in the blood stream. Two important requirements are that the bubbles must ring within the heart chambers and that the bubbles must be extremely precise in order to obtain accurate measurements.

Method

Gas microbubbles are encapsulated under pressure in a fused saccharide sphere. The strength of the saccharide shell contains the pressurized microbubbles. Carbon dioxide has been selected as the bubble gas because it is nontoxic, has low damping and is rapidly absorbed by the blood. The blood gradually dissolves the saccharide shell in the blood stream. At some critical point the shell becomes thin and is unable to tolerate the built-up stresses

caused by the pressurized bubble and suddenly fails. The freed microbubble rapidly expands and rings ultrasonically at its new pressure, the blood pressure. A compression wave is propagated to the chest wall where it is detected by a hand-held transducer. The ringing frequency of each bubble is a direct measure of its pressure at that point in time. Pressure histories are determined by timing the signals relative to the electrocardiogram.

The method that is envisioned in the future is quite simple. The physician would place the transducer on the chest of the patient at the appropriate location. The pressurized saccharide encapsulated microbubbles suspended in a viscous slurry would be delivered into a large vein. The particles would than be carried into the heart by the flush and the venous return. This process would spread out their arrival in the heart over a few heart beats. Cardiac dynamics would thoroughly mix the slurry with the blood exposing all the particles which would then begin dissolving. Shortly thereafter, and for the next few heart beats, free ringing signals would be detected by the hand-held transducer placed on the patients chest. The ultrasonic signals would be decoded electronically and converted into pressure with the use of Eq. (4). Note that the detection system would only be a receiver system. Hence, conceptually, it would be simpler than conventional echographic equipment which involves both transmitter and receiver.

Experimental results

Before carrying the technology past the research stage into the development stage, three key questions should be answered.

First, can bubbles be made to ring in compressional oscillation? If so, is there a unique, and preferably linear, relationship between this ringing frequency and ambient pressure? If the answers to these first two questions

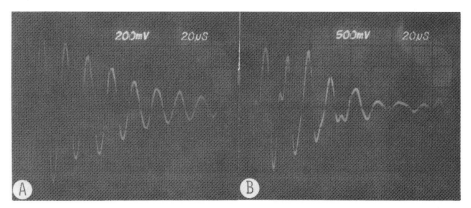

Figure 1. Oscillograph tracing showing free ringing bubble signal. *a)* Ideal damped sine wave signal; *b)* Damped signal with secondary oscillations.

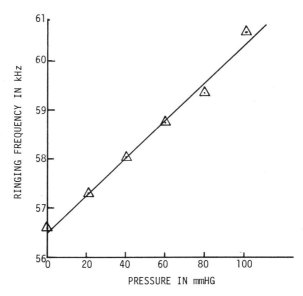

Figure 2. Variation of free ringing bubble frequency with pressure.

are positive, then the third question becomes, is the accuracy of the technique adequate for clinical use?

The first question can be answered by examination of Figure 1a and b. The two oscillographic tracings were taken of two different free ringing bubble signals. Pressurized particles were placed under the surface in a container of water which was being stirred. An ultrasonic transducer was placed on the surface to record any signal that would be created. Figure 1a shows the case of a classic damped sine wave of a 148 micron microbubble. Figure 1b also shows a free ringing bubble signal, but one which is not perfect. This imperfect signal is believed to be caused by the bubble rupture mechanism, which introduces shape oscillations that distort the compressional dynamics. This effect is thought to be the primary source of error. Because this effect exists, numerous data samples are required to obtain statistically significant results. Each particle is extremely small, being approximately 10^{-6} cc in volume, so additional particles are not believed to be a problem for delivery or toxicity. Naturally, toxicity tests must be performed to confirm this.

The same liquid chamber was employed to answer the second question. This time the liquid vessel was placed within a pressure chamber. The pressure within the chamber was varied from 0 to 100 mmHg at 20 mmHg multiples. Data were recorded on magnetic tape and reduced for frequency content at a later time. The results of this test are presented in Figure 2. A linear regression curve was employed to fit the data. This yielded an error in the pressure measurement of ±16 mmHg. The correlation coefficient for these data was computed to be 0.995. Clearly, the results derived in Eq. (4)

were achieved. If the zero reference frequency is determined, then Eq. (4) can be used to calculate the absolute cardiac pressures. This zero reading is made by placing some of the free ringing material into a beaker of water exposed to the atmosphere and determining the average f_0. The mean frequency is associated with the sum of small beaker pressure and the measured barometric pressure p_0.

The third question still remains to be answered and will be answered as testing progresses. Clearly, there are two routes to take to obtain more accurate pressure measurements. First improve the accuracy of the particles so that they ring more precisely. Second, sample more signals before computing the pressure. For example, injecting four times as many particles would decrease the error by a factor of 2 and would only introduce approximately 0.03 cc of additional material.

FLOW MEASUREMENTS

Background

Cardiac output is often measured using some form of dye dilution technique which involves threading one or two catheters into the heart of a patient. The echocardiographer can see within the heart using various noninvasive devices but cannot utilize existing dyes to measure cardiac flow. It would be highly desirable to echo a "dye" within the heart and thereby eliminate the requirement for catheters. Bubbles have been shown to be superior ultrasonic reflectors [4, 5] and therefore should act as an excellent ultrasonic dye.

In 1978, Bommer, DeMaria et al. [6] suggested a method whereby cardiac output measurements could be made from dilution type curves created from photo-densitometric sampling of the image brightness created by microbubble reflections using two-dimensional echo systems. Their data indicates considerable promise for the approach.

Another potential method also exists and is presently being developed in our laboratory. This approach is based upon the attenuation of an ultrasonic signal passing through a bubbly medium. When sound waves are propagated through a medium containing microbubbles, scattering and absorption remove energy from the incident beam giving rise to an exponentially decreasing sound energy with distance (attenuation). Attenuation is generally expressed in terms of an attenuation coefficient α. Previous investigators [7, 8] have shown that suspensions of sand and clay particles and lycopodium spores increase the attenuation coefficient linearly with volume concentration or particle concentration. Oceanographers [9, 10, 11] have observed the comparable effect with microbubbles. In the past few years, Medwin [12] has used this effect and has developed instrumentation to

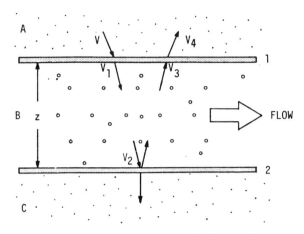

Figure 3. Schematic drawing showing reflection of plane waves.

measure bubble size distributions within the ocean. The bubbles' contribution (α_1) to the attenuation coefficient is then given as

$$\alpha_1 = k\varphi, \tag{5}$$

where k is a bubble constant which is a function of bubble gas, diameter, and ultrasonic excitation frequency and φ is the bubble concentration by volume.

The total attenuation coefficient is

$$\alpha = \alpha_0 + \alpha_1, \tag{6}$$

where α_0 is the attenuation coefficient for blood. It will be shown that this simple relationship can be used to measure bubble concentration.

In order to demonstrate this point, consider a plane wave V passing through medium A as shown in Figure 3. It will encounter two interfaces, walls, identified as 1 and 2, before continuing into medium C.

Medium B, lying between the two interfaces, is blood which may or may not contain the microbubbles. The amount of energy which is propagated through the interfaces depends upon the acoustic impedance of the media [13] and upon the attenuation of the signal by the bubbly medium B. The ratio of the signal strength between 1 and 2 is given by

$$V_2/V_1 = e^{-\alpha z}, \tag{7}$$

where z is the thickness of the medium.

It can be shown that the ratio of the backwall signal V_r for the case with bubbles to the case without bubbles is

$$V_r = e^{-2z(\alpha - \alpha_0)} \tag{8}$$

It also can be shown that, if the ratio of V_r remains near unity when bubbles pass by, Eq. (8) is further linearized and becomes

$$V_r = 1 - 2zk\varphi. \tag{9}$$

The bubble volumetric concentration φ is determined from Eq. (9) because k is known and z and V_r are measured during the test. Also, because precision microbubbles are used, the bubble volume v is known so the bubble concentration C, which is the number of bubbles per unit volume, is simply computed by $C = \varphi/v$.

For steady infusion, cardiac output CO [14] is computed by

$$CO = I/C_{max}, \tag{10}$$

where I is the known bubble infusion rate (bubbles/ second) and C_{max} is the equilibrium (plateau) value of the bubble concentration curve.

For bolus injections, the cardiac output equation takes the form

$$CO = \frac{N}{\int_0^\infty C(t)\,dt} \tag{11}$$

where N is the total number of injected bubbles. It is thus postulated that attenuation of an ultrasonic radio-frequency (rf) signal can be measured in vivo and used to determine bubble concentration and, with the aid of dye dilution technology, cardiac output.

Method

The basic approach lends itself to either the bolus injection or steady infusion method for measuring cardiac output. Consider here the steady infusion technique. Following the preparation of the bubble-containing syringe or dye-tube and insertion of an intravenous catheter into the median cubital vein of the patient, the ultrasonographer examines a backwall cardiac surface with a cardiac echo unit and, when satisfied with the signal and its stability, starts an infusion pump to deliver microbubbles at a constant and known rate into the vein. When bubbles arrive in the heart, the backwall signal becomes attenuated. This reflected signal decreases with time until equilibrium has been reached and then stabilizes at a constant value. The associated electronics converts the signal into a measurement of mean flow.

Microbubbles

Microbubbles of gases such as nitrogen and carbon dioxide ranging from 10 microns to 300 microns in diameter have been produced in various encapsulation materials. The encapsulation materials used most often are saccharides and gelatins. The saccharide agents consist of solid spherical precision particles, containing precision bubbles, and are packaged in a sealed container until ready for use. The agent is then mixed with a delivery vehicle on site. Gelatin encapsulated microbubble agents are packed and centered along the axis of a syringe or dye tube and refrigerated until ready for use. A gelatin matrix surrounds these bubbles during storage. All excess gelatin dissolves from the bubbles when injected into the blood stream, leaving only a thin layer of gelatin around each microbubble. The gelatin microbubbles can be made to be very precise, with a standard deviation of ± 0.7 microns. Exact precision of the saccharide encapsulated microbubbles has not been determined yet but is believed to be approximately equal to that of the gelatin agents.

Because the microbubble itself is the echo source, and not the shell, either encapsulation material is acceptable for cardiac output measurements. From a practical standpoint, the gelatin appears to be easier to deliver at slow steady infusion rates and appears to be somewhat more difficult to deliver for bolus injections.

Experimental results

The prospect of noninvasive cardiac output measurements depends upon the demonstration that (1) a unique and preferably linear relationship exists between bubble concentration and the dimensionless backwall signal level; (2) homogeneous distributions of bubbles exist within the heart; (3) all injected bubbles flow into the heart and do not recirculate; and (4) a stable and suitable echo source can be found within the heart. If these four conditions are achieved, then a device can be designed which would take a modified form of the rf signal from an ultrasonic unit and automatically convert the signal into a measurement of cardiac output.

Previous work [11] strongly suggested that high intensity, long duration ultrasonic pulses are attenuated linearly by bubble concentrations. However, present units have relatively low level signals which are of short duration. Additionally, our own research [15] indicates that a minimum pulse duration of more than ten equal amplitude cycles is required to excite bubbles into steady-state oscillation. Hence, it remained to be shown that bubbles respond to present day ultrasound pulses in a predictable manner. To do this, we used a SKI Ekoline 20A as our ultrasound source. The rf receiver signal was taken from the unit after amplification and before other processing. Tapping this signal did not alter the normal response of the unit. Our cardiopulmonary model was employed for the study. The model was to human scale and had a 2.5 cm diameter "pulmonary artery". Seventy-six micron diameter gelatin-

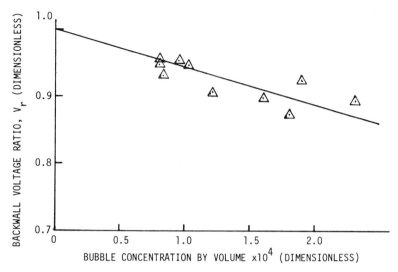

Figure 4. Variation of backwall signal as a function of bubble concentration using gelatin encapsulated microbubbles of 76 micron diameter.

encapsulated microbubbles were infused at a steady rate by a syringe pump into a vein in the model, and the pulmonary artery was insonated from above. The backwall portion of the rf signal was separated from the total signal and its steady-state peak value recorded for five different infusion rates. Figure 4 presents the dimensionless backwall voltage as a function of bubble concentration. A least-squares linear fit with an intercept at unity was made to these data. The correlation coefficient for these data was found to be 0.92. This particular form of a linear fit was chosen because it matched Eq. (8). Our preliminary results look quite promising and suggest that Eq. (8) is valid and can be used to obtain bubble concentration.

Experimental verification of the homogeneous distribution of bubbles was achieved by examination of many M-mode records of the pulmonary artery. One such record is shown in Figure 5. The reader will note a uniform opacification of the lumen by the microbubbles.

An integration effect occurs as sound waves pass through a bubble field. This is characteristic of the microbubble attenuation approach. Hence, even if small areas of inhomogeneity exist, they are averaged by the sound wave. It appears that the requirement of homogeneity can be relaxed somewhat for our particular approach, although our preliminary data do not indicate that it is necessary.

An electronic circuit was developed which would take the reflected backwall signal and convert it into a direct current voltage so that time variations could be recorded. One such recording was taken on the cardio-pulmonary model in pulsatile flow (Figure 6). The time of injection was also noted. One can observe a steady decrease in signal level as more bubbles

322

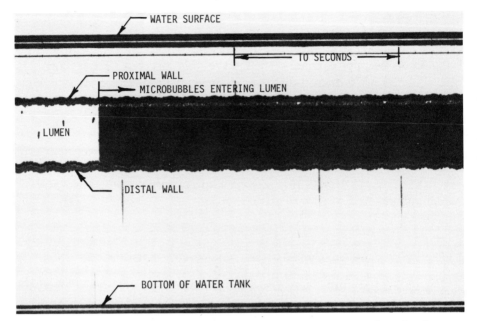

Figure 5. M-mode tracing showing distribution of bubbles in lumen of cardiopulmonary model.

enter the pulmonary artery until equilibrium is reached and a plateau is observed. Note that the lungs of the model capture the gelatin microbubbles as do real lungs so recirculation does not occur. The slight oscillations in the curve are caused by the pulsatile nature of the flow. Note that the baseline does return to its initial no-bubble level following the test.

The fact that a plateau is observed indicates that the bubble infusion rate is constant and that the bubbles are passing below the transducer at a constant rate, i.e. bubbles are not being trapped somewhere within the system. This was easily verified experimentally because much of the model was fabricated from clear plastic.

Testing has shown that there is a specific range of bubble densities which can be used. High concentrations ($\varphi > 10^{-3}$) virtually eliminate the backwall signal as observed by Meltzer et al. [4] and preclude determination of bubble concentration. Somewhat lower concentrations cause the effects to be nonlinear. Further, small bubble concentrations ($\varphi < 10^{-5}$) do not cause significant

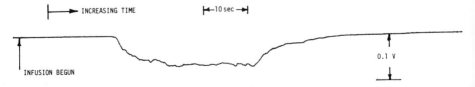

Figure 6. Demodulated backwall signal variation with time for constant infusion rate.

changes in backwall signals, resulting in measurement errors. Laboratory tests are currently underway to optimize delivery rates, bubble gas, size, density and other basic parameters. Currently, we find bubble concentrations by volume of approximately 10^{-4} serve this purpose. Fewer than 435 microbubbles of 76 micron diameter in one cubic centimeter blood volume are then sufficient for measurement. This can be accomplished by selecting the bubble delivery rate relative to the anticipated mean flow.

Peripherally injected microbubbles are trapped by the lungs. The lungs filter microbubbles larger than 8 microns and bubbles smaller than this dissolve in the blood stream before they can traverse the pulmonary circulation [16, 17]. Hence, microbubbles do not recirculate to cause what is sometimes referred to as recirculation error.

Conclusions

Bubbles are known to be very echogenic and hence act as superior ultrasonic contrast agents. They also exhibit the potential for noninvasive right heart side pressure and flow measurements. Theoretical considerations and preliminary experimental results indicate their potential. Encapsulation materials and bubble gases appear nontoxic. Detailed animal and toxicity studies are planned to insure the efficacy and safety of the materials. Microbubbles now appear to be a key part of a noninvasive "cath-lab." It may even be possible to make one peripheral injection of our pressurized microbubble dispersion and obtain right heart ultrasonic contrast, pressures and flows simultaneously.

ACKNOWLEDGEMENTS

Much of this work would not have been possible without the technical assistance, encouragement and candid comments from various people. The author is grateful to Drs. N. Rasor and H. Rugge for their guidance and foresight throughout this effort, and to D. Griffin, T. Nyren, J. Rasor, and T. Sahines for making many technical contributions. Additionally, the author expresses his thanks to Drs. W. Bommer, A. DeMaria, H. Feigenbaum, G. Goetowski, E. Kinney, R. Meltzer, R. Popp and N. Silverman for their encouragement and medical inputs at various times during the development. Part of this effort was supported by a contract from the National, Heart, Lung, and Blood Institute, Division of Lung Diseases.

324

REFERENCES

1. Devin C: Survey of thermal, radiation and viscous damping of pulsating air bubbles in water. J Acoust Soc Am 31:1654, 1959.
2. Plesset M, A Prosperetti: Bubble dynamics and cavitation. Am Rev Fluid Mech 9:145, 1977.
3. Minnaert M: On musical air-bubbles and sounds of running water. Phil Mag, 16:235, 1933.
4. Meltzer R, G Tickner, T Sahines, R Popp: The sources of ultrasound contrast effect. J Clin Ultrasound 8:121, 1980.
5. Lubbers J, J Van den Berg: An ultrasonic detector for microgasemboli in a bloodflow line. Ultrasound in Med. and Biol. 2, 301, 1976.
6. Bommer W, A DeMaria, et al.: Indicator-dilution curves obtained by photometric analysis of two-dimensional echo-contrast studies. (Abstract) Am J Cardiol 41:370, 1978.
7. Urick RJ: The absorption of sound in suspension of irregular particles. J Acoust Soc Am 20:283, 1948.
8. Stakutis V, R Morse, M Dill, R Beyer: Attenuation of ultrasound in aqueous suspensions. J Acoust Soc Am 27:539, 1955.
9. Urick RJ: Principles of Underwater Sound, p 203 McGraw Hill Book Co., New York, 1967.
10. Gavrilov L: On the size distribution of gas bubbles in water. Sov Phys-Acoust 15:22, 1969.
11. Medwin H: Counting bubbles acoustically: a review. Ultrasonics 15:7, 1977.
12. Medwin H: In-situ acoustic measurement of microbubbles at sea. J Geophys Res 82:971, 1977.
13. Wells P: Physical principles of ultrasonic diagnosis, pp 9–14. Academic Press, New York, 1969.
14. Hamilton W: Measurement of the cardiac output. Handbook Physiology Sec. 2 Circulation 1:551 (Hamilton W, ed.). Amer Physiol Soc, Washington, D.C., 1962.
15. Tickner G, N Rasor: Noninvasive assessment of pulmonary hypertension using the bubble ultrasonic resonance pressure (BURP) method. Annual Report #HR-62917–1A, NHLBI, 1977.
16. Butler B, B Hills: The lungs as a filter for microbubbles. J Appl Physiol 47:537, 1979.
17. Meltzer R, G Tickner, R Popp: Why do the lungs clear ultrasonic contrast. Ultrasound Med Biol 6:263, 1980.

27. MICROBUBBLE TRACKING WITH ECHO DOPPLER

STANLEY J. GOLDBERG, LILLIAM M. VALDES-CRUZ, and HUGH D. ALLEN

INTRODUCTION

Two major problems encountered with detection of microbubbles by M-mode echocardiography are 1) microbubbles generally produce weak echoes, and these weak echoes can be eliminated by echo processing adjustments, and 2) generation of sufficient microbubbles for tracking is not always possible. Since echo Doppler is designed to function with low level signals, the possibility of microbubble detection by echo Doppler merits investigation. The purpose of this investigation was to determine if range gated echo Doppler is useful for detecting microbubbles for flow tracing.

METHODOLOGY

Microbubble detection by range gated Doppler was investigated in patients during routine cardiac catheterization. Microbubbles were created by saline injections in volumes of 2 ml in children under 10 kg and 5 ml in larger patients. Injection sites included peripheral veins via needles and catheter sheaths, and specific chambers through various types of lengths of catheters. Two Doppler systems were utilized to image the passage of contrast material. The first was an ATL 500 equipped with a second generation time interval histographic frequency output and another trace which indicated the strength of the Doppler signal. The ATL 500 also had electro-cardiographic and M-mode outputs which were recorded simultaneously with the frequency analysis. Initially, studies of the M-mode output of the ATL 500 and a SmithKline 20A were performed in duplicate for the purpose of comparing results of microbubble detection. After eight injections in three patients demonstrated virtually identical results, the ATL 500 was used exclusively in the remainder of the studies. The settings of the ATL 500 Doppler are critical, and standardization was accomplished as follows. Threshold was set to maximal. Doppler gain was adjusted so that full scale strength indicator peaks were achieved only on strong signals, but during weak or no signal conditions, the signal strength indicator fell to or near zero. If a frequency dispersion was present in the cardiac area of interest, Doppler gain for that area only was decreased until the time interval histogram no longer demonstrated a frequency dispersion. The second Doppler instrument used to record results of injections was a prototype two-dimensional echo Doppler device produced by Honeywell. This instrument was operative in two modes. The first was a two-dimensional or M-mode presentation with a movable cursor for range gating. Once the range gate location was determined. the seond mode could be entered, but it consisted of only a Doppler output with an ECG reference signal. Accordingly, simultaneous display of an M-mode or two-dimensional image and Doppler frequency output was not possible with this version of the instrument. Doppler frequency output was accomplished by fast Fourier transform which required no adjustment.

Two general types of injection studies were performed. The first consisted of an injection into a chamber or great vessel with range gate sampling from a great vessel or chamber that was not in the direction of flow. This type of study tested the selectivity of the range gated Doppler. As an example of this type of study, an injection might be made into the aortic root of a patient with a normal aortic valve. If the Doppler range gate was the left ventricle, no microbubble detection would be expected. The second general type of study was one in which an injection was made into a chamber or great vessel and the range gate was placed in the direction of blood flow as determined by catheterization results and angiography. For example, in a patient with aortic stenosis, , an injection could be performed into the left ventricle and the range gate placed in the aortic root. Microbubble detection in the aortic root would be expected.

All records were evaluated without knowledge of the diagnosis of the patient. If microbubbles were detected by M-mode or Doppler in the direction of flow, this was scored as an appropriate result. An appropriate result was also scored if microbubbles were not detected in vascular or cardiac areas where catheterization indicated that they should not enter. An inappropriate result was detection of microbubbles in areas where flow should not have entered, or failure to detect microbubbles in areas where flow should have carried them.

M-mode contrast results were identified according to original descriptions [1–3]. ATL Doppler records were judged positive if 1) the frequency dispersion was greater than 1 cm vertical distance after microbubble injection [4] and 2) a rise occurred in the Doppler signal strength indicator. Records recorded with the prototype Honeywell echo Doppler machine were evaluated for additon of a spectral dispersion overlying the standard velocity pattern.

RESULTS

Eighty-eight studies were performed in 16 children, 78 with the M-mode system and ten with the prototype two-dimensional Doppler system.Complications were not encountered. Three M-mode studies were discarded because of equipment failure. For the ATL instrument, reflection from microbubbles caused a frequency dispersion and a marked rise in the Doppler signal strength indicator. M-mode contrast had the expected characteristics [1–3]. Microbubble detection was quite simple with the time interval histographic technique. However, M-mode contrast appearance frequently produced weak signals, although in some instances, very strong signals were noted. In 36 instances, the contrast effect was detected only with difficulty by M-mode while the Doppler registered a very strong signal (Figure 1). Comparison of M-mode and Doppler studies indicated that, in all instances (n = 20) in which microbubbles were not expected, none were detected by Doppler, but one error occurred for M-mode. In this instance of error, microbubbles were detected in the right ventricular outflow tract during injection into the left ventricle of a patient with no left-to-right shunt demonstrated by angiography. In this instance, the Doppler range gate was placed into the left ventricle and thus did not test the right ventricular outflow tract. This result was not repeatable. No explanation was found for this error.

In instances in which microbubbles were expected (n = 55), five failures occurred

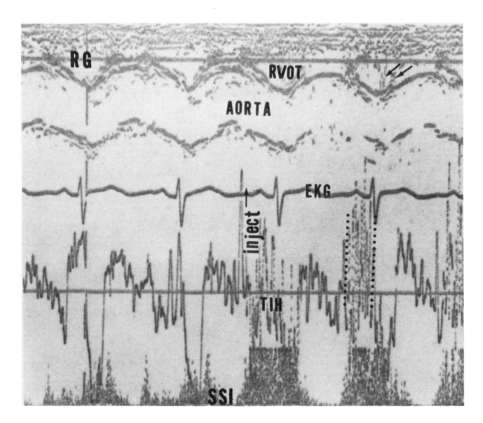

Figure 1. The range gate (RG) is in the right ventricular outflow tract (RVOT). An injection was performed in the pulmonary artery of a patient with pulmonary valvular insufficiency. Injection time is marked on the EKG. In the M-mode, several images of microbubbles are designated by arrows. A marked frequency dispersion, bounded by linear dots, occurs on the time interval histogram (TIH). The signal strength indicator (SSI) shows an increased signal magnitude.

328

for Doppler and 15 for M-mode. Three of the five Doppler failures occurred when injection and range gating were in the same chamber, and this result may have been due to streaming. No reason was apparent for the other two failures. For 15 M-mode failures, no obvious reason or pattern was detectable.

For the two-dimensional echo Doppler system with fast Fourier spectral analysis, microbubbles were depicted as a background haze or wide bandwidth noise overlying the original wave form. Appropriate detection occurred in eight out of ten instances (Figure 2). Positive identification of contrast was not made in two in-

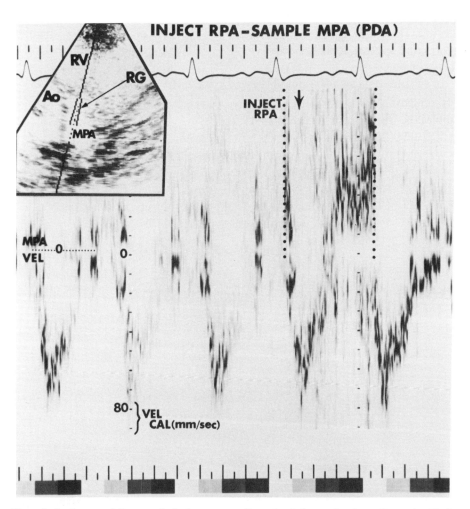

Figure 2. In the upper left corner is the locator two-dimensional short-axis echocardiograph with the range gate (RG). The RG is in the main pulmonary artery (MPA). RV = right ventricular outflow tract; Ao = aortic root. The main portion of the figure is the velocity tracing. The calibrated velocity is depicted for the main pulmonary artery (MPA VEL). Immediately following injection of saline in the right pulmonary artery (RPA), designated by the lines of dots, a background frequency dispersion is added to the waveform. Maximal dispersion occurs just after the arrow.

stances in which it was expected and, in both of those instances, the injection site and range gating were in the same chamber. These failures may also have been due to streaming.

DISCUSSION

The results of this investigation demonstrate that echo Doppler has significant clinical utility for detection of microbubbles. Spectral outputs, time interval histography and fast Fourier transform, are significantly different, but each has advantages and disadvantages. The time interval histography is extremely sensitive for microbubble detection, but the velocity wave form is lost during microbubble passage. Fast Fourier transform is less sensitive to microbubble passage, but velocity wave forms remain recognizable and reasonably intact.

In this investigation, no effort was made to maximize the generation of microbubbles. Had a major effort been made to enhance microbubble production, M-mode contrast detection surely would have improved. However, the specific intent was to determine if low level, low density microbubbles were efficiently detected by Doppler, and the result was in the affirmative.

We conclude that echo Doppler is an efficient tool for tracing blood flow and that signals reflected from microbubbles are more readily detected by Doppler than by standard M-mode echocardiography if no effort is made to maximize microbubble production.

REFERENCES

1. Gramiak R, PM Shah, DH Kramer: Ultrasound cardiography: contrast studies in anatomy and function. Radiology 92:939–948, 1969.
2. Valdes-Cruz LM, DR Pieroni, J Roland, PJ Varghese: Echocardiographic detection of intracardiac right-to-left shunts following peripheral vein injections. Circulation 54:558–562, 1976.
3. Sahn DJ, HD Allen, W George, M Mason, SJ Goldberg: The utility of contrast echocardiographic techniques in the care of critically ill infants with cardiac and pulmonary disease. Circulation 56:959–968, 1977.
4. Areias JC, SJ Goldberg, SEC Spitaels, VH de Villeneuve: An evaluation of range gated pulsed Doppler echocardiography for detecting pulmonary outflow tract obstruction in d-transposition of the great vessels. Am Heart J 96:467–474, 1978.
5. Meltzer RS, EG Tickner, TP Sahines, RL Popp: The source of ultrasound contrast effect. J Clin Ultrasound 8:121–127, 1980.

INDEX OF SUBJECTS

332

INDEX OF AUTHORS